W9-BXG-779

RESEARCH AND THE INDIVIDUAL

Human Studies

The author is a member of

The Trustees' Committee on Research and the Individual
Massachusetts General Hospital

and

First Chairman of the Subcommittee on Human Studies
Massachusetts General Hospital

Chairman of the Standing Committee on Human Studies
Harvard Medical School

Chairman of the *ad hoc* Committee to Define Irreversible Coma
Harvard Medical School

RESEARCH

TH

Little, Brown and Company

Henry K. Beecher, *A.M., M.D., Dr. (hon.), M.D. (hon.)*
Henry Isaiah Dorr Professor of Research in Anaesthesia
Harvard University

AND
NDIVIDUAL
HUMAN STUDIES

ston

Library of Congress catalog card No. 79–101753

First Edition

Published in Great Britain by J. & A. Churchill Ltd., London

British Standard Book No. 7000 0168 9

Printed in the United States of America

Margaret Swain Beecher

Searching for a phrase,
I found none to stand beside her name

Preface

While it might be pretentious to describe this book as a study of the impact of science on society or of the impact of society on science, in a very limited sense the work *is* the modest record of a struggle to recognize the problems involved in human studies, to state them, and to grasp their meaning insofar as they relate to experimentation in man. Human experimentation is as old as civilization, but only in recent decades has it achieved a scope and a usefulness not previously envisioned. This broad development makes it necessary to define the possibilities, the pitfalls, and the degrees of freedom permissible. The principals are the investigators and their subjects in their interrelationships, not only with each other, but also with their internal and external environments. Legal and ethical considerations are emphasized throughout this book.

A question that often arose during the writing of this book revolved about the character of its audience. It is designed to be read by everyone who deals with or is interested in medical studies in man. In addition to the investigators and their subjects, this audience embraces physicians, scientists, psychologists, sociologists, lawyers, students, and all who wish to examine a crucial phenomenon of our times. It is regarded as crucial because the very growth and development of medicine depends upon the conduct of our responsibilities in this experimental field. One irresponsible investigator can do grave harm, not only to himself, to his human subject, to his project, and to his institution, but also to the area of medical experimentation and, indeed, to the entire field of medicine.

While it is true that certain sections could be greatly expanded, it is my conviction that little would be gained by doing so; if I have failed to deal with the serious questions involved in experimentation, insofar as the available material warrants, then my major purpose has failed. I hope and trust that this is not the case. The length of the present exposition seems appropriate to the situation as it now exists. With the extraordinary recent expansion of medical studies in man, it seems unquestionably clear that old problems will change in relative importance and that new and unsuspected questions will arise. I have tried to provide a satisfactory basis for an understanding of future as well as present problems.

There is an evolving philosophy of experimental medicine. To some extent, this can be seen in the changing emphasis over the years in the sequential material on codes, in Appendix A. I must, perhaps, state the obvious: I am not a philosopher; neither have I any pretensions in that direction. I grant that there is a pressing need for a philosopher's approach, but only by one so wise that he can competently resolve the enormous complexities of the problems involved. I am an investigator, one who has been studying man for nearly 40 years—sometimes successfully, sometimes not—and continues to do so with relish. I mention this only as a passing answer to those who may profess to think that the criticisms I have made are an attempt to denigrate the subject.

Some who have read the manuscript have questioned the fact that its form is similar to that of a medical review. That is exactly what it was intended to be: a readily available guide to pertinent material in the field of human experimentation. I make no apology for it. The other approach, that of the philosopher, is both beyond my competence and certainly outside my intention.

As I mentioned earlier, experimentation in man for scientific purposes is as old as recorded history. There is little new in terms of principle. What is new is the rapid increase in the magnitude of the problems. There is great need for constant reexamination of the ethical aspects of the procedures involved. This need is imposed by progress in science and by the advance in moral and ethical standards. In the several decades just passed two developments emerged that especially pointed up the need for a new examination of the subject. First, there were the medical outrages of Hitler's Germany. While the philosophical problems raised by those gross actions are not within the scope of this work, they nevertheless indicate the need for a long, straight look at our current practices. Second, there is the recently recognized fact that some types of basic scientific advances can be achieved only in the presence of disease. This will be discussed later.

The Hippocratic Oath says nothing about preventive medicine; neither was prevention of disease a particular concern for thousands of years, except as the Biblical concept of "clean" and "unclean" states might be construed to be related thereto. In the last century, however, it has become evident that the physician has a duty to go beyond the patient's immediate complaint—a duty, not only to relieve or cure, but to prevent disease. With this concept, the horizons of medicine have broadened immeasurably, and the need for searching out causes, for treating, for testing, for comparing, and for experimenting is no longer a privilege; it has become a duty. This is to say that the medical profession must accept as its responsibility not only the prevention of disease and the care of the sick, but also the advancement of knowledge on which both depend, a view stressed by McCance [293]. He also has emphasized the importance of impressing patients with the fact that the very best hospitals carry out experimental work, not only for the immediate benefit of the ill, but also for the benefit of mankind, and that the patients themselves owe incalculable advantages to such work that has already been done on others. One hopes that eventually the public will understand that if they are to have the privilege of entering these leading hospitals they will be expected to collaborate knowingly and willingly in developmental procedures.

The American public has an intense interest in and a considerable understanding—or at least an awareness—of medical research. Research is increasing in geometric progression, supported by both financial and cultural factors in our society. It is evident that this situation prevails far more commonly in the United States than in other Western or in Asiatic societies. It is essential that the medical profession make clear to its members and to a watchful public the necessity for human experimentation. The medical experimenter has grave responsibilities; he also has remarkable opportunities for advancing the welfare of mankind.

The Federal Food, Drug and Cosmetic Act of 1906 charted a course for the United States. Not much was done to alter it or improve it until the appalling effects of a new sedative were reported a few years ago. This agent produced tragic maiming of embryos. The reaction of the public was swift, and in 1962 the Kefauver-Harris amendments were swept into law. A new era of federal control was at hand. The remarkable power of public pressure was once more exhibited. Although the thalidomide effect was neither foreseen nor could reasonably have been anticipated, it nevertheless led to drastic action. When unethical experimental procedures are exposed, an even more violent public reaction against them can be expected, with the possibility that extreme legislation will ensue, to the detriment of sound and ethical procedures. There is a further urgency, then, to correct existing abuses. Scientists are thus obliged to ponder the necessity for proceeding thoughtfully and carefully and ethically in the complex field of human studies.

The breaches of ethical conduct that have come to my attention were usually owing to ignorance or thoughtlessness; they were neither willful nor unscrupulous in origin. It is hoped that the material presented here will help those who would do so to protect themselves from the errors of inexperience, "to exercise those wise restraints that make men free."

Wherever there are major concentrations of power, moral questions arise. This is as true of the power that comes from knowledge as it is of other forms of power. The extraordinary advances in medical knowledge are a case in point, for these can lead to "the power to control, to manipulate, to alter human life as well as cure human disease" [401]. We are brought face to face with the central question: What are the permissible limits to and the proper conditions for experimentation on human beings?

At a recent conference on human experimentation at the American Academy of Arts and Sciences, only about eight of the thirty or so participants present could be described as experienced investigators in man. This is excellent. Clearly, the investigators are in for an abundance of advice, some of which will be very good. This seems to parallel the view that war is too important to be left to the generals.

The well-being, the health, even the actual or potential life of all human beings, born or unborn, depend upon continuing experimentation in man. Proceed it must; proceed it will. "The proper study of mankind is man."

The title of this book is purloined from a phrase of Bishop Henry K. Sherrill—with his permission. My debt to the clergy goes far beyond this. The many questions I directed to the Archdiocese of Boston were promptly answered, not by the librarian's assistant, as I had expected, but by His Eminence, Richard Cardinal Cushing, who also at one point arranged for two theologians to examine my statements concerning the views of the Roman Catholic Church. Two scholars of another faith have likewise been of help to me: Rabbi Jerome D. Folkman of Cleveland and Rabbi Irving M. Levey of Princeton.

Professor Joseph Fletcher of the Episcopal Theological School (Cambridge, Mass.) and Dr. Joachim S. Gravenstein of Case Western Reserve University (Cleveland) read the entire manuscript, made many suggestions, and saved me on occasion from grievous error. Dr. Arthur J. Dyck of Harvard has given me help with Chap. 7, gratefully received. Mr. Kenneth Ludmerer of the Department of the History of Science, Harvard University, kindly read the brief section on history and made some valuable suggestions.

Miss Genevieve Cole, Librarian of the Treadwell Library at the Massachusetts General Hospital, was tireless in running down the last obscure reference.

I consulted Professor William J. Curran, Harvard School of Public Health, and the Harvard Medical School, on matters of the law so many times that I am embarrassed to meet him on the street. Professor Curran is one of the foremost legal authorities in the area of human experimentation.

I must express my gratitude to Mr. Ralph Lowell, Trustee of the Lowell Institute, who has contributed so much to the cultural wealth of his times. My thanks are not only for the opportunity of being three times a Lowell Lecturer, but also for the opportunity of drawing seven Lowell Lectures from the material contained here.

Miss Ada Wing, secretary during the later stages of work on this book, contributed greatly to my peace of mind by her painstaking skill and accuracy.

Last, but at the same time foremost, I must acknowledge my debt to Miss Ruth M. Studley, my secretary for nearly a quarter of a century, who has put up with my vagaries and my compulsive rewriting with infinite patience. Her devotion to her task, and her skill, are legendary.

Over the years I have dealt with many publishers. The editorial staff at Little, Brown—Mr. Fred Belliveau, Mr. Richard Bickford, and Mrs. Anne N. Merian—through many amiable conferences, always have been pleasant and invariably helpful to a degree not heretofore experienced.

To all of these persons I express my gratitude. If there is error here, it is mine.

Henry K. Beecher

Acknowledgments

I appreciate the privilege granted of quoting directly the material on codes; specifically:

Mr. Leo E. Brown for the statements on "Penal Institutions of the American Medical Association House of Delegates (1952)."

Mr. Caspar W. Buckley, Superintendent of Documents, Food and Drug Administration (1966), for its statement of requirements concerning study of new drugs.

Mr. Kamleshwar Das for Article Seven: Draft covenant on civil and political rights, United Nations (1966).

Dean Robert H. Ebert (M.D.) and Dr. Dana L. Farnsworth for the Harvard Codes.

Dr. Lee J. Gehrig, Acting Surgeon General of the United States Public Health Service (1966), for its policy on investigation involving human subjects.

Mr. James E. Hague, American Hospital Association (1957), for its "Statement of Principles."

Dr. J. D. J. Havard for the British Medical Association Code on experimental research on human beings (1963) and human experimentation—code of ethics of the World Medical Association (1964).

Sir Austin Bradford Hill and the proprietors of the *British*

Medical Journal for "A Code for the Clinical Trial" and his critique of the World Medical Association Code.

Mr. Edwin J. Holman for "Ethical Guidelines of the American Medical Association, for Organ Transplantation, 1968."

Mr. Magnus Marshall, Medical Alumni Association of Western Reserve University School of Medicine, for "Human Experimentation as Exemplified by the Career of Dr. William Beaumont" (Beaumont's Code) and Dr. Wiggers's Code, 1950.

Dr. Jack Masur for the National Institutes of Health Codes (1966, 1968): "Group Consideration and Informed Consent in Clinical Research."

National Academy of Sciences Board of Medicine, 1968, for its statements on Heart Transplants.

Miss Margaret L. Natwick, Executive Secretary of the World Medical Association, for the "Declaration of Geneva (1948)," "International Code of Medical Ethics (1949)," "Principles for Those in Research and Experimentation (1954)," and the "Declaration of Helsinki (1964)."

Miss Helen Orr, American Psychological Association (1963), for its "Ethical Standards."

Mr. Edward J. Pollock, Catholic Hospital Association of the United States and Canada, for its "Ethical and Religious Directives."

Miss Maude Rix for the Director of Publications, Medical Research Council of Great Britain (1963), statement on "Responsibility in Investigations on Human Subjects," published by permission of the Controller of Her Britannic Majesty's Stationery Office.

Mrs. E. Schrama-Coster for the statement of the Public Health Council of the Netherlands (1955).

Dr. John H. Talbott for the American Medical Association Codes, 1846, 1847, 1946, 1949, 1958, 1966, 1967.

General K. G. Wickham, the Adjutant General, United States Army, Army Regulation No. 70–25: "Use of Volunteers as Subjects of Research (1962)."

Dr. Wolf Wolfensberger and *Science* for "Wolfensberger's Code" (1967).

Dr. Dale Wolfle, Executive Officer, American Association for the Advancement of Science, for remarks quoted.

Also, I thank Dr. John Talbott, Editor, *Journal of the American Medical Association,* for permission to reproduce as Appendix B the Harvard *ad hoc* Committee's "Definition of Irreversible Coma" (*J.A.M.A.* 205:337–340, 1968).

Contents

RESEARCH AND THE INDIVIDUAL

Human Studies

1
Research and the Individual

In a modest way, this entire book is concerned with the impact of research on society and, conversely, with the impact of society on research. Several particular points in these basic relationships can and should be spelled out at the beginning of this examination if a firm foundation for subsequent considerations is to be established.

DEFINITION AND SCOPE OF EXPERIMENTATION IN MAN

In experimentation in man, one asks a question of Nature; a hypothesis is made; it is tested in a human being. The test is attended by doubt and uncertainty. Even the *efficacy* of treatment can be assured only by experiment. Experimentation involves (1) observation and (2) systematic changes in conditions, accompanied by observation before, during, and after these changes are made. Although the word experiment is at times used loosely to cover only observation, in Lord Moulton's words, "When we are reduced to observation, Science crawls." Sound experimentation has as its purpose the advancement of knowledge by the discovery of some truth or in the attack on or substantiation of some hypothesis. Record keeping is usually a part of the procedure. One shares

Lord Kelvin's view: ". . . when you can measure what you are speaking about, and express it in numbers, you know something about it; but when you cannot measure it, when you cannot express it in numbers, your knowledge is of a meagre and unsatisfactory kind; it may be the beginning of knowledge, but you have scarcely, in your thoughts, advanced to the stage of *Science* whatever the matter may be." Today, sound experimentation often requires the protection afforded by probability theory and associated statistical techniques to guard against erroneous interpretation of data. It must be remembered that to do nothing can, at times, also be an experiment, even a fatal one.

McCance believes that the definition of an experiment may depend on the mental approach of the man who makes the tests; he regards collecting an extra specimen of urine or taking an extra few milliliters of blood from a vein puncture as falling within the range of the term *experiment* [293]. He says, "I would certainly regard weighing a baby 'unnecessarily' as an experiment. Some people may think I am taking up a ridiculous attitude over this, but if an experiment is not defined in this way, where is the line to be drawn: All experiments involve some risk. It may be an infinitesimally small one, but it is always there—you, or the nurse, may drop the baby."

Since the early 1940s Bradford Hill has held that the general emphasis on careful planning in advance really constitutes a new development [209]. Such planning requires (1) two or more similar groups of subjects studied at the same time, but differing in their treatment; (2) random distribution of the subjects; and (3) withholding treatment from one group or the other. A placebo or a "standard" agent may constitute the treatment of the control group. Through the controlled clinical trial thus arranged, one hopes to avoid the situation Cheever spoke of more than a hundred years ago [64]: "Effects are ascribed to drugs which really flow from natural causes, and are but the usual succession of the morbid phenomena; sequences are taken for consequences, and all just conclusions confused. From the want of this knowledge [of the natural history of disease]; from defective observation, rash generalizations, and hasty conclusions *a priori,* have arisen the thousand conflicting theories which have degraded Medicine from its true position as a science, and interfered with its advancement as a practical art."

Bradford Hill says with wry honesty, "To be fair to Dr. Cheever I should add that he thought the experimental approach to be of 'doubtful application in the therapeutical art' and had this to say of statisticians in 1861: 'All the theorists say to the practitioner at the bedside, Do not try, but think; reason, argue, deduce!' Empirical Hunter said, 'Do not think, but try!' So the modern disciples of the numerical method would say to us, 'Neither think, nor try; but calculate!' Meanwhile the patient dies."

One hopes that with the carefully planned clinical trial patients will die less often than without it. This subject is of such importance that it deserves treatment in a later section (page 269).

There are many good reasons for a careful consideration of the scope of experimentation in man: protection of the subjects, the investigators, their research and their institutions, and the sound development of medicine. These all require a level-headed approach. Comparatively recent developments in medicine and changes in emphasis give added weight to the importance of an examination of human experimentation at this time. The truly basic scientist has developed a new interest in human experimentation.

Such experimentation, especially since World War II, has been extraordinarily successful; it has also created some difficult problems because of the increasing employment of patients, prisoners, children, and other individuals as experimental subjects, especially when it becomes apparent in some cases that they would not have participated if they had been truly aware of the uses to be made of them. Although a belief prevails in some sophisticated circles that attention to these matters would impede progress, in the words of Pope Pius XII, ". . . science is not the highest value to which all other orders of values . . . should be subordinated."

There are several kinds of experimentation in man: self-experimentation; experimentation in patient volunteers and in normal volunteer subjects; and, unfortunately, occasional experimentation in unwitting subjects. Probably most common of all is experimentation in an ailing subject to establish a diagnosis and needed therapy. These subjects may be employed in studies of preventive medicine, in diagnosis and therapy, and in physiologic work. *Experimentation on a patient not directly for his benefit, but for that of patients in general, presents especially complex problems;* they will be discussed.

JUSTIFICATION FOR THE HUMAN TRIAL

Several points related to this subject have been presented in the Preface. They will not be repeated here.

As mentioned, clinical research involves observation or experimentation, or both. The value of Bacillus Calmette-Guerin (BCG) was shrouded in doubt for 25 years because no controlled study of its worth was carried out. Sir George Pickering believes that after tens of thousands of sympathectomies for hypertension we still are uncertain of its value [340]. He has contrasted our ignorance in this area, owing to lack of controlled experiment in man, with our dependable knowledge, based upon controlled experimentation, of the usefulness of drugs in tuberculosis.

The importance of the project undertaken must be commensurate with the risk involved. The assurance of this is a cardinal responsibility of all who undertake experimentation in man. Having stated that important principle, there remains a vast area in which judgment—one hopes, sound judgment—will operate. Only the fanatic denies that animal experimentation must usually precede that on humans. As Sir Geoffrey Jefferson put it, "Man is too rare, too expensive, altogether too valuable an animal" to be the first used in studies of technical procedures or trials of even therapeutic agents.

It must be evident that human experimentation that has already proved its essential usefulness must increase. There is thus a need for clarification of the limitations on and the freedoms of such work.

A BRIEF HISTORICAL RÉSUMÉ[1]

Those who do not know history are doomed to repeat it.
SANTAYANA

The oldest world literatures contain references to experimental work with both animals and man. It was the practice in ancient Persia for the king to hand over condemned criminals for experimental purposes in science. The Ptolemies used criminals in Egypt, and so did Fallopius in Pisa during the Renaissance. Lord Platt recalls: "A Persian prince at the time of Avicenna was giving advice to a young man who was going to join the medical profession. He said, 'Once you embark on a career as a physician if you wish to gain experience and a reputation you must experiment freely, but you had better not choose people of high rank or political importance for your subjects' " [346].

Hippocrates, in stating firmly that epilepsy is no more divine than any other disease, cleared the way for the study of neurologic and mental disease. He was the great observer, the excellent clinician. Galen added experimentation to observation; Galen is therefore generally considered the father of the experimentalists. It is better to remember him for this than for his "Galenic" preparations!

There are two aspects to Galen the scientist: his philosophy of research and the results of his research. Viewed in retrospect, much of his philosophy, which emphasized the importance of empiric investigation, proved sound, even though many of his findings were later recognized as invalid. Unfortunately for medicine, it was his experimental *results,* not his experimental *philosophy,* that had extraordinary impact on the European world for fourteen centuries after his death.

Galen somewhat formalized medical experimentation about 1800 years ago, but this fell under a cloud for the 1,400 years of the Dark and Middle Ages until Vesalius in the sixteenth century

[1] A rounded, detailed discussion of this subject is not relevant to the purposes of this book. A few illustrative examples will be used.

overrode the tradition against dissection of the human body and demonstrated certain errors in Galen's concept of the circulation of the blood. Curiously, Galen's dominance of medical thought was terminated by William Harvey who, in a sense, was a follower of Galen in his physiological demonstrations. Harvey, after carrying out controlled experiments in animals and in man, demonstrated the circulation of the blood, in particular that it must all pass through the heart and lungs (for there was no porous septum), if his calculations of volume and velocity were correct. Thus, the first idea of measurement in biologic investigation bore fruit in 1616, with publication in 1628 [176].

The iatrophysicists were a school of sixteenth-century Italian scientists who viewed man as a machine and who attempted to adapt the methods of the physical sciences to biologic research. Their work was characterized by two main features: (1) their concern with quantifying results and (2) their emphasis upon the importance of empiric findings, with a corresponding disdain for theoretical work. Iatrophysicists often studied man in this way. Santorio, for example, of the University of Padua made a study of the amount of water a person loses a day through perspiration. Santorio weighed his subjects daily, as well as their total intake and output, and then determined the amount of perspiration by finding the difference between their food intake and their urination and fecal excretion.

Lind, in 1757, carried out a wonderfully controlled study and demonstrated that oranges and lemons could cure the scurvy.

In 1722, inmates of the infamous Newgate Prison volunteered to be inoculated for smallpox—as an alternative to hanging, it might be added. All survived, and hence all were released. In 1798, three-quarters of a century after this, Jenner, after controlled experiments in man, published his proof of the value of vaccination against smallpox. In the early part of the eighteenth century, in the United States, Cotton and Increase Mather and other clergymen supported Dr. Zabdiel Boylston, who was charged with "scandalous" experiments: inoculating against the smallpox, with his own son the subject. Benjamin Waterhouse, an American physician, reported in 1800 how he inoculated his child and two of his servants with the pox in an experiment on inoculation [420]. The attack on and the defense of inoculation were moral issues. Great excitement and great protest were aroused, with the result that the first hospital for inoculation at Cat Island, off Marblehead, Mass., was set afire and burned down [192].

The origins of the use of such agents as the soporific sponge to depress the central nervous system are lost in prehistoric mists. Modern anesthesia could have begun in 1799 with the young Davy, who at the age of 20 carried out beautifully planned studies on himself and concluded, "As nitrous oxide in its extensive operation appears capable of destroying physical pain, it may probably be used with advantage during surgical operations . . ." Someone, probably Faraday, editorializing in the *Lancet* in 1818, evidently knew about anesthesia. Indeed, anesthesia is defined as "a defect in sensation" in Bailey's dictionary of 1724. In January, 1842, three months before the later much-publicized activity of Crawford Long, Clarke carried out anesthesia in a girl; the self-experimentation of Horace Wells in 1844 is also to be noted. All of this interest culminated in the epoch-making first public demonstration of anesthesia by Morton at the Massachusetts General Hospital on October 16, 1846. Little animal experimentation preceded the introduction of human anesthesia.

Radiology (1895) grew out of a chance observation and was developed into a useful clinical tool in a few weeks of human experimentation by Röntgen. In 1896, *Science* printed a communication concerning the physiologic effects of x-rays. Dr. William L. Dudley was interested in the possibility of locating a bullet in the head of a child with the use of x-rays. Before doing so, he tried the technique on himself first, exposing himself to radiation for one hour. "The plate developed nothing, but yesterday, 21 days after the experiment, all the hair came out over the space under the X-ray discharge. The spot is perfectly bald, being 2″ in diameter . . . the skin looks perfectly healthy and there has been no pain nor other indication of disorder" [378].

After reading about this case, Leopold Freund, a German doctor, decided to use x-rays as a therapeutic tool to remove hair on moles. In 1898 he tried this procedure for the first time on a young girl and successfully removed the hair from her mole, although he nearly killed her in the process. This example is interesting for two main reasons. In his autobiography, Röntgen said that Freund's use of x-rays on a girl was the first case he knew of in which radiation was used therapeutically. Also, the whole story involves both a doctor experimenting on *himself* (Dudley) and a doctor experimenting on his *patient* (Freund).

The world was ready for two of its greatest experimentalists, Claude Bernard (1813–1878) and Louis Pasteur (1822–1895). Although Bernard is usually considered the modern father of experimental medicine, he certainly had distinguished predecessors in Galen, Harvey, Jenner, Hunter, and Lind.

All was not smooth sailing for the eager investigator. Experimentation on other men implies a willingness to experiment upon oneself as evidence of good faith, although in a given case self-experimentation may be wholly impracticable. When it is carried out, it must be done with the same safeguards that are applied to other subjects. Ivy cites a number of examples to indicate that willingness without the discipline of proper controls can be misleading or devastating, or both, to the self-experimenting participant [226]. There was the case of John Hunter, who inoculated himself in 1767 (*Treaty on Venereal Disease,* 1786) with gonorrheal pus to prove that the disease was thus transmissible. He succeeded, but from the same inoculum he also acquired syphilis and concluded that gonorrhea and syphilis were merely manifestations of the same disease. Purkinjé gave himself enough digitalis to kill nine cats in order to study its visual effects in himself. He suffered cardiac pain and irregularity and vomited for a week. Hales, enthusiastic about the marvels of intravenous injection, received a half ounce of castor oil by this route and lived to describe its remarkable effects. In 1830, in order to convince the French Academy of the extraordinary powers of charcoal to adsorb alkaloids, Tonery took, with this safeguard, a dose of strychnine that would have been lethal without it. In 1857, carbon tetrachloride was tried out as an anesthetic in man; a few animal experiments would have shown it to be unsuitable. In 1894 Oliver told Schafer that he had made extracts of all the endocrine glands and injected them into his own son. Schafer altered the experiment and was first to demonstrate the pressor effect of epinephrine in dogs and cats. Ivy concludes that "these experiments may be a tribute to the enthusiasm and bravery of these early medical scientists, but they clearly show the limitations and dangers of uncontrolled self-experimentation."

Clearing a hundred years in one leap, we come down to the present and find able men still involved in difficulties. When one shifts from a study of objective manifestation of disease to subjective effects—specifically, for example, to a quantitative study of the effect of drugs on symptoms—it becomes apparent that added controls are mandatory [20]. Chief among these is the use of the "double unknowns" approach to eliminate bias, not possible when the experimenters are also subjects who, as drug experience and sophistication grow, cannot remain in ignorance of the "aura" produced by opiates, for example. The scores of studies that have been lost because of a failure to recognize and employ adequate controls have been reviewed by Beecher [20].

Observation is the tool of the practitioner. Oliver Wendell Holmes, although Professor of Anatomy at Harvard, was not divorced from patients and their problems. Thus observation and empiricism gave him and Semmelweis a new understanding of puerperal sepsis and how to control it long before Koch and Pasteur achieved better insight into the disease through "scientific" means. As mentioned, in his almost perfectly controlled study, Lind had set a high standard for such inquiry and discovered how scurvy could be prevented a century and a half before "the facts, dangling before the averted eyes of chemists and physiologists . . ." offered a rational explanation [13]. Long before those in the laboratory knew anything about the filterable virus causing yellow fever, Walter Reed discovered the manner in which it spread to cause epidemics. For a long time before the missing factor was isolated, physicians knew that they could treat pernicious anemia with liver. The concept of the controlled clinical trial may have done more to make modern medicine a reality than any other single factor. In 1814, La Place suggested application of statistics with the use of two groups, one treated, the other serving as a control. The world owes a remarkable debt to Sir Austin Bradford Hill for his pioneering work in developing this area.

Medical science is economical; every new fact is multiplied—not divided—as it is disseminated and utilized down the years. It is not possible for medical research to stand still. If it fails to progress, it will regress; one need only recall how knowledge fell away in the Middle Ages.

Today, there is perhaps too much of a tendency to adopt a patronizing attitude toward empiricism. While empiricism requires an extravagant waste of time and human material, by no means has it been barren. In addition to the examples just mentioned, there is castor oil as a cathartic, opium as a pain reliever, squills for the dropsy, digitalis for the failing heart, Rauwolfia for hypertension, and the treatment of skin disease with sulfur and mercury. The last two have had a good medical reputation for nearly 4,000 years.

Historic matters are only briefly germane to the purposes of this book. One reason for mentioning them at all is to delineate changing or changed attitudes toward human experimentation. Celsus, practicing in Alexandria in the third century B.C., cried out against dissection of living men. Certainly, while sweeping generalizations are not indicated, it may be interesting to sample some of the activities going on at the end of the nineteenth and in the early part of the twentieth centuries. At that time nutritional studies were of special interest.

Beriberi was a particular problem. In December, 1905, William Fletcher took the lunatics in an asylum at Kuala Lumpur, marched them to the dining room, and numbered them off. The odd-numbered patients were given the regular hospital diet of uncured rice, and the even-numbered received cured rice, containing sufficient vitamin B to prevent beriberi. Some 43 of the 120 patients on uncured rice developed the disease, and 18 of them died. No patient of the 123 on the cured rice died, and only 2 developed beriberi. (They had it on admission.) The study was important, and is often cited [162]. Brieger has sought unsuccessfully for any comment on the ethics of the situation [46].

In 1913 Vedder, in describing experiments on beriberi by Fraser and Stanton, said: "Finally I have been authoritatively informed that Fraser and Stanton in the course of their work on beriberi, performed a large number of human experiments, in which they tried by every conceivable method, including insect transmission, to infect healthy individuals from beriberi patients. The experiments were all negative, but were unfortunately suppressed by the government for political reasons." Perhaps twinges of conscience explain the final comment [414].

At about the same time (1902), a series of experiments was carried out on food preservatives. A dozen volunteers recruited from the civil service were called the "Poison Squad" and were the subject of considerable amusement to the press; no evidence of ethical concern for their welfare is to be found.

In 1908, President Roosevelt appointed a board of eminent scientific experts, headed by the distinguished Ira Remsen, to carry out various human experiments with benzoic acid and saccharine. On this occasion, unlike the others, the board was severely criticized by the medical and scientific communities and by industry. Alas, Professor Remsen's main concern was addressed to methods of payment for the subjects. Other similar examples are cited. One group, however, raised questions of morality: the antivivisectionists! Brieger concludes that the experiments of 50 and 100 years ago simply did not strike many as unethical [46]. Others also began to be concerned, as cited by Stevenson [396].

One can grant the value of empiric observation without in the least obscuring the role of planned medical research in bringing medicine out of the realm of folklore, superstition, and philosophical speculation to today's science. There are still some who have "humanitarian" qualms about the value and propriety of medical research. In the words of McCance, the answer to inhuman research is "humane research, not no research" [293].

Paradoxically, in the last half century at least, those who experiment on man have been freer of attack than those who carry out animal experimentation; in this one can see a wry commentary on present times and culture in the Western world. It has been estimated that until 1940 Americans spent more on funeral flowers than on medical research!

The foregoing examples illustrate the ancient origins of human experimentation. The burgeoning of a *general awareness* that experimentation in man can create ethical problems is of rather recent origin, although its antecedents are ancient.[2] One of the first, if not the first, symposia on the subject of the ethics of human experimentation was that on human pharmacological experiments. This was held at the meeting of the Federation of American Societies for Experimental Biology at Atlantic City, on March 15–19, 1948. The first multidisciplinary symposium to express concern was held at the University of California in 1951. On that occasion a medical investigator, a physician, a lawyer, and an administrator participated in a medical staff conference that was published two years later—see Shimkin [383] and Guttentag [196]. The development of this first multidisciplinary conference was furthered, one can believe, by the Nuremberg Trials and the Nuremberg Code (1946–1949) and by four rather notable papers: Ivy's study

[2] One can find here and there evidence that in ancient times the thoughtful physician recognized that experimentation in man created some ethical problems. Indeed, the Oath attributed to Hippocrates (470–360 B.C.) can be construed to advise on experimental diagnosis and therapy, especially when one takes into account Hippocrates' aphorism concerning "experiment perilous, decision difficult." From this one vaults over 2,000 years to Percival's code, 1803, followed by William Beaumont's code, 1833, Claude Bernard's personal code, 1856, and the American Medical Association's recurrent statements on ethics (1846, 1847, 1946, 1949, 1958, 1966, 1967, to mention a few). (The details of the codes mentioned are recorded in Appendix A.)

It seems evident that the astounding German material uncovered at the Nuremberg trials, which led to formulation of the Nuremberg Code, 1946–1949, was directly responsible for the interest in human experimentation recorded in the two decades just after World War II. For example, there is Wiggers's code, 1950; the American Hospital Association's code, 1957; Bradford Hill's code for the clinical trial, 1963; Harvard University Health Services code, 1963; the Harvard Medical School code, 1965; the Declaration of Helsinki, 1962–1964; the National Institutes of Health code, 1966; Wolfensberger's code, 1967; and Beecher's "Guiding Principles," 1966 and 1967, to mention some typical examples.

of "History and Ethics of the Use of Human Subjects in Medical Experiments" [226], von Weizaecker's "Euthanasie und Menschenversuche" [415], Wiggers's "Human Experimentation as Exemplified by the Career of Dr. William Beaumont" [425], and finally McCance's "The Practice of Experimental Medicine" [293].

An important further influence was that derived from the thorough collection by Ladimer and Newman and republication in 1963 in a single volume of a vast amount of material on legal, ethical, and moral aspects of human experimentation. This fine compendium [263], a product of William Curran's Law-Medicine Institute, made easily accessible the principal modern papers.

Three other very different events and their consequences resulted in a wide awareness of the existence of ethical problems. First, the widely publicized injection of live cancer cells into 22 patients who were not informed as to the nature of the injection. A startling aspect of this was the origin of the study in one of the most celebrated laboratories and hospitals in the world. Second, governmental action as in the Kefauver-Harris Amendments to the Federal Food, Drug and Cosmetic Act (1962) and the February 1966 requirement by the Surgeon General of the United States Public Health Service that all applications for grants from the Public Health Service must be examined by a committee in the originating institution and approved on the basis of consideration for the "rights and welfare of human subjects in research . . . the risks and potential medical benefits . . ." Third, the careful editorial study and subsequent acceptance in 1966 by the *New England Journal of Medicine* of Beecher's paper, "Ethics and Clinical Research" [28].

It may seem presumptuous to place the Beecher article in relationship to the other two events; however, the thousand requests for reprints, the heated comments for and against, the subsequent references to it in published papers, and the sudden emergence of many symposia dealing with it and the subject of the ethics of experimentation in general—all of these indicate that it was responsible for creating an increased awareness that ethical problems exist in this area, a primary purpose of the publication. Curran has suggested that the clarification of the Food and Drug Administration's stand as presented in Goddard's August 24, 1966, regulations, coming as they did two months following the publication of Beecher's article, were influenced by the paper [126]. Lasagna says, "While it is not evident how much of the impetus for the new regulations has come from Congressional prodding of the FDA, doubtless some of the force for change derived from the widespread publicity given two events: the injection of cancer cells into some aged residents of a Brooklyn Hospital, and a speech (later published) by Dr. Henry K. Beecher, Professor of Anesthesia at Harvard" [268]. M. M. Katz of the National Institutes of Health has said, "The drug research field, as noted, has been much affected by these disclosures. They have already led to legislation in the area and may lead to more" [240].

Other critics clearly imply that "these ends justify these means" or that "the most good for the most people" is the goal sought, ignoring the fact that if the individual is sacrificed, so also will current standards of justice for the masses be lost. One can only conclude from their clear statements, as well as inferences, that some critics hold that science, not morality, is the highest value. Without for a single moment holding any belief in anyone's infallibility in any area, I conclude that some of the criticism of the article mentioned is based upon such surprising attitudes that it is evident that the article or one like it was necessary. Fortunately, many competent observers have concurred in that view, not the least of them the distinguished editor of the *New England Journal of Medicine,* the then dean of the Harvard Medical School, and the then president of the Massachusetts Medical Society, to mention a few, all of whom were consulted prior to publication.

Curran has presented some interesting data on the decline of "problem projects" [127]. One wonders if the discussion precipitated by Beecher's 1966 paper may have influenced the 65 percent decline in problem projects in man in two years' time [26], as shown in Table 1.

TABLE 1
NATIONAL INSTITUTES OF HEALTH PROBLEM PROJECTS—
HUMAN EXPERIMENTATION *

Month and year	*Total applications received, number*	*Projects involving human subjects, estimated number*	*Problem projects,%*	
			Number	*Percent of those involving humans*
June 1966	4100	1230	81	6.6
March 1967	4001	1200	27	2.2
June 1967	3931	1180	38	3.2
November 1967	3677	1100	35	3.2
March 1968	3651	1095	37	3.4
June 1968	4078	1250	40	3.2
November 1968	3393	1118	26	2.3

* Data provided by the Division of Research Grants, courtesy of Eugene A. Confrey, Ph.D.

REASONS FOR URGENCY OF STUDY

Possibilities for ethical errors are increasing, not only in numbers, but in variety; for example, the recent problems arising in transplantation of organs (Chap. 5). Serious attention to the general problem is urgent for a number of reasons. Of transcendent importance is the enormous and continuing increase in available funds, as shown in Table 2.

TABLE 2
MONIES AVAILABLE FOR RESEARCH EACH YEAR

	Massachusetts General Hospital *	*National Institutes of Health* †
1945	$ 500,000	$ 701,800
1955	2,222,816	36,063,200
1965	8,384,342	436,600,000

* Approximation, supplied by Mr. David C. Crockett of the Massachusetts General Hospital.

† The National Institutes of Health figures are based upon decade averages, excluding funds for construction, kindly supplied by Dr. John Sherman of the National Institutes of Health.

Since World War II the annual expenditure for research—in large part in man—in the Massachusetts General Hospital has increased a remarkable 17-fold. At the National Institutes of Health, the increase has been a gigantic 624-fold. This "national" rate of increase is over thirty-six times that of the Massachusetts General Hospital. These data, rough as they are, illustrate vast opportunities in terms of support and concomitantly expanded responsibilities in the use of human subjects.

Taking into account the sound and increasing demand of recent years that experimentation in man must precede general application of new procedures in therapy, plus the great sums of money available, there is reason to fear that these requirements and financial resources may be greater than the supply of competent, responsible investigators. In 1955 the Public Health Council of the Netherlands stated its belief that "there has been some deterioration of ethical standards in experimentation which it wants to check, insofar as possible, by preventive and educational measures." All this adds to the urgency of the problems under discussion.

Medical schools and university hospitals are increasingly dominated by investigators. Every young physician knows that he will never be promoted to a tenure post, to a professorship in a major medical school, unless he has proved himself as an investigator. If the ready availability of money for conducting research is added to this fact, one can see how great are the pressures on ambitious young physicians. Implementation of the recommendations of the President's Commission on Heart Disease, Cancer and Stroke means that further sums of money will become available for research in man.

In addition to the foregoing three practical points, there are others. Lord Platt has discussed them: a general awakening of social conscience; greater power for good or harm in new remedies, new operations, and new investigative procedures than was formerly the case; new methods of preventive treatment, with their advantages and dangers, now applied to communities as a whole, as well as to individuals, with multiplication of the possibilities for injury [345]. Medical science has shown how valuable human experimentation can be in solving problems of disease and in its treatment; one can therefore anticipate an increase in experimentation. Finally, there is the newly developed concept of clinical research as a profession—for example, clinical pharmacology—and this, of course, can lead to unfortunate separation between the interests of science and the interests of the patient. Beyond these matters, perhaps owing in part to current widespread concern for civil rights, one senses a new awareness of the importance of an ethical approach to the individual involved in medical and scientific studies.

FREQUENCY OF UNETHICAL OR QUESTIONABLY ETHICAL PROCEDURES

Nearly everyone agrees that ethical violations do occur. The practical question is, how often? A preliminary examination of the matter was based on 17 examples, which were easily increased to 50. These 50 studies contained references to 186 further likely examples—on the average 3.7 leads per study. Violations at times overlapped from paper to paper, but this figure indicates how conveniently one can proceed in a search for such material. These data are suggestive of widespread problems. However, there is need for another kind of information; this was obtained by examination of 100 consecutive human studies published in 1964 in an excellent journal; 12 of these seemed to be unethical. If only one quarter of these are truly unethical, this still indicates the existence of a serious situation. In England, Pappworth has collected more than 500 papers based upon unethical experimentation [330]. It is evident from such observations that unethical or questionably ethical procedures are not uncommon.

CONSENT IN CLINICAL EXPERIMENTATION

Consent,[3] variously characterized as informed, valid, or understanding, is the central issue on which hang most of the ethical problems in human experimentation. This is the principal condition that must be satisfied as far as possible if activities in this field are to be both ethical and lawful. Any law requiring consent requires *informed* consent, insofar as this can be achieved, whether it deals with personal injury, mistake, fraud, or contract, for example. Informed consent is characterized by appreciation, not only of known risks, but also of suspected risks. The patient, if he is aware of and understands the risks involved, has the right in giving consent, to determine what factors are significant to him. This is not the province of the investigator. There is no right to withhold facts that the subject might consider relevant to his consent or its withholding.

Dykstra [141] contends that the subject, in consenting to experimentation, has a right to assume (1) that the proposed study has in view legitimate and justifiable ends; (2) that the investigator is well qualified; (3) that the investigator will supervise the experiments and will follow them closely and discontinue them if serious unanticipated risks develop; (4) that, where pertinent, preliminary tests have been conducted; and (5) that the investigator has in mind possible side effects and is prepared to cope with them.

There are some exceptions to spoken consent. For example, a sick man goes to his physician for relief or cure of his ailment.

[3] Defined by the FDA as follows: "'Consent' or 'informed consent' means that the person involved has legal capacity to give consent, is so situated as to be able to exercise free power of choice, and is provided with a fair explanation of all material information concerning the administration of the investigational drug, or his possible use as a control, as to enable him to make an understanding decision as to his willingness to receive said investigational drug. This latter element requires that before the acceptance of an affirmative decision by such person the investigator should make known to him the nature, duration, and purpose of the administration of said investigational drug; the method and means by which it is to be administered; all inconveniences and hazards reasonably to be expected, including the fact, where applicable, that the person may be used as a control; the existence of alternative forms of therapy, if any; and the effects upon his health or person that may possibly come from the administration of the investigational drug" [127].

There may be no known standard treatment. His physician is obliged to experiment for the sake of this specific patient. As already pointed out, most diagnosis and therapy require experimentation. The patient has put his trust in his doctor; in the act of coming, he has given consent to reasonable efforts to relieve him. In many cases, it would not be to the patient's advantage to go into a detailed exposition of what the physician thinks and proposes to do. For one thing, such an approach might alert the patient to the *possibility* that his disease was a fatal one, whether true or not. There are rather tedious arguments as to the interpretation of the law concerning the possible obligation to inform the subject and gain his consent when there is no discernible risk and when to do so would possibly so distort the results as to make them of questionable value. This has been discussed elsewhere (page 176).

The law relies on penalties to force compliance; how can these be invoked when the subject and his next of kin do not know that experimentation is involved and could not prove it even if they knew it? The subject who is in a diagnostic or therapeutic relationship with the physician often may not be aware that he is the subject of experimentation. When he knows this and has consented to it, he still may not know that the information on which he based consent was either misleading or not adequate for his decision. Cavers believes that gradations in degree make the judicial decision between permissible and impermissible action so difficult as to make unlikely a successful civil damage suit, not to mention a criminal suit [62].

GENERAL COMMENTS

The roots of the word consent (*con-sentire, con-sensum*), when translated, are particularly appropriate to defining present needs: *"to feel together," "to agree."* When it comes to experimentation in man, the word is further qualified. What is sought is "informed" or "valid" consent; it is on this rock that many if not most of the ethical problems come to grief. Some of the difficulties of achieving this will be discussed shortly, and some of the inherent impossibilities will be circumvented if what one obtains is "risk appreciation" or if one accepts Freund's sensible suggestion that the best one can achieve in many cases is *informed participation* [171] or Ritts's *agreement to participate* [361]. Clearly, these fall short of the ideal goal, but in all honesty they often represent as nearly accurate a description of the true situation as possible. The idea that the truth, the whole truth, and nothing but the truth can always be conveyed to the subject is false. It is what Whitehead has called the fallacy of the misplaced concreteness.

Before we can arrive at an acceptable consent, the investigator must disclose to his subject all the information he has concerning purposes, possibilities, uses, and value, as well as all risks, present or possible. Frequently, the difficulty is that no one knows what the risks or the benefits really will be. The heavy mass of codes presented in Appendix A is a reflection of the difficulties and unease most investigators feel when confronted by the need for "full" disclosure to a subject when matters for study are even moderately complicated. In short, it is necessary to discard the belief that a rational, intelligent man is capable of imparting information fully and accurately. Aristotle notwithstanding, every man is not sufficiently eloquent for that which he knows, and in the present context he often does not even *know*. On the other hand the subject, rational and intelligent though he may be, is often not capable of understanding, of grasping the meaning of the hazards of what is proposed to him. More than this, the situation is full of "irrational," unknown determinants, and these, as Jay Katz [238] has pointed out, may lead the subject to act in ways that others might interpret as misinformed, uninformed, incompetent, or irresponsible.

Despite all this, consent seeks increased respect for the individual by providing him with opportunities for self-determination; at the same time, it seeks to reduce assaults on the integrity of the man through hidden interventions by others, however benevolent they may be. The final decision as to the degree of acceptable risk belongs to the subject. As mentioned above, the difficulty is that often he is not competent to understand; indeed, on many occasions, no one knows the risks involved. In such a case, this must be made clear insofar as it is possible to do so.

Jay Katz has stated that only a little over 30 years ago [238]:

> The Supreme Court of Michigan explicitly introduced consent as a prerequisite for "experimentation." [If] the general practice of medicine and surgery is to progress, there must be a certain amount of experimentation . . . , but such experiments must be done with the knowledge and consent of the patient or those responsible for him, and must not vary too radically from the accepted method of procedure. Here the Court acknowledged the need for experimentation, circumscribed by consent and progress in small steps. A few other recent opinions similarly emphasized that patients must be informed about and consent to novel intervention. This suggests that law would look with disfavor on research with uninformed subjects and decisions from other areas of law would support such a conclusion.

Curran holds that the courts have also determined in the diagnostic or therapeutic situation that the requirement of informed consent can be measured by the standards the community sets for medical practitioners [126]. The community standard is now being extended in some states. Doubtless this is owing to improved communications and also to broadened medical competence.

A strict interpretation of this view would forbid all research not for the patient's direct benefit if the patient remains uninformed. Some have held that in the absence of risk and when the potential benefit to science is great, the investigator may proceed without the subject's knowledge. This is hazardous territory. It can be considered remotely only in therapeutic situations when a procedure is undertaken for the subject's welfare.

One must agree that to eliminate one group—in this case, uninformed subjects—may bias the results and check scientific growth. Whenever such situations arise, they should be carefully documented. Some believe, as this writer does not, that eventually lawmakers may resolve the conflict by ruling in favor of progress in science.

In some reflections on consent, Freund has emphasized the

effects of the requirement of consent on the investigator [170]. He suggests that too much attention may have been focused on the "isolated act of communication between the experimenter and his subjects." When the investigator knows that he must explain his proposal to the subject, he is not likely to take too casual an attitude toward his procedure. The immediate result of this can be a more penetrating insight into his own motives and the revelation of discreditable aspects he may have suppressed from his own thought. The need for communication can reveal these things and sharpen understanding of the risks and benefits present. One must always bear in mind the inequality between subject and investigator. The latter is usually more competent than the subject and better informed.

Wolfensberger [428] has summarized the types of rights the subject may yield to the investigator: "(i) Invasion of privacy; (ii) donation or sacrifice of personal resources such as time, attention, dignity, and physical, mental, or emotional energy; (iii) surrender of autonomy, as in hypnotic, drug, or brain-stimulation studies, or in studies entailing restriction of movement and action; (iv) exposure to procedures entailing mental or physical pain or discomfort, but no risk of injury or lasting harm; and (v) exposure to procedures that may entail risk of physical or emotional injury."

Suppose, for example, that true understanding and valid consent have been obtained and recorded. What is the protection that is thus afforded and what significance and meaning may be attached to it? Ladimer has answered. *First,* consent is legal authorization to proceed. The subject cannot later claim assault or battery. *Second,* depending on the extent of the consent, it gives legal authority to use the data obtained for professional or research purposes. Invasion of privacy cannot later be claimed, although commercial use would not ordinarily be included, unless specifically granted. *Third,* failure to benefit would not be a basis for a charge. *Fourth,* consent is a defense to an injury arising from the inherent risk of the procedure understood and consented to. *Fifth,* consent is a defense to an injury owing to the subject's failure to follow instructions for safety or for after-care, if the orders were well explained and reasonable [262].

It must be understood that consent to experimentation will not protect the investigator if he is guilty of negligence. The consent agreement covers adversity created by proper, but not by improper, conduct. (See page 38 concerning liability insurance.)

MYTH AND REALITY

As mentioned earlier, the patient who goes to a physician for relief consents, in the very act of going, to reasonable efforts to treat him, and very often this inevitably involves experimentation; our concern at this time presents more difficult problems than this. The present discussion is directed to experimentation on one individual, not for his benefit, but for that of patients in general.

There is a disturbing and widespread myth that codes—all of which emphasize, above all else, consent—will provide some kind of security. While there is undoubted value to be gained from examining them as guides to the thinking of others on the subject, the reality is that any rigid adherence to codes can provide a dangerous trap. No two situations are alike; it is impossible to spell out all contingencies in codes. When an accident occurs in the course of experimentation, it will be easy for the prosecution to show failure to comply fully with a code's provisions, and an endless vista of legal actions opens up. It is a curious thing that lawyers for even the greatest institutions are much more likely to cripple themselves and their institutions with inevitably imperfect codes than are the investigators involved, who usually understand the possible pitfalls presented in the codes. Security rests with the *responsible* investigator, who will refer difficult decisions to his peers. Morally responsible action is the result of making the best choice among several possibilities.

Most codes dealing with human experimentation start out with the bland assumption that consent is readily obtainable. This is a myth. The reality is that informed consent is often exceedingly difficult or impossible to obtain in any complete sense. The difficulties inherent in this complex situation are no excuse for giving up the effort: *informed consent is the goal toward which we strive.* This necessity is based upon reasons in at least three categories. (1) *Ethical:* No man has the privilege of choosing participants for a risky procedure without the knowledge and agreement of the subject. There may be a modest exception to this in circumstances where there is no discernible risk and where discussion with the patient would vitiate any possibility of success as, for example, where one compares a placebo with a pain-relieving agent. However, opinions and interpretations of the law in this area differ. (2) *Sociological:* Society will not long tolerate the investigator's domination of another, with the possible expenditure of his subject's health or life. Studies that do not have at least the tacit support of the public will not flourish. (3) *Legal:* The law, as Professor Freund [168] has put it, "is deeply protective of human integrity and life. An offensive touching or invasion of the body, if not consented to, is a trespass against the person, a battery, redressible in an action for damages." The Bill of Rights holds that a man shall be safe in his person. Imperfect as our attempts to obtain informed consent may be, an important reality nevertheless invariably emerges from such effort: the patient involved then knows that he is to be the subject of an experiment—too often, not otherwise the case—and knowing, can reject the opportunity if he chooses to do so.

It is often contended that patients who trust their doctor will accede to almost any request he cares to make: "My doctor would not ask anything of me not for my good." In too many cases this, too, is a myth. The experienced clinician-investigator knows that if he has rapport with his patients, they will often knowingly submit, for the sake of "science," to inconvenience and even to discomfort, if these are not too long continued. However, except in rare cases, the reality is that patients will not knowingly put their health or their lives in jeopardy for a scientific experiment. It is erroneous to assume otherwise. When serious risks are taken and more than a few subjects are involved, it is accurate to assume that informed consent has not been obtained in all cases.

A different kind of myth is that perpetuated by some critics; namely, that if the investigator *says* he has consent, then all is well. Far more dependable evidence of right or wrong is to be found in examination of a given investigation. It is clear that a good many published studies should never have been undertaken.

The problems are compounded by the reality that some studies bearing moderate risk may be entirely ethical when fully informed consent is obtained, but are otherwise unethical. Such studies, unlike those mentioned in the preceding paragraph, may appear proper in published form and yet be suspect, depending on the understanding reached by investigator and subject before the experiment was initiated.

A particularly pernicious myth is the one that depends on the view that the end always justifies the means. A study is ethical or not at its inception; it does not become ethical merely because it turned up valuable data. Sometimes an experiment is rationalized by the investigator as having produced the most good for the most people. This is blatant statism. Whoever gave the investigator the god-like right to choose martyrs for science? (Kety)

Is the patient, then, without hope for honest, responsible care? Not at all. One must never minimize the importance of striving for truly informed consent, but the patient's greater safeguard in experimentation, as in therapy, is the skillful, informed, intelligent, honest, responsible, compassionate physician. One hopes and believes these are in the majority.

Kety's discussion [246] of consent is, as usual, to the point:

> In studies on normal individuals where there was no intent or little possibility of helping the subject, the rule of voluntary consent is, of course, absolutely essential and the necessity of complete explanation equally important. The completeness of the explanation, however, need refer only to that information which will enable the subject to make a judgment upon hazards and need not include other scientific information irrelevant to the question of risk and knowledge of which on the part of the subject may be prejudicial to a controlled experiment. In other words, if one were giving a potent drug or a placebo, it would be necessary to explain to the subject only the risks involved in the taking

of the drug. [For another view when deception is involved, see page 112.]

In the case of patients there are important justifications for clinical research in addition to those which hold for normal controls. In the first place, if the research is relevant to the clinical condition from which the patient is suffering, and I feel that it should be, there is the clear possibility of personal benefit to the patient from the research itself, and there, perhaps the criterion might be the chance of harming the patient versus the chance of helping him. Even though both of these chances may be low, in most clinical research the chance of personal benefit is usually considerably greater than the chance of harm to the individual patient.

With regard to the justification for using a placebo instead of a drug in the treatment of a disease, this can, of course, be justified if the purpose of the study is to evaluate a new and untried drug, since one can hardly be criticized for withholding an agent of unknown potential for good or harm. With regard to the question of withholding a drug of known benefit temporarily, the concept of greater harm versus greater good to the patient may still apply, in addition to which it may be perfectly possible to get the voluntary consent of the patient to cooperate in a research problem in which certain parts of the treatment may be delayed or withheld temporarily in order to make certain observations. In fact, in any case where the element of hazard is greater than the chances of benefit, the patient may still consent with full knowledge of the risk.

When a patient places himself in the hands of a physician for relief of a symptom or cure of a disease, this act implies consent to the physician to carry out all necessary and acceptable means to relieve or cure. If the problem is pain, for example, we know that a placebo will often relieve half to two-thirds of the pain relievable with an optimal dose of morphine [18, 218, 241]. Surely, it would be carrying matters too far to require a dissertation to the patient on grades or degrees of relief anticipated, when real value could be expected from the use of a placebo. Such use of a placebo could reveal, for example, whether a powerful narcotic was actually necessary and thus be for the patient's good.

Originally, perhaps, before its power to relieve was established, the use of a placebo in such work might have been challenged on ethical grounds more effectively than at present. This is true of many, if not most, standard therapeutic procedures in wide use today. Cardiac catheterization—whose wide usefulness has been recognized by a Nobel Prize for three men—could, in its early days before its value was known, have been challenged on serious grounds as jeopardizing the immediate subject's life. Even now, this sometimes proves to be the case. However, it is now generally recognized that the demonstrated value of the technique outweighs the risk. Ladimer has described in chilling detail the probable fate in a court of law of the conscientious but bold investigator who takes such risks and experiences initial failures [255]. In most cases, neither true risk nor benefit can be initially assessed, and therefore they cannot be adequately described.

AN UNORTHODOX APPROACH

In a recent paper published in *Anesthesiology* [280], Long, Dripps, and Price stated:

> The problem of obtaining valid consent always exists in an experiment performed on human beings. Despite the fact that all of our subjects were interviewed before the study and the procedure explained, we believe that an informed consent cannot be obtained for a study of this type, because of the impossibility of transmitting to a patient both the relevant information and the *background* needed to analyze and evaluate such information. Instead, *we have accepted the role of guarantor of the patient's rights and safety* . . .

This statement comes from distinguished and senior members of a renowned university and commands attention. Theirs is a revolutionary approach to the complex problem faced by all clinical investigators.

First, since there is no indication to the contrary, one must assume that the editor and the editorial board of the journal, or at least a majority of the members of its editorial board, approved of the authors' statement. This in itself is rather remarkable, for in sounding out a number of experienced investigators, the writer has not found a single one who agreed with the authors.

Second, the "role of guarantor of the patient's rights and safety" in lieu of informed consent is outside the law, violating the Kefauver-Harris amendments to the Federal Food, Drug and Cosmetic Act of 1962 and the rulings of the National Institutes of Health, which have the effect of law.

Third, granted that "fully informed consent" is a chimera—an impossibility in many instances and probably in the majority of complicated studies—the fact remains that informed consent is a *goal toward which we must strive.* This point probably has less relevance to volunteers than to patients subjected to experimentation not for their direct benefit; however, honest striving for informed consent even with volunteers would undoubtedly best bring to their attention the hazards involved, insofar as these are known.

Fourth, this writer cannot agree—a view he shares with many others—that the deliberate evocation of ventricular extrasystoles is a safe procedure. There is much evidence to show that when ventricular extrasystoles appear, ventricular fibrillation sometimes follows. It is not always possible to restore a normal beat to a heart in ventricular fibrillation. The procedure, therefore, is not without serious danger.

Fifth, as pointed out elsewhere, after nearly 40 years of investigation in man one of the clearest lessons to emerge from this experience is that patients will usually agree to participate in experimentation, if their doctor approaches them agreeably and asks them to do so, as long as only discomfort and inconvenience are involved and provided these do not last very long. On the other hand, patients in general will never willingly agree to risk their health or their lives for the sake of science alone, except rare individuals who perhaps seek martyrdom or devoted investigators such as Walter Reed and his colleagues, whose lonely exploit is still celebrated 70 years or more after the event. In the ordinary case, when *post hoc* it becomes evident that the health or life of several subjects has been jeopardized, it is usually clear that they did not all understand what they had agreed to.

In discussing these matters, Fink [157] has said, ". . . there is an obvious inconsistency between the claim to guarantee the patient's rights and the failure to honor the foremost of those rights, the right to exercise informed consent or dissent. A guarantee of this sort is nugatory. Further, the role itself implies infallibility, as if the investigator can always guess correctly whether the patient would consent to the procedure if she fully understood the nature of the experiment."

Sixth, it is clear from the context and from personal knowledge of these responsible investigators that their intent is the consequence of an honest recognition of what they regard as an impossible requirement. They have adopted a defeatist attitude. In fact, they promise something they cannot guarantee; if the subject believes this guarantee, he is deceived. This is certainly not an intentional result, but nevertheless the inescapable consequence of their policy.

Seventh, an adoption of the paternalistic view recommended really leaves all decision-making to the investigator; what should be a joint enterprise between subject and investigator becomes a monopoly of the investigator, who is thus unhampered by personal discussion with the subject of the latter's wishes and interests. There would be no limitations—not in the case of these responsible, careful workers, but with others less careful and less scrupulous—if the policy stated here were to be generally adopted. It should not be adopted, notwithstanding the wide experience and distinction of those who have suggested it. This critique is presented in some detail, for the proposal, or something like it, will probably be suggested by other sorely tried investigators. It is very likely that many others have in effect assumed the role of "guarantor," but have lacked the forthright candor of Long, Dripps, and Price.

GRADATIONS OF CONSENT

When the Public Health Service first turned its attention to matters of consent, it held that fully informed consent is an essential feature of all research activities involving human subjects. There is now a growing conviction that *gradations* of consent must be considered. Consent may be fully informed and freely given, or consent may be implied, as in the case of a man going to his physician for relief of an ailment. There is the case in which no discernible risk to body, to mind, or to privacy is involved and where the obligation to obtain informed consent would destroy the possibility of deriving dependable data. This is not, it must be pointed out, the interpretation of the law by the Food and Drug Administration. In some limited circumstances, of course, full information to a subject would alert him to the fact or the possibility that he has a fatal disease. It would be easy to misapply the cautious liberalization suggested in the preceding remarks and conclude that these ends justify these means. The purpose of the present comments is to indicate that the concept of consent is in an evolving state, and this is desirable.

CONSENT COERCED

The foregoing material has touched on most of the problems concerning valid consent and, by implication at least, includes consent effected through coercion; this, of course, is a contradiction in terms and no consent at all. Valid consent is a contract between equals as far as it involves freedom to accept or reject. The investigator, with his superior knowledge, must overcome any tendency to adopt an overbearing approach. In this situation, superior power of whatever kind must be curbed. It appears variably in the relationship of teacher to student, of jailer to prisoner, of physician to patient, and of scientist to subject. It can be "engineered" in a host of subtle ways. Whatever the mechanism, coercion nullifies consent. It is against our democratic tradition [161a].

Edmond Cahn has had some penetrating comments to make on this [56]:

> One of the major malpractices of our era consists in the "engineering of consent." Sometimes this is effected simply by exploiting the condition of necessitous men, as in certain Indian states where thousands of consents to sexual sterilization have been purchased by offering a trivial bounty to the members of a destitute caste. Then again, consent may be "engineered" by the kind of psychologist who takes it for granted

that his assistants and students will submit to experiments and implies a threat to advancement if they raise objections. Or the total community may "engineer" a consent, as when the president, the generals, and the newspapers call with loud fanfare for a heroic crew of astronautical volunteers to attempt some ultrahazardous exploit.

It is worth considering that the destitute Indians who accept payment for sterilization can at least know what they are consenting to; the psychological and astronautical subjects cannot. Moreover, though the astronauts are fairly certain of winning some species of glory, the lady who submits to hypnosis in the interest of science is certain of scarcely anything. Fortunately, there is evidence that responsible psychologists are becoming aware of the problem and are seeking to cope with it. Even a free consent must have moral limits in a society that honors human dignity and, honoring it, puts a ceiling-price on truth.

Lord Henley [206a], as long ago as 1762, clearly saw the problem: "Necessitous men are not, truly speaking, free men, but, to answer a present exigency, will submit to any terms that the crafty may impose upon them."

PROBLEMS OF PUBLICATION

In the view of the British Medical Research Council [49], it is not enough to ensure that all investigation is carried out in an ethical manner; it must be made unmistakably clear in the publications that the proprieties have been observed. This implies editorial responsibility in addition to that of the investigator. The question arises, then, about valuable data that have been improperly obtained.[4] It is the writer's belief that such material *ordinarily* should not be published. There is a practical aspect to the matter: failure to obtain publication would discourage unethical experimentation. How many would carry out such experimentation if they *knew* its results would never be published? Admittedly, there is room for debate. Others believe that such data, because of their intrinsic value, obtained at a cost of great risk or damage to the

[4] As far as principle goes, a parallel can be seen in the recent Mapp decision by the United States Supreme Court. It was stated there that evidence unconstitutionally obtained cannot be used in any Prosecution, no matter how important the evidence is to the ends of justice. *Mapp v. Ohio* 367 U.S. 643, 81 S. Ct. 1684 (1961).

subjects, should not be wasted, but should be published with stern editorial comment. This would require exceptional skill, if an odor of hypocrisy is to be avoided.

Publication is both a privilege and a responsibility. This fact might be used to require the investigator to report whether consent had been obtained; whether it was oral or written; what inducements, if any, were offered; and whether the objectives and hazards were discussed with the patient. If the author was reporting on the results of an accepted treatment and specific consent was not required, this could be stated. In such a situation, the editor would not be responsible for the author's veracity. Certainly much of the information an investigator would need to disclose—for example, his description of his consent procedure—would merely be that required in any new drug study. If the records did not contain adequate consent data or acceptable reasons for their omission, the Food and Drug Administration could refuse to accept the investigator's report in support of the sponsor's New Drug Application, "to the acute embarrassment of the former and the costly discomfiture of the latter." Whenever suspicions were aroused and investigation showed that false statements were present, criminal prosecution could be instituted. This is provided for in Section 1001 of Title 18 of the United States Code, applicable when false reports are made to an agency of the United States.

The requirement of a "consent" addendum to published reports could provide a continuing flow of cases out of which a "common law" of consent could grow [62]. Better by far than dependence on legal limitations would be a consistent professional practice that would go well beyond the minimum requirements of the law. The editorial practice suggested would promote this [62]. In 1955, the Public Health Council of the Netherlands stated, "Publication of articles describing human experiments that are contrary to medical ethics is strongly criticized; and it is recommended that medical journals refuse to publish articles based on unethical experiments." This view is shared by Thomson [407] and by the distinguished former editor of *The Lancet,* T. F. Fox [166].

2
The Subject

The subject, when interviewed by an investigator, should listen first, for what the investigator wants to tell; second, for what he does not want to tell; third, for what he cannot tell [206].

The rights of the individual have come more and more to the front in recent years. The Supreme Court of the United States has emphasized this. The Court has been charged with "coddling" criminals and thereby encouraging lawlessness. It seems evident that what the Court is attempting to do in this era of growing federal power is to protect the helpless individual, to guarantee his fundamental rights in the belief that it is better to go easy on a few criminals than to subject millions of blameless citizens to the rude power of a police state where bugging, wiretapping, spying, nighttime search, seizure, and arrest are common. The individual's liberty and constitutional safeguards are not to be jeopardized. In all of this, the fact must not be overlooked that society also has its rights (see page 47).

PRIOR ANIMAL WORK

Before turning to the human subject for experimentation, the possibilities for learning from animals must be exhausted. Animal experimentation tells us much about anatomy, physiology, biochemistry, and to a considerable extent about pharmacology and toxicology; for definitive treatment, however, human experimentation is indispensable. Some codes state categorically that animal work must always precede experimentation in man. This, of course, is absurd: many human diseases do not spontaneously occur in and cannot be produced in animals. In study of psychologic and psychiatric problems, man is usually the only possible experimental subject; however, when drug studies are undertaken in those conditions, it is sometimes possible to obtain information of value from animals as to the side effects of the drugs. Many concepts can be discovered and tested in animals; their establishment in man can be effected only by experimentation in man. The proof is found here, and it very often is found best, most economically, accurately, and rapidly in the controlled clinical trial. Man is the "animal of necessity."

THE AWARE, UNDERSTANDING, AND CONSENTING SUBJECT

This has been dealt with in some detail in the section on Consent, page 18. These matters can scarcely be overemphasized, nor can we overlook our frequent inadequacies in achieving these states.

Lay subjects, sick or well, are not likely to understand the full implications of complicated procedures, *even after careful explanation.* If a subject dissents, he is not to be used in experimentation. The British Medical Research Council has stated [48]:

> To obtain the consent of the patient to a proposed investigation is not in itself enough. Owing to the special relationship of trust which exists between a patient and his doctor, most patients will consent to any proposal that is made. Further, the considerations involved are nearly always so technical as to prevent their being adequately understood by one who is not himself an expert. It must, therefore, be frankly recognized that, for practical purposes an inescapable responsibility for determining what investigations are, or are not, undertaken on a particular patient will rest with the doctor concerned. Nearly always his judgment will be accepted by the patient as decisive.

McCance has expressed the same view [293]. Or, as Guttentag [196] has put it, ". . . one has only to think of present-day specialization in medicine in order to realize that the patient is frequently not able to grasp all the implications of a certain procedure so far as his health is concerned." To some, this complexity leads to a strong admonition concerning volunteer work: At one time Pfeiffer [338] held the view that one should ". . . never use anyone except a volunteer who is at least at the level of a graduate student and who has investigated for himself the nature and possible dangers of the drug or procedure involved." Many would not completely endorse this view. For some types of investigation, especially when subjective factors are involved, it is essential to have subjects who know nothing about the expected results and have no vested interest in the outcome. Certainly, Pfeiffer's early requirement for a knowledgeable subject cannot be adhered to in the case of the diseased subject seeking relief. Such difficulties, however, give emphasis to the increased responsibility of the investigator when the subject cannot truly understand the full implication of the study contemplated. This is mentioned in some detail, for comparison with this idealistic, yet thoughtful and practical, investigator's current views. Pfeiffer [339] states his present view: "My quotation from 1951 must certainly be modified as of this date since we are using prisoners at the Atlanta Penitentiary who are not graduate students! We do screen our prisoners for psychiatric difficulties by having them complete a Rorschach examination, IQ assay and MMPI tests. We also go over their psychiatric history very carefully. My statement of 1951 represents the ideal situation rather than the practical situation."

There are, of course, many possible approaches to study of the experimental subject. They are rather obvious and need not be mentioned here, save for one example: Shimkin separates human experimental subjects into three groups, depending on their condition [383]: (1) The normal healthy subject; (2) the subject with reversible, non-fatal disease; and (3) the patient with fatal disease. The types of experiment can be classified as (1) "Passive" research, a study of human tissues outside the body; (2) "late active" research, studies in man following animal or in vitro studies; and (3) "initial active" research, studies initially undertaken on man as the only possible subject.

It is probably best to avoid the use of doctors or medical students in experiments that involve exposure to any kind of radiation, since in the course of their careers they are likely to have considerable exposure of this kind, and it would not be wise to add to this load in experimental procedures.

THE SUBJECT IN SELF-EXPERIMENTATION

While this matter is appropriate to the theme of this chapter, it has been sufficiently discussed for present purposes in Chap. 1; it will not be repeated here. (See also Code on Self-experimentation, National Institutes of Health, 1968 [94].)

LIMITATION ON CONSENT OF A PERSON TO EXPERIMENTATION ON HIMSELF

The first question to be examined is: how far can one go in consenting to severe injury to himself? For example, consent to abortion, except for therapeutic reasons, is a crime and not allowable. The fact that the woman gave consent is no defense for the doctor. Neither can a person consent to his own death; it is still murder by the man who kills him.

The situation is presumably different when the motive is advancement of science rather than the direct advantage of the person who permits the injury. Even so, an individual cannot *legally* consent to a serious injury that amounts to maiming.

PROTECTION OF THE SUBJECT AND THE INVESTIGATOR

There is a curious conflict to be found in what the law *says* about research—"a man experiments at his peril" [1]—and the almost universally held credo of Western civilization that advancement of medicine is desirable. This requires research; much of this research must be carried out in man; it is wrong to place a man in jeopardy or to penalize him for attempting to help his brother.

The law's statements concerning experimentation are really based on a considerable misunderstanding of the procedure. The

[1] Notwithstanding this, the FDA *requires* human experimentation!

phrase about peril goes back to the English case, *Slater v. Baker* (1767), the New York case, *Carpenter v. Blake* (1871), and many following cases. In both of these cases the attack was based upon the lack of consent of the patient to the use of a new procedure, construed as negligence. The patient's presumed expectation was that he would be treated in accordance with the accepted practices of the community. In each case, the courts' judgment was that a physician experiments at his peril. Notwithstanding their slight, if any, connection with the kind of human experimentation of particular interest here, they are often referred to. These factual situations, erroneously labeled experimentation—except as nearly all therapy involves trial and error—have done much to confuse legal concepts.

According to Ladimer, the position taken by legal writers and jurists who have summarized the issue's present position is as follows [255]: In treating the patient, "there must be no experimentation . . . we find that legal encyclopedias have unwaveringly set forth that while it is the duty of the physician or surgeon to keep up with advancements in his profession, it is also his duty not to try to forge ahead of it by trying experiments." Evidently nothing shall ever be done for the first time! The doctrine is, "the physician experiments at his peril." Many similar examples could be given. In this harsh stand the law seems to close its eyes to reality for, as every able physician knows, the adequate practice of medicine involves continual experimentation. No two patients respond precisely alike to any therapeutic procedure. There is no "standard" patient. Even in ordinary practice, the able doctor experiments until his treatment is successful, or until the patient goes elsewhere, or until he dies. Nonetheless, "the trail blazing practitioner is always courting a brush with the law" [404].

The need for a redefinition of human experimentation becomes apparent as one encounters [55] the many court rulings in which experimentation is equated with "rash action" or "ignorant and unskilled departure from approved methods" and one hears the low esteem of the court expressed in such phrases as "rash or experimental methods," "mere experiment," and "reckless experiments." It may be added that all the acts so castigated could by no means be labeled as foolish; neither were they always the work of incompetents. The remarks quoted, which are quite typical in cases of this kind, reveal the association in the judicial mind between experimentation and professional disregard or negligence. Needless to say, "this represents either a complete misconception of scientific experimentation or the singular use of the term so that it partakes of reckless behavior or quackery . . ." [55]. "The term 'experimentation' has been used loosely by the courts" [255]. According to Ladimer [255], the precedents, the cases of record, have usually "dealt not with major problems baffling to medicine and science on which basic research or applied clinical study was required, but with questions which confront the regular practitioner."

Little existing law deals explicitly with human experimentation. However, Jaffe points out that the common law, the law devised and administered by the courts, has developed and continues to develop doctrines that are applicable. The physical touching of an individual without his consent may be actionable, even when no physical injury has been sustained. Manipulation of an individual by deceit may be actionable as fraud. Carelessness in experimentation, if it leads to injury, may be actionable as negligence [229].

The Kefauver-Harris Amendments to the Federal Food, Drug and Cosmetic Act (1962) have legal force, for the first time directly concerned with human experimentation. The rulings of the National Institutes of Health have the force of law. We seem to be well on our way to the formulation of a body of laws that will apply directly to human experimentation.

In an examination of liability, the *Duke Law Journal* in 1960 offered, as a partial solution to the perils of the investigator, the concept of "liability without fault." This view should be compared with that of Wolfle [429]. If, in the course of an experiment a subject is damaged, he would be entitled to be made whole, by treatment or rehabilitation, or if not completely restored, to receive compensatory damages. The subject and the investigator would be protected. In this view, the investigator would not be considered to be at fault, for he had acted in the interests of society. Society, then, through government channels, would assume the costs of restoring or compensating the experimental subject; this is similar to the arrangement whereby society, through government channels, supports most of the experimentation for which the concept of liability without fault would be fitting. Society already has accepted the view that risk is reimbursable and that those who engage in hazardous pursuits deserve extra pay. While the first purpose is to protect the subject, the investigator must also be freed from unjust liability [cf. 31a].

One cannot deny that difficult problems are present; for example, answers to many psychological as well as physical problems can be found only in the response to stress. What are the limits? At what point will the subject break down? Will he sustain lasting damage? Screening of astronauts requires such testing as, for example, in study of G factors. One can take the view that some experiments are not ethical and never can be ethical. Alternately, as suggested above, one might possibly arrange a system of monetary compensation, "liability without fault," with the understanding and consent of the subject. Coordinated with such recompense, every effort to make the subject whole through treatment and rehabilitation would be carried out. The intention is to protect both subject and investigator. Society, through appropriate governmental channels, would bear the cost just as government now supports great areas of medical research.

There can be no question that the exposure of human experimental subjects to test situations can involve risk of injury even in some necessary procedures. Granted that all reasonable precautions have been taken to protect the subject from physical damage and the investigator from unethical practices, the possibility for injury may still remain. It is unreasonable to expect that the society, in profiting actually or potentially, should not share in the responsibility for what was done. This it can do, not only in requiring a sound and ethical approach to experimentation, but also by arranging for rehabilitation and restoration of the possibly injured subject and by providing financial recompense, when this is indicated, to relieve both subject and investigator of economic jeopardy.

There is uncertainty whether the physician's liability insurance will protect him, for experimental procedures, if valuable, can hardly be in accord with the usually required "accepted standards of the community": they of course go beyond, and are outside of, such standards.

Under the present circumstances, in the case of accident the injured subject would, if he sought recompense, have no recourse in most cases except to sue for damages. He might proceed against the investigator and his staff, against the hospital, against the laboratory, against the governmental agency or other source of funds, or against the hospital's review boards—that is, the research committee or the committee on ethics that had approved the research plan. The action would be based upon negligence or some other defect on the part of the investigator or sponsor. If the plaintiff won, payment might be required from any or all of the defendants.

Considerable injustice could thus be inflicted; there is the contention of Ladimer [259] that "Studies on human beings, because they involve some intervention, exposure, manipulation or deprivation, are not intentional assaults and batteries . . ." It is not appropriate that either the subject or the investigator alone should be required to face the consequences described. The injured subject has the right to expect to be "made whole" insofar as medical care and money can make this possible. There is no right to expect the careful and responsible investigator to bear the brunt of suit alone.

On some occasions federal agencies have already established precedents whereby funds for liability insurance have been included in the grants made. Examples are the allowances made by the National Institutes of Health under the 1957 Price-Anderson amendments to the Atomic Energy Act. The Congress has not made similar provisions for other hazardous programs. In a 1963 report, the Columbia University Law School, through its Legislative Drafting Fund for the National Security Industrial Association, recommended extension of advance protection. In another instance, the

National Foundation for Infantile Paralysis purchased liability insurance for its Salk vaccine field studies. In a study of seat belts under N.I.H. Project R.G. 6284, accident insurance with $100,000 maximum liability and $100 per week for a year of incapacity was purchased. The need for protection thus has been recognized on occasion.

Ladimer [259] has summarized the situation:

> The Report on Harm in Government Programs states that "Compensation for members of the public injured in a catastrophic accident would depend to a large extent upon their ability to recover damages by means of a lawsuit. Such suits would be governed by the law of torts which, generally speaking, holds an actor whose conduct injured another—either through carelessness or, in exceptional situations, even in the absence of fault—liable for compensatory damages to the injured person." The application of liability without fault, although growing, particularly where there is a "substantial risk . . . regardless of the degree of care" is still generally restricted to cases of injury arising out of the direct operation of a defendant, as opposed to indirect cause. When and whether the doctrine may apply depends on legal action and local law.

As Freund [171] has put it:

> The question is an instance of a pervasive confrontation between two social philosophies—the one putting primacy on responsibility, blameworthiness, rewards, and penalties for behavior, the other stressing security of the victims against the impersonal dooms of modern life. The conflict marked the early days of unemployment compensation, when debate centered on employer or plant funds versus pooled funds—the former providing an incentive to a firm to regularize employment, the latter providing greater assurance of compensation to the unemployed. . . .
>
> A combination of the two forms of liability . . . is possible, as the current Keeton-O'Connell plan for automobile accident compensation demonstrates. Under that plan, compensation would be due, without inquiry into fault, for expenses and loss of wages, up to $10,000; recovery for pain and suffering would require a lawsuit involving proof of the defendant's fault. In the field of experimentation, a similar combination might be tried, perhaps with the variation that the recovery based on fault would require proof not simply of fault but of gross fault, in

order to discourage speculative claims while retaining some extrinsic deterrent against recklessness. The existence of the basic compensation plan might serve, furthermore, to improve the general attitude of judge and jury toward the experimentation itself.

Ladimer suggests the feasibility of application of the principle of the workmen's compensation concept rather than employer liability or the malpractice approach [259, 261]. In the approach to these matters, it should "not be necessary to show fault, negligence or lack of caution." To take another approach, limited health and accident insurance could be written on each subject.

Practical problems remain. Which experimenters would be protected? How would psychological or physical damage be assessed? There are already legal precedents, of course, for reimbursement for injury. It would seem probable that something like these could be applied to this new area. Wolfle [429] has observed that ". . . the fact that such details and the underlying legal and moral issues are being seriously considered constitutes somber evidence that scientific inquiry will prove increasingly powerful in gaining knowledge of man himself." In this process those responsible for the growth of knowledge must be protected.

THE "TOO CASUAL" VIEW OF THE PATIENT AS SUBJECT

The "too casual" view is not a universal, but when it exists, it is in part owing to the defective education of clinical investigators, with background and purposes inadequately informed. In earlier years, research in the clinic was carried on by physicians whose field was often general practice. Problems arising in a puzzling patient were the incentives to study and analysis and discovery. The focal point was the patient, not science. Nowadays, we have a new generation of physicians whose primary interests are scientific; this is good only as long as the scientist proceeds and coordinates his activities with those of the patient's physician; only thus will any "too casual" view of the patient as subject be avoided.

"SENSITIVITY" OF SUBJECT-PATIENT CARE

It is essential that one's respect be communicated to all patients, experimental as well as others. Richmond [360] has discussed measures of sensitivity of patient care: There is respect for *identity,* achieved by a personal relationship with one staff member, perhaps best exemplified by Guttentag's [196] phrase, "physician-friend"; so to say, "one patient–one doctor." There is respect for *privacy* regardless of economic status; this is effected by private interviews, physical examinations where modesty is preserved as far as possible, and avoidance of an inordinate number of examinations for teaching purposes. There is respect for *time* when the inevitable delays between hospital admission and comfortable establishment in bed are reduced to a minimum. Care here makes a subtle but great impression on the patient-subject.

DIFFICULTIES IN THE TRANSFERENCE OF DATA FROM THE WELL TO THE SICK

It is often not possible to transfer observations made in normal individuals directly to the sick. The complexities here are so great that only one or two suggestive examples need be mentioned:

1. It is exceptionally difficult, sometimes impossible, to reproduce usefully in normal subjects symptoms that ordinarily arise in disease. Pain is an example. Beecher [20] compiled evidence that supports this view when he and, later, 14 other groups of investigators failed to show a dependable relationship in man between pain *threshold* and the action of analgesic agents, notwithstanding scores of papers to the contrary; nevertheless, even small doses of narcotics nearly always lessen pain of pathologic origin, that caused by disease or injury. In more recent studies, Smith, Egbert, Markowitz, Mosteller and Beecher (1966) again failed with experimentally contrived pain, for reasons not altogether clear, to show a dependable effect of narcotics on slight pain; however, they achieved increasingly reliable effects with increasing severity of pain [391]. These observations illustrated the complexity encountered and incidentally threw a revealing light on the pain process.

2. Morphine produces a higher incidence of nausea in normal volunteers than in patients with pain of pathologic origin. Notwithstanding the array of difficulties encountered in this area, the fact remains that there is often great need for "normal" baselines, for definition of the limits of normality, in order to determine where abnormality begins.

Information obtained in normal subjects can lead to dangerous effects when applied to the sick. Consider, for example, the substitution of lithium for sodium when a low sodium diet was sought. For the individual in normal sodium balance, lithium posed no threat; when, however, lithium was administered to individuals in sodium imbalance, the effect was disastrous.

DEATH AND SUBJECTS THREATENED WITH SUDDEN DEATH

The remarkably increased average length of life indicates that the time of dying has been greatly postponed. Even the characteristics of dying often differ from those of earlier years. The changes have been brought about by a variety of factors: antibiotics, potent drugs, intravenous fluids, transfusions, pain suppression, and artificial and transplanted organs. Sometimes the ancient prerogatives of the patient—his right to be let alone and to die in comfort and dignity seem to be overlooked. Individuals who may die suddenly or who seem to be in imminent danger of death should not, under ordinary circumstances, be chosen as subjects for experimentation, however harmless the planned procedure may be. Obviously, if death occurs during such an experiment, it could cast a shadow over a potentially valuable agent or useful technique, not to mention placing the investigator in an unhappy predicament where although innocent, he may have the appearance of guilt.

INTERCURRENT DISEASE

It is usually unwise to study a therapeutic procedure in an individual who has also a disease unrelated to the expected therapeutic effects.

OTHER UNDESIRABLE SUBJECTS

In general, the very young, the very old, and pregnant women are not desirable subjects for research, unless directly concerned with these states.

THE SICK MAN AND BASIC SCIENCE

There exists a newly recognized fact that some types of basic scientific advance can be made *only* in the presence of disease. There is little point in discussing extensively questions involving basic *versus* applied science. To this writer, science devoted to the discovery and establishment of new concepts is basic, and all else is applied science. In this sense, basic science can and does emerge from clinical studies. It is regrettable that the relatively new field was called clinical pharmacology instead of human pharmacology, which in truth it is. "Clinical" connotes downstream activity, whereas, as mentioned, it can be basic in the truest sense of that word. The scientist working in the clinic has advantages over those who like to call themselves basic scientists. The latter have in general been limited to animal studies, except through an intermediary. The scientist in the clinic is not so limited: In 1960 the writer planned and participated in a series of Lowell Lectures that had for its theme *Disease and the Advancement of Basic Science* [24]. A score of busy and distinguished scientists—four were Nobel laureates—participated, demonstrating with their own work that truly basic, conceptual science can have its origins at the bedside. Nature presents us with bolder experiments than we would ever dare to perform ourselves. We profit from a study of them; *basic* science profits.

An abundance of examples comes to mind. Pauling's interest in "molecular disease" arose in part from work with abnormal forms of hemoglobin. While neurophysiologists have long been interested in the biochemistry of the potassium ion, recent basic advances in knowledge of this ion have come from studies of dehydration. Knowledge of the physiology of the endocrine glands is largely indebted to the fundamental leads found in diseased glands. The anatomy of the central nervous system has in significant part been learned by study of cerebrovascular accidents. Such diverse matters as the discovery and understanding of vitamins, the development of microbiology, even the advance of genetics in the study of hereditary factors in disease—all of these leave no room for doubt that truly basic science can be advanced by a study of disease processes.

This thesis need not rest alone on such objective matters. It has now been found possible and rewarding to make a quantitative approach to subjective phenomena. If the so-called behavioral sciences are ever to be put on a really sound basis, a quantitative approach would seem to be essential. Technical measurement of subjective responses to various factors—drugs, for example—has depended in very large part upon the study of pain as prototype [22]. The presence or absence of anxiety can greatly alter certain drug effects [20, 135]. Some of the greatest stresses are present in disease within the hospital. This area has hardly been tilled.

While the university hospitals have long been recognized as fields where already discovered concepts are applied, it has now become evident that they are the *only* places where certain discoveries basic to the advancement of pure science are likely to be made. Such institutions are indispensable units in the advancement of some aspects of conceptual science. In short, a new role for the great teaching hospital is emerging.

This awareness leads to a further extension of human experimentation. Having seen what fundamental ends can be achieved by human experimentation, the investigator is led to carry on where Nature leaves off. The purposes of human experimentation thus become deeper and more complex than ever before, and so also do the ethical problems surrounding it; this furnishes justification for this study.

Ladimer [256] expounds this point as follows:

> Properly conducted experimentation [in the sick man] by qualified scientists must therefore be considered an integral branch of biologic and medical science, but it does not thereby become customary medical practice. Nor does its essentiality and acceptance establish clearly its

character or place the methods employed beyond scrutiny. The responsible professions have a duty to delineate for their own members and for a critically vigilant public the nature of medical research and the limits within which it may be properly undertaken.

Prevention of experimentation can also be an experiment, even a very dangerous one, as, for example, withholding treatment. If experimentation is to be withheld, as Shimkin [383] points out, ". . . it should be demonstrated that the proposed experiment is more dangerous or more painful than the known [or probable] results of inaction." This is often the expression of an ideal rather than a practical possibility.

SOCIETY AND THE INDIVIDUAL IN HUMAN EXPERIMENTATION

A clear issue emerges from all of the current charges and countercharges. It rises above personalities and above legalistics. It is simply this: In experimentation in man, is the individual subject the first to be considered, or does society have priority? It is essential that the debate now be directed to this fundamental issue.

Society certainly has rights, recognized in law and by thinking men in the invasion of the individual's privacy by the census; in the legal requirement of certain standards of education and of hygiene; in the required reporting of venereal disease; in vaccination; in maintenance of civil order; and in the required acceptance of the military draft, in wartime a life-or-death issue. It is evident that at times society properly acts against the welfare and the wishes of the individual, without his consent. Thus, while freedom of choice and of consent must stand very high, the freedom cannot be total, as illustrated in the examples just given. At times, to protect society, the decision must go against the individual. This is a grave and crucial problem.

Notwithstanding these and other exceptions where society must come first, there are, it seems to me, cogent reasons why, *as a general principle,* the individual must have priority in human experimentation. We can examine these reasons. We shall do this in the hope that advocates for the preeminent position of society will also attack this complex problem and attempt to substantiate *their* points of view.

A healthy society requires moral treatment of individuals. A great discussion, a truly divisive debate on this theme, has been going on; like an iceberg, seven-eighths lurks below the surface, and only one-eighth appears above it.

Unfortunately, those who espouse the good of society—"the most good for the most people," as they say, sometimes in justification of untrammeled experimentation—tag those who believe in the supremacy of the individual as "zealots," "one-track zealots," "zealous crusaders," or "extremists."

Curiously, the competence of anyone who dares to criticize the morality of some experiments, is questioned if he is not an expert in the field of cardiology, or immunology, or toxicology, or an authority on liver disease, or an endocrinologist. The "zealots" have unfortunately disturbed some who evidently assume the right to choose martyrs for science, to adopt Kety's phrase. Such acts involve far more than annoyance: they embody the serious possibility of delaying progress of medicine.

In the hospital, physicians are constantly required to make decisions whereby some lives are saved and others lost. The control of these decisions is the issue; where research is involved, it becomes particularly difficult to be certain of one's judgments. While society has a direct oversight of such decisions through the hospital's committee on research and in its committee on ethics, such groups nevertheless usually place greater emphasis on concern for the individual than on the welfare of the masses of future lives comprising society. The wish of the individual cannot be the *single* controlling element in deciding which life will be saved, which lost. The interests of society, as well as the interests of the individual, must be considered here; the question is which should have *first* consideration. When it comes to research, the more the risking of lives becomes official or societal, the more important becomes the valid consent of the subject. He must not be pressed, coerced, or tricked into a collaboration he would reject if he were fully informed.

As Calabresi has put it, we want a decision that reflects a societal choice and society's control over the conditions under which subjects are to be risked for the common good; at the same time, however, we do not want society to lose its role as protector of individual lives [57]. These are conflicting desires, but both are essential to a decent society. In clinical investigation, the physician presently has the power to determine which shall prevail at a given time; however, it remains undetermined that he has this right. A rigid and pedantic adherence to existing customs, rules, codes, and laws could easily lead to the untenable conclusion that the only supreme interest is that of society. This is false: the individual also has his rights, and *these*, barring a few exceptions, must predominate.

Calabresi puts the matter well [57] when he says:

> Consent, though very useful in preserving the appearance that society hardly ever condones the sacrifice of an individual against his will, is unlikely to suffice where a too obvious societal choice to take victims is involved . . . Even more important, consent cannot serve as the general control item which determines when the future good requires the taking of present lives. Therefore, it is to the development of a workable, but not too obvious, control system which can use various forms of consent as an adjunct that scholars seriously concerned with the problem of saving future lives and at the same time not undermining our commitment to the sanctity of individual present lives ought to be devoting themselves.

The extraordinary preoccupation of individuals and groups with codes appears to be an attempt to place on society the responsibility for what may happen during human experimentation. If these "guides" are accepted by society and if the individual experimenter has followed them, then if an accident occurs, the responsibility is not that of the investigator—or, at least, not his alone—but that of society. Man is not willing to take the responsibility for mankind in the mass, only for individuals; rather unfairly, he expects mankind—society—to protect him! One difficulty here is that the individual experimenter cannot know how much risk society wants him to take for future benefit; however, consultation with his peers can provide some help.

As mentioned, society is the protector of individuals, but society must also maintain control over situations that inevitably lead to sacrifice of some for the common good. Consider the decisions made regarding allocation of the artificial kidney: the widow whose children are grown will be rejected by society's committee in favor of the father of several young children. The widow will be allowed to die, while the other is saved by dialysis. It is more comfortable to look at this from a positive and general approach. Society has acted to save the young father rather than acted to sacrifice the widow; life has been sustained. The situation is different when specific lives are jeopardized or sacrificed, as in the numerous examples described in my paper on questionably ethical or unethical human experimentation, with no immediate gain for a specific individual [28]. In this case, the gain is for faceless mankind in the future, and the bystander is uneasy.

There is some quiet opposition to respect for the patient's rights —more than a casual observer might suppose. Not long ago a distinguished scientist heatedly said to me, "The individual is not infinitely valuable." This clashes with Guttentag's view [196] and my own that: "the use of force is not justified on a single person, even if millions of other lives could be saved by such an act. [One realizes] the act would not just save millions of lives but that, as an amoral act from the standpoint of democratic brotherhood, it might create millions of amoral sequels, and that the moral history of mankind is more important than the scientific" [196]. The act also clashes with Reston's [358] view: "If there has been a decline of decency in the modern world and a revolt against law and fair dealing, it is precisely because of the decline in the belief in each man as something precious."

Jaffe [228] argues that "the ethics of human experimentation is governed by the proposition that the individual is an end in himself and must not figure as a means to an end beyond his own interest. This proposition is said to derive from our Judaic-Christian tradition. The absolute priority of each individual is according to this thesis central to our public philosophy. I question this thesis both as history and as a reading of our present public philosophy. It is true that we do not exalt the state above the individual."

If the individual does not have "absolute priority" and if "we do not exalt the state above the individual," who, then, does have first consideration? It seems to me that he cannot have it both ways in terms of principle. The practical fact that the individual's immediate welfare must sometimes be sacrificed to the public good—in vaccination or in the military draft, for example—does not alter the validity of the general *principle* of the individual's priority. The danger of the opposing view was documented more than two decades ago in Nazi Germany.

Jaffe asks for "a more flexible, a less obsessive application of general propositions which we all accept." In the first place, all do *not* accept. Would he grant that the health and the life of individuals could properly be jeopardized without their consent or even their knowledge? It is not difficult to find hundreds of examples where this has been done in human experimentation and done, moreover, in the "best" institutions.

In a subsequent communication Professor Jaffe prefers the phrase "the group" to "the state," where neither has priority [230]. His view is that "in each situation the claims of each are considered and a tolerable adjustment is made . . . it is what we in fact do today and I do not find it shocking. You [Beecher] state that 'the practical facts that the individual's immediate welfare has, sometimes, to be sacrificed to the public good,' e.g., vaccination, draft, 'does not alter the validity of the general principle of the individual's priority.' But I think it *does* alter its validity. I do not, however, see most situations in terms of all or none. I see them as resolved by compromises in which the interests of the individual and the group are both given due weight." My respect for Jaffe's views does not entirely relieve discomfort at the thought that equating the group's rights with those of the individual can lead all too easily—to those who vote for the group—to condoning as a goal the-most-good-for-the-most-people when the cost is the sacrifice of the individual's rights. The "group's rights" suggest to me totalitarian "rights." I suppose that is my main difficulty with Jaffe's point of view.

The individual is concrete; society is an abstraction, apart from its existence as an aggregation of numbers of individuals. The numbers game is a dangerous one, as Jonas [234] points out, ". . . it may well be the case that the individual's interest in his own inviolability is itself a public interest such that its publicly condoned violation, irrespective of numbers, violates the interest of all . . ." While in abnormal times, as when the nation is threatened, the primacy of the individual very often must be temporarily suspended for the common good, in normal times denigration of the primacy of the individual threatens the whole of society. The close relationship of these matters to "statistical morality," discussed in Chap. 7, is evident.

THE VOLUNTEER [2]

GENERAL

The volunteer may be sick or well, in hospital or not, normal or abnormal.

SOURCES OF "NORMAL" VOLUNTEERS

Smith [390] suggests:

1. United States Employment Service. No more difficulty was found with applicants from this source than with students. As a matter of fact, subjects from this source were more amenable to experimental procedures than were students; they do not attempt to anticipate the goals, as students often do. They were available for extended periods of time. The Employment Service has even been willing to select subjects according to specified variables such as age, sex, type of occupation. The cooperation with this Service was obtained by explaining the objectives and their relevance to

[2] Fox [166] holds that the word volunteer should imply much more than passive participation in an experiment, and that its meaning, though debased, would still seem odd when applied to "a group of volunteer mice," as was the case in a recent journal article.

national goals. It is helpful to point out to the Service, when such is the case, that governmental support is behind the project.

2. Military Reserve Units. At many military centers, men meet in the evenings and on Sundays to drill and to attend classes. These men are usually good and cooperative subjects. In obtaining men from several centers, Smith was never required to go through official channels. Again, a word as to governmental sponsorship of the activity is helpful, when appropriate. An advantage of this population is the possibility of generalization, with application to military situations. A disadvantage is the desire of a good many officers to observe the experiments. Further possible disadvantages are the varying group sizes and the diversity of civilian backgrounds and occupations.

3. Operational Military Units. Use of men from such units requires an approach through channels; the approach can be facilitated by stressing the pertinence to military interests and military support, when these are present. In the Army, the channels route requires about 60 days, but much less time in the Air Force. Subjects from some of these units are especially useful for certain research studies, as, for example, the stress of isolation, as on mountain tops and at other isolated places. Assurance that the research will not interfere with the primary tasks of the military man helps, plus the fact that credit will be given to all concerned in official communications. The military subjects are superior to students in their greater naiveté concerning research, in better motivation, and in availability often for longer periods. In studies of social psychology, they constitute useful established groups.

In the military world, Johnson points out that a soldier is prohibited from volunteering if such an act would interfere with performance of his primary duties [233]; if requested through channels, however, permission for such action may be granted. (Specifically, see Department of the Army, Special Regulation 70–30–1, 24 January, 1949. Subject: "Research in Human Resources and Military Psychology.") "Unduly" hazardous or "unnecessary" experimentation will not be tolerated. Presumably, Walter Reed's triumph would not now be possible!

According to Karsner [237], "Studies [in naval hospitals] that are of no direct benefit to patients cannot be condoned. Any experiments that may be dangerous cannot be permitted, and any that may disturb the cordial patient-physician relationship common in naval hospitals are excluded . . . [There] is the necessity for impressing on the public the fact that in the naval hospitals every advantage is taken of facilities to improve the care of the patients. The naval hospital should take its place among all other medical institutions in providing for progress—progress for the welfare of the whole structure of medicine, both military and civilian." Apparently the Navy, at least as described by Karsner, fails to see the obvious contradiction in the above statements: "progress for the welfare of the whole structure of medicine, both military and civilian" can hardly be effected without experimentation not limited to the immediate benefit of the subject. Naval medicine, if the above is an accurate statement, is doomed to a limited, dependent role.

4. Prisons. See the separate section on prisoners, page 69.

5. Fire Departments. Large numbers of men are on duty, with little to do for long periods of time. They have been found to be very cooperative. Permission to approach these individuals has not been difficult to obtain by describing the importance of the research for the achievement of national goals, when this is the case. Sometimes there is a parallelism between the scientist's goals and problems needing solution in the fire departments. Attention to such a possibility is, of course, helpful. Advantages of this group are the great time spans often available, the willingness carefully to fill out tedious questionnaires and personality inventories, and work at group tasks. In social psychological research, there are ready-made groups who know each other well, not only under simple conditions of eating and communal sleeping, but under circumstances of occasional great stress and danger.

6. Other Sources. The use of students, hospital and laboratory personnel, and patient volunteers have been discussed elsewhere (page 77). Finally, certain religious groups, particularly the Mennonites and the Quakers, cooperate gladly as volunteers in scientific studies. Conscientious objectors are also in this category.

CONCLUSION

Professional men sometimes act as though cooperation of the subject with the scientist is the latter's inborn right and that his problems and objectives are more important than those of other men. The result is easily anticipated. On the other hand, a tactful and understanding approach by which the scientist can possibly help nonscientific organizations with *their* problems can lead to a symbiotic, productive relationship on both sides. The mutual-need-satisfaction basis is the approach, not the everyone-should-help-science stance [390].

WILLINGNESS TO VOLUNTEER AS SUBJECTS FOR EXPERIMENTATION

Investigators, however earnest, able, and ambitious, would not proceed without subjects. The motivation of volunteers for such work is therefore relevant to present considerations. The role of volunteer may serve as a means of achieving certain goals of importance to the subject. The research may illuminate the volunteers' own medical problem without financial cost because of the availability of free medical care and a free "research" bed. Participation as a volunteer may relieve a lonely or tedious existence. Financial rewards are important to some volunteers. Conscientious objectors as volunteers can in some cases fulfill a military obligation by contributing to the maintenance of the national health. Pacifists or members of religious groups participate as volunteers for experimentation for other reasons, to be discussed. For these individuals, as well as for others, volunteering leads to spiritual rewards that are approved, not only by individuals, but also by society. The volunteers are honored by the investigators.

There are some rather striking differences among various social groups in their willingness to volunteer as subjects for experimentation. These matters have been studied by Arnold, Martin, and Richard [7]. Prisoners in a Missouri jail, incarcerated for misdemeanors and with sentences of one year or less, were offered participation in a malaria study project. They were to be paid, but were told they could expect no shortening of sentence. The risks and expected discomfort were described, and an "informed consent" form was presented for signing.

A follow-up interview with 36 inmates who acquired malaria and were successfully treated was compared with that of 24 inmates who had not volunteered. The responses of the two groups were compared concerning: "(1) understanding of and information about malaria, the risks in taking it and chances of being cured; (2) demographic characteristics; and (3) reasons for volunteering or not and the role of probable inducements to volunteer."

There was no difference in level of understanding between the two groups. One third of the nonvolunteers mentioned risk as a reason for not volunteering. The volunteers were evenly split between "altruism" and money as their motivation. One quarter of those who mentioned money gave altruism as an additional reason. Of those who did not volunteer, nearly all described the enterprise as an "act of courage"; they expressed or implied respect for those who did volunteer. The authors conclude that the quality of informed consent was a far more complex matter than simply giving understandable information and asking for "free consent."

The behavior of individuals is constrained by the circumstances under which they live. The values and attitudes of their social group, and how well they live up to them, can be controlling. This applies not only to prisoners, but also to clergymen, doctors, janitors, lawyers, salesmen, nurses, and machinists (Table 1).

Following the studies in prisoners, the investigators decided to carry out work in free-living social groups as to their thoughts

TABLE 1

WILLINGNESS TO VOLUNTEER OF SEVERAL SOCIAL GROUPS [7]

	Malaria		*Drugs*		*Cold*		*Poison*	
Volunteers	*Yes*	*No*	*Yes*	*No*	*Yes*	*No*	*Yes*	*No*
Prisoners	40	20	44	16	49	11	50	10
Helping hand, welfare, and housekeeping	7	19	9	17	10	16	17	9
Fire and police	3	37	5	35	11	29	28	12
Professional	0	28	1	27	2	26	26	2

about and willingness to participate as subjects in medical experiments. Willingness to volunteer was also studied among groups with widely varied backgrounds and responsibilities. The experimental conditions were such that it was evident that there would be different degrees of risk, time demands, interruptions of standing obligations, and degrees of social importance.

All groups responded similarly; i.e., with increased willingness as one progressed from left to right. It is also evident that groups with different socioeconomic characteristics have different degrees of willingness to volunteer; those in the lower socioeconomic groups show the greatest willingness to volunteer. When the data were arranged according to age, sex, race, and living arrangements, the age and race categories showed no differences. When the prisoner group is removed, sex showed differences in willingness to volunteer, and so did the "living arrangement" group.

Table 2 shows the comparative responses of "free-living" (not prisoners) men and women.

In all cases, women showed a greater willingness to volunteer than did men.

Subjects not obligated to others show a greater willingness to volunteer than others. The closeness of obligation also seems to be important. When the subject has responsibility for a spouse and children, the willingness is lowest (Table 3).

The preceding material has been presented in some detail for, notwithstanding the fact that the numbers are not large, interesting trends are shown in this fresh approach to old problems;

TABLE 2
COMPARISONS OF "FREE-LIVING" (NOT PRISONERS) MEN AND WOMEN ON WILLINGNESS TO VOLUNTEER [7]

	Malaria		*Drugs*		*Cold*		*Poison*		*Group*
Volunteers	*Yes*	*No*	*Yes*	*No*	*Yes*	*No*	*Yes*	*No*	*total*
Men	4	65	7	62	13	56	49	20	69
Women	7	18	8	17	11	14	22	3	25
Total	11	83	15	79	24	70	71	23	94

TABLE 3
COMPARISONS OF THREE GROUPS WITH DIFFERENT LIVING ARRANGEMENTS ON WILLINGNESS TO VOLUNTEER [7]

	Malaria		*Drugs*		*Cold*		*Poison*		*Group*
Volunteers	*Yes*	*No*	*Yes*	*No*	*Yes*	*No*	*Yes*	*No*	*total*
Self (alone)	17	17	20	14	24	10	26	8	34
With others (not family)	19	26	22	23	27	18	35	10	45
Nuclear family	15	60	17	58	22	53	55	20	75

clearly it merits extension. It is to be hoped that Arnold and his colleagues will do this.

Arnold has said [7]: "Those of 'more privileged status,' particularly men, seem least apt, not only to express the [helpful] sentiment, but to show willingness to operate on it. This fact is of some concern since those presently discussing and conferring about use of human subjects in clinical research—who will, in all likelihood, eventually decide the fate of this major enterprise [human experimentation] for generations to come, are of this group." While there may be some reason for concern, it seems likely that the basis for the reluctance mentioned may be quite simply the time factor: the successful man is too busy to participate. He has a place in society; his life is filled with meaning, whereas the lower groups, especially prisoners, have time and boredom on their hands.

The stake in medical progress involves all classes of people. There is reason to believe, in fact, that the lower socio-economic groups are the most acutely concerned. Although the stake in medical progress involves all groups, the willingness to contribute is not uniformly equal in all groups. It is of great concern that policy decisions not be restricted to a self selected few, but that all segments of our society be considered. It seems particularly important to respect the rights of potential volunteers to make their own decisions on the basis of their own motives once they have proper information. Great care should be exercised to make certain that decisions on the use of human subjects are not falsely based and truly reflect the sentiments of those people who might be willing to make significant contributions to the betterment of mankind [7].

REWARDS

Some have taken the view that when a student with scientific curiosity or a scientist with a project is involved as a volunteer in an experiment he should not be paid. On the other hand, when the subject derives no scientific or intellectual information from his participation, he should receive a reward; this may be financial or it may be satisfaction at having performed a service. Although responsibility is already present, payment may increase the legal obligation. For further comment on rewards see Prisoners, page 69.

PSYCHOPATHOLOGY IN VOLUNTEERS

Very often the furtherance of experimentation in man requires the use of volunteer subjects. Sometimes these are useful because some abnormality requires study. At other times "normal," well individuals are needed so that a standard of reference can be determined in order to make comparisons between the normal and the abnormal states. There is a seldom recognized pitfall here: volunteer subjects may not truly represent the general population.

Lasagna and von Felsinger have studied certain drug responses in a normal volunteer population: their psychological make-up, the reasons for volunteering, and finally the interaction between the first two factors and "primary" drug effects in a determination of total drug responses [270]. Fifty-six male college students, from 21 to 28 years of age, were studied. Certain psychological tests not relevant in detail to the present discussion were applied and it appeared that an unusually high incidence of severe, psychological maladjustment was present in the volunteer group. No attempt was made to achieve precise diagnoses; rather, general categories were utilized. Without question, most of the subjects listed in Table 4 would have qualified as deviant regardless of the exact label given by examining psychologists or psychiatrists.

The report on homosexuality[3] refers only to those volunteers freely describing overt and continuing homosexual practices and

[3] Alfred Kinsey expressed to the writer indignation at this report. He asserted that the incidence of homosexuality reported was no higher than in the general population and said he would write a rebuttal. He died a little later, and evidently did not carry out his plan.

TABLE 4
INCIDENCE OF PSYCHOLOGIC MALADJUSTMENT IN 56 VOLUNTEERS

Psychosis	3
Psychoneurosis:	
Under treatment	1
Seeking treatment	6
Others	5
Psychopathic personality	3
Alcoholism	1
Overt homosexuality*	6
Peptic ulcer, severe	1
Stutter, severe	1

* Two of these are also represented in psychotic group above.

was not based upon presumptive or laboratory data. The question must be raised as to whether this "normal" sample was representative of anything. The subjects here differed from other students by reason of volunteering for participation in experiments. Examination of volunteers in other similar studies is therefore in order.

Other data derived from personal communications to Lasagna and von Felsinger support the above view and tend to indicate that volunteer group data are likely to be unrepresentative of the population as a whole. Specifically, their group seemed to show an incidence of serious psychologic difficulties twice as high as that to be expected in an unselected college population. Reasons for volunteering in the Lasagna-von Felsinger study varied: money, "free" professional advice, solution of personality problems, "new experiences," "thrills," "kicks," escape from personal problems, escape from "drives," relief from boredom, "sexual gratification in a guilt-free environment," and satisfaction of self-destructive urges.

In another study, the performance of 59 volunteer psychology students was compared with that of 149 students who participated in the same psychomotor experiments as a course requirement. Significant differences between the two groups were identified by

Brower, who believed that incentive—"differential motivation"—accounted for the differences [52]. Maslow, in studying the sexual habits of women, found that the volunteers rated higher in sexuality, in "dominance people," than the nonvolunteers [291]. Maslow and Sakoda deal with what they call "volunteer-error": volunteers are higher in self-esteem and in "unconventional" sexuality than nonvolunteers [292]. Thus, the use of volunteers alone may give a false picture of the general population.

Perlin, Pollin, and Butler made a psychiatric examination of 29 youthful volunteer subjects (15 female, 14 male), age range 18 to 30, median, 21 years; and 54 in an aged group of men volunteers, 65 to 92, median, 72 years [337]. Nineteen of the fifty-four older subjects had no diagnosable psychopathology. In thirty-five (65 percent), psychopathology was found. In the young group (15 female, 14 male), 52 percent showed psychopathologic symptoms.

Data derived from volunteer groups are not necessarily unrewarding: they must, however, be used with caution and whenever possible pitted against data derived from nonvolunteers.

Psychiatric screening of "normal" volunteers would introduce its own kind of bias. The old assumption that "healthy" volunteers are normal mentally is clearly not always tenable. Esecover, Malitz, and Wilkins have studied 56 such volunteers who agreed to participate in hallucinogen studies [148]. Psychopathology was discovered in 46 percent of the group; 41 percent needed treatment. The "better adjusted" subjects generally volunteered for financial or scientific reasons; those with psychopathology tended to volunteer for reasons "frequently related to their maladaptive patterns." The personality pattern of members of this group covered a wide range, with obsessional and schizoid types predominating.

There is already a considerable literature to indicate that "normal" volunteers are, in a high percentage of cases, far from normal. The several examples given are sufficient for the present purposes. Those who wish to pursue this aspect of volunteer subjects can easily do so by giving attention to the references contained in the original material described here.

A VOLUNTEER CORPS

Hogben and Sim [217] have this to say:

> If we approach the problem [of human experimentation] against a background in which the major advances of medicine occurred in the social setting of pestilences, practical difficulties of enlisting volunteers without violence to ethical standards are easy to exaggerate; but a wholesome regard for the sanctity of life becomes increasingly less relevant to a statement of the priorities of medicine in western communities with a life expectation well above 60 years at birth. There is indeed an ever more pressing need for knowledge about many once-thought *minor* evils. We cannot effectively tackle them by group methods; but we might well do so with the help of individuals now willing to risk life or limb on the speedway or in the ascent of Mount Everest, if we could institutionalize a not uncommon appetite for adventure consistent with acceptable moral standards. It is not beyond the reach of social engineering to create a new corps of civil defense with that end in view. The voluntary response to the appeal for blood donors disposes of doubts about the feasibility of such an undertaking, if sponsored by an adequately accredited organization.

I have observed that there are in this country the beginnings of such a corps in the group of conscientious objectors to military service who volunteer [22].

It has been estimated [4] that 4,000 Quakers, Mennonites, members of the Assembly of God and the Church of the Brethren, or other pacifist sects follow this course each year. According to Ladimer, the Clinical Center of the National Institutes of Health has a more or less permanent corps of normal volunteers as the result of contractual agreements, made by Ladimer, with these "peace churches" [257].[5] In addition to these groups, under some circumstances volunteer groups are derived from the armed services, prisoners, technical aides, students, nurses, patients—especially ward patients—and physicians.

[4] *Time,* Sept. 27, 1954.

[5] See also Beaumont, W., and St. Martin, A. (footnote, page 219).

CHILDREN

GENERAL

Parents have the obligation to inculcate into their children attitudes of unselfish service. One could hope that this might be extended to include participation in research for the public welfare, when it is important and there is no discernible risk. There is, of course, useful legislation to protect children from mistreatment. Society depends on the integrity, mental stability, and good faith of the parents for the protection of their children. If the parents fail, the law steps in. In any case a child would be used, if ever, only when adults are not suitable.

A great deal has been said recently about infringement of the right to privacy. Surely the right to privacy entails the right of the citizen to the use of his privacy as he sees fit, within the laws of the land. Sometimes this means sharing it with an investigator.

THE ENGLISH VIEW

When experimentation in children is for diagnosis or treatment for the direct benefit of the child, the ethical problems are few as long as the consent of the parent or guardian has been obtained. The situation is more complicated when the experimentation is not for the patient's direct benefit. A strict interpretation of English law declares this to be illegal, even with the approval of the parents, according to the Medical Research Council, 1962–1963.

> The situation in respect of minors and mentally subnormal or mentally disordered persons is of particular difficulty. In the strict view of the [English] law parents and guardians of minors cannot give consent on their behalf to any procedures which are of no particular benefit to them and which may carry some risk of harm. Whilst English law does not fix any arbitrary age in this context, it may safely be assumed that the Courts will not regard a child of 12 years or under (or 14 years or under for boys in Scotland) as having the capacity to consent to any procedure which may involve him in an injury. Above this age the reality of any purported consent which may have been obtained is a question of fact and as with an adult the evidence would, if necessary,

have to show that irrespective of age the person concerned fully understood the implications to himself of the procedures to which he was consenting.

In the case of those who are mentally subnormal or mentally disordered the reality of the consent given will fall to be judged by similar criteria to those which apply to the making of a will, contracting a marriage or otherwise taking decisions which have legal force as well as moral and social implications. When true consent in this sense cannot be obtained, procedures which are of no direct benefit and which might carry a risk of harm to the subject should not be undertaken.

Even when true consent has been given by a minor or a mentally subnormal or mentally disordered person, considerations of ethics and prudence still require that, if possible, the assent of parents or guardians or relatives, as the case may be, should be obtained.

Investigations that are of no direct benefit to the individual require, therefore, that his true consent to them shall be explicitly obtained. After adequate explanation, the consent of an adult of sound mind and understanding can be relied upon to be true consent. In the case of children and young persons the question whether purported consent was true consent would in each case depend upon facts such as the age, intelligence, situation and character of the subject and the nature of the investigation. When the subject is below the age of 12 years, information requiring the performance of any procedure involving his body would need to be obtained incidentally to and without altering the nature of a procedure intended for his individual benefit.

Curran and Beecher [31b] have examined the legal principles in the United States and England regarding the use of children in clinical investigation. Misconceptions abound in this area concerning the restriction on the use of children as subjects. In point of fact, neither in the United States nor in England is clinical investigation limited to studies where there is a potential and direct benefit to the child. The stern English restriction on the use of children was not really based on English law as the Medical Research Council states but rather on the opinion of Sir Harvey Druitt, K.C.B., [138a] who was the referee for the Medical Research Council. Sir Harvey has kindly permitted quotation of his letter in which he asserts that the legal position taken in the statement of the Medical Research Council was based upon his advice. He says, "I am confident about the correctness of that statement but I cannot cite any Statute or decided case which is exactly to the point."

IN AMERICA

Two American precedents are remotely relevant. Curran cites the decision of the Supreme Judicial Court of Massachusetts in the case of identical twins, one with kidney failure, one well [122]. The question was the propriety of permitting the well twin to give his kidney to his ailing brother. The decision evaded the central issue by declaring that the well twin would also profit from the transaction in a negative sense; i.e., he would be permanently injured psychologically if he were not permitted to give his kidney to his ailing brother. The other "precedent" (*Bonner v. Moran* 126 Fed. 2d 121 [D.C. Cir. 1941]) concerned the use of a minor as a donor for skin grafts to a cousin who had been badly burned. The donor's mother was ill and had not been informed before the first grafting. The matter was brought to court and the judge *implied* that if the mother had been informed the grafting would have been acceptable.

Although American law often follows English law, it is so far not very explicit on this issue. Too many decisions in the field of experimentation are now made in this country by default. It would be much sounder to achieve group agreement and then forthrightly to formulate a policy to cover the situation, as we have attempted in 127a. It is quite possible that such statements, made by thoughtful and responsible individuals, would powerfully influence judicial decision and lead to the establishment of a valuable legal precedent in the final test.

DEFINITION OF A CHILD

Since physical and psychological growth generally reach a plateau at age 16 to 21, it has been suggested that 18 should be the age dividing child and adult in the United States. The law, however, very often takes into account *understanding*. The courts of Great Britain will not regard a child of less than 12 years of age as being capable of consenting to any procedure that may do him harm. In Scotland it is age 14.[6] In the United States, the age is generally 16 or more. If self-supporting, if a high school graduate, if married, or if in military service, a child in the United States can be considered to be capable of understanding and consenting to experimentation that may entail some risk, provided it is properly approved by his parents and by the investigator's peers. A recent law concerning voluntary commitment to psychiatric institutions in Massachusetts uses age 16 as the dividing line. The voting age in Georgia is 18; the draft age in the United States is also 18. Since a "child" of 18 may be required to give his life in military service, it seems reasonable to conclude that at such an age he may make independent judgments concerning his welfare. While such matters may enter into a court's consideration, the *legal* age is still 21 years, after which the individual is unquestionably capable of consent to participation in research if he is mentally sound.

RESEARCH ON NORMAL CHILDREN

I believe that the following statements are tenable and reasonable.

1. The informed consent of the parents, or that of the legal guardian, and that of the child, when this is feasible, shall be required for all subjects under 21 years of age. The nature of *informed* consent and the complexities often surrounding its attainment are such that sometimes it becomes only a goal toward which we strive. It would be wrong to suppose, as most so-called codes seem to, that this goal is easily attainable. A great advantage to be derived from striving to obtain truly informed consent is that the parents and subjects, if at the age of understanding, are then alerted to the fact that they are indeed to be subjects of an experiment. Unfortunately, this has not always been the case in the past.

2. If the subject is too young to give consent, the consent of the parent or guardian is sufficient when no risk is involved and the safety and value of the proposed study are supported by the investigator's peers. When the child is capable of understanding, he

6 Medical Research Council, 1962–1963.

shall never be forced to cooperate in experimentation by overzealous or unstable parents or guardians.

Discussion with children of sexual attitudes or practices is especially likely to bring down a storm on the head of those who investigate such matters. Another delicate area is the privacy of the home; parents often discuss their attitudes quite candidly in the house, but object when an investigator puts relevant questions to the children. In the parents' view this, in effect, puts the child in the position of spying on the parents. There is another troublesome area: when local issues on which there are strong feelings are present, the research worker can have trouble with the parents, especially if he allows his own bias to be evident.

3. Many thousands of psychomotor tests and sociological studies have been carried out in children during the child's development; they have revealed much of value. It would be difficult to fault this work on any sound basis, provided all required anonymity is preserved. Sound nutritional studies without risk have been carried out, as have certain blood studies.

Limitation of research in children to studies directly beneficial to them is not necessary. For example, such a restriction would greatly hamper behavioral studies, as well as studies of inborn errors of metabolism. Such work is *potentially,* and sometimes unexpectedly, of direct benefit to the subject. Considerable valuable research can be carried on without discernible risk.

These and other useful and essentially risk-free endeavors are jeopardized by studies such as those at Willowbrook, where 250 mentally defective children, many 5 to 8 years old, were deliberately infected with hepatitis virus; by studies proving the hepatotoxic effects of "Tri-A" in mentally defective subjects and juvenile delinquents; by the thymectomies in infants carried out in a transplant study, and by the repeated biopsies of testicles in normal prisoners (see Chap. 4; also reference 28, and footnote 8, this chapter).

4. Parents still have the right to decide whether their children will participate in experimentation, even if not for their direct benefit, provided the studies contemplated have no discernible risk

and have been approved by a high-level review committee as necessary and valuable for human progress and do not unfairly take advantage of the child.

Some investigators—Edsall, for example, in a recent communication to the author—regard it as an unwarranted intrusion for an impersonal body, such as "the law," to intervene between parent and child and prohibit such a procedure. He goes on to say, "Laws have a tendency to be unintentionally rigid and short-sighted, and they require extremely careful thought and farsighted planning if they are to be written in such a way that they will really serve their purpose."

5. Research that entails discernible risk may not be performed on subjects too young to give mature and informed consent, unless for their direct benefit.

RESEARCH ON SICK CHILDREN

The child brought to a physician for relief of an ailment has, in the act of coming, given his and his guardian's consent to reasonable efforts to relieve him. This usually requires experimentation; sometimes it requires going beyond "standard" therapy. In this case the guardian—and the child, if feasible—should be informed and should consent.

If studies other than those required in therapy are to be undertaken, no discernible risk shall be the rule; and if the studies are carried out, they should be discussed at length and approved by the child's parents or guardian and by a high-level review board. The Golden Rule should be adhered to. Any appreciable risk should be reserved for those occasions where the subject promises to profit directly.

IN CONCLUSION

As long as the law is not well formulated on experimentation in children, legal responsibility rests with the parents or guardian. The issues are (1) no risk, if the subject is below the age of understanding; (2) screening and approval by a review board; (3) purposeful, useful goals; and (4) no coercion or deception of the parents, but their full understanding and consent. Here, as in other problem cases, an additional safeguard is to be found in the child's physician rather than in the physician experimenter.

PRISONERS

The use of prisoners in experimentation has a long history. Included as civil "prisoners" are the inmates of orphanages [182] and asylums for the insane [281, 282] and prisoners in jail [72, 182–184, 189, 190, 398]. During World War II, both federal and state prisoners made important contributions to studies of malaria, to studies of the use of blood plasma, plasma fractions and plasma substitutes, and to trials of various new drugs.

CIVIL PRISONERS

During World War II the Governor of Illinois and its Department of Public Safety allowed penitentiary prisoners to serve voluntarily, but without any promise of pardon or reduction of sentence, in certain medical experiments. Governor Green appointed a committee to advise him on the ethical problems involved: first, the conditions under which prisoners might be permitted to serve as subjects in medical experiments and, second, under what conditions a reduction in time in prison might be granted as a reward for collaboration. The committee report was published in 1948.

The ethical rules under which prisoners were allowed to participate were similar to those later enunciated in the Nuremberg Code. This is not surprising since Ivy was the leader in the Illinois decisions as well as a consultant at Nuremberg (page 227). These rules were adopted in essence by the House of Delegates of the American Medical Association in 1948.

The rules embodied the following provisions. It is essential that the subjects truly volunteer because, as with other captive groups, there will always be lingering belief that coercion was involved. It is imperative that the subjects be informed of all hazards and that they freely consent; to the life-termer, even the remote possibility of a reprieve after years of imprisonment may be an overwhelming coercive force. (The difficulties inherent in this complex field have been discussed elsewhere; see page 75.) The experiment should be based upon knowledge of the natural history of the disease under study. The experiment "must be so designed that the anticipated results will justify the performance of the experiment." The results must be unprocurable by any other method and must be "necessary for the good of society." (This has an unfortunate totalitarian sound.) The investigator must be scientifically qualified, and the experiment must be conducted so as to avoid all unnecessary suffering. It may be undertaken only after prior animal work has indicated that serious injury or death are unlikely; in addition, if known hazard is present, the investigators should serve along with the nonscientific personnel as subjects. In commenting on the Green Report, Shimkin [383] observed that "research on human beings is too hazardous and implies too many responsibilities to be undertaken by lone investigators. It should be a group effort supported by a proper consultative body."

In the past, either a reduction of sentence or a pardon has been offered as inducement to the prisoners to participate—*before* the work was undertaken. This amounts to a questionable bargaining. Specifically, both in New Jersey and in Illinois the possibility of a reduction in sentence was considered before the work was undertaken. Whether or not definite promises had been made, it is likely that the prisoners recognized the possibilities and that this influenced their decision. One can only hope that prisoners who decline to participate in experiments will not be discriminated against.

Among the five usually accepted purposes of imprisonment—punitive, expiative, deterrent, protective of society from criminals, and reformative—the last is especially important in the present consideration. Under the parole system, a reduction of prison sentence is recognized as encouraging and rewarding good conduct and industry, and it is also allowed for exceptional bravery or fidelity in a good cause. The purpose of the use of prisoners in medical research is reformative to the prisoner and constructive in terms of the advancement of medical knowledge. It is assumed that service in a medical experiment is consonant with the parole system's statutory "good time," "merit time," "industrial credits."

The Green Committee took up the question of what sort of volunteer is acceptable. Service as a subject in a medical experiment is considered to be an act of good conduct, for such activity is often unpleasant and sometimes hazardous and is thus a demonstration of social consciousness of a high order when it is carried out primarily as a service to society. The purpose is to balance the subject's social consciousness against the obvious desire for reduction of sentence, but it is not at all clear how such estimates can be made. The committee concluded that whatever the motivations, habitual or notorious prisoners guilty of heinous crimes are not acceptable as volunteers for medical experimentation. The House of Delegates of the American Medical Association in 1952 passed a resolution disapproving "the participation in scientific experiments of persons convicted of murder, rape, arson, kidnapping, treason, or other heinous crimes" by inmates of penal institutions.

A further point of importance is that the reward should not be excessive; as such, it would constitute a bribe and violate the principle of the free volunteer. If the prisoner is motivated to contribute to human welfare, a reduction in sentence would be perhaps an excessive reward, but how can such a judgment be properly made? The question of what constitutes a reasonable reward must be considered in each individual case. As Freund [170] has put it,

> I would suggest that the amount paid should not be so large as to constitute undue influence—that is, so large as to obscure an appreciation of the risk and weaken the will to self-preservation. We ought not be put in the business of buying lives. . . . Next, bearing on the problem of consent, is the category of prisoners, a relatively favored group for obvious reasons. I suggest here that the experiments should not involve any promises of parole or of commutation of sentence; this would be what is called in the law of confession undue influence or duress through promises of reward, which can be as effective in overbearing the will as threats of harm.

Newman has pointed out that prisoners as normal volunteers are clearly useful for medical research because one deals with large numbers of individuals in a controlled environment [319]. Requests for their collaboration in such studies are so regularly oversubscribed that one may justifiably assume that such participation is voluntary and not the result of coercion, however subtle. It is the opinion of officers in correctional institutions that ongoing programs of medical research provide useful educational and training programs that not only result in rehabilitation of attitude, but furnish specific training to potential research assistants and laboratory technicians. This has value to those who participate, when they are discharged and must make their own way in life. Such studies are directly useful within the prison when they are directed toward better understanding and treatment of the personality and behavior problems of criminal offenders. Newman considers the elements of scientific "necessity," ethical propriety, correctional coordination, and maximum individual rehabilitation as forming a basis for useful prison research programs that benefit, not only the investigator, but also the prisons and the volunteers [319].

In addition to the difficulties that have already been pointed out, other problems and needs have arisen. There is the initial problem of choosing among the studies presented for consideration by outside investigators. More attention must be given to the process of proper selection among volunteers. There is need for further study of the rewards to be given for meritorious service as volunteers. Discussion between the administrators of correctional institutions and the investigators should be helpful here. Before a project is undertaken, the same officials should decide what the legal arrangements are to be; parties to such decisions may be the state or the prison warden, the sponsor of the research, the clinical investigator, and the prisoner subjects. In Newman's view, too often the consent forms are such "that . . . the prisoner signs away his rights and absolves the researcher of any responsibilities."

A considerable segment of society considers the use of prisoners in individual experimentation as exploitation, even though undertaken for a good cause; while there doubtless have been such cases, they are by no means the rule. It is important, therefore, to find out who in prison life volunteers and why. McDonald has addressed himself to these questions in a New York prison [295]. The inmate has the right to volunteer, just as he has the right to be let alone, if he so chooses. He also has the right to be protected. Society, on the other hand, has the less concrete right to expect progress in medicine. Some very important progress has been made through the participation of prisoners, a pragmatic reason for continuing. It is not always easy for those who have not worked in prisons to grasp the viewpoint of those within the prison walls; this creates the need for scrupulously cautious judgment on the part of outsiders and concern for the welfare of the insiders.

While McDonald agrees that an inmate does not necessarily volunteer because he expects his sentence to be shortened or to receive financial reward, the Illinois and New Jersey cases referred to earlier throw a shadow of some doubt on this general rule. In McDonald's view, the prisoner volunteers for "much more immediate reasons, which are quite apparent to him and which seem quite sound." He recognizes advantages in these programs.

In connection with McDonald's work 2,000 men were given a circular calling for volunteers. In three days 350 petitions were handed in. After that no more were accepted. Fifty individuals were chosen for a 12-week study of three successive skin allografts. Only one subject dropped out of his own accord.

Reasons for the prisoners' participation are described as trust in the doctor's sense of responsibility, a favorable image, a break in the monotony of prison life, and the opportunity to participate in a stimulating, exciting adventure. As the men say, "It breaks the time." The inmates like to be involved in "positive action," in "doing something." They have something to talk about. The volunteers were subjects of interest to their colleagues, as well as to prison employees; "they were no longer nonentities—suddenly, they were important!" The experiment bolsters the ego. The prisoner proves to himself, to his family, and to friends that he can do something admirable. The inmate has a desire to be a part of society; since the experiment originated outside, he is a participant in outside, useful activity; it is a "good thing" to do. Since no one is now dependent on them, prisoners dare to accept risks they would not wish to assume if they were free and carrying responsibilities. As the experiment progressed, a considerable group spirit developed. The prisoners' minds were taken off themselves as their interest in each other and in the experiment grew.

As evidence that administrative pressures were not present in his prison work, Starzl [394] placed a notice on the bulletin board of a Colorado prison where it could be seen by 4,000 prisoners; fewer than 100 expressed interest in donating a kidney, and in the end "only a fraction of this group ultimately underwent nephrectomy." This can be construed as evidence for lack of coercion. Most of these prisoners were incarcerated for relatively minor crimes such as car theft; in many cases, their sentences would terminate in a few weeks or months. No pay was involved, and no reduction of sentence was offered. The prisoners did not know the potential recipient. Starzl therefore suggests that prisoners may be freer of pressure than are members of families in a transplant situation. Starzl finally became convinced "that the use of penal volunteers, however equitably handled in a local situation, would inevitably lead to abuse if accepted as a reasonable precedent and applied broadly." The transplantation committee at the University of Colorado agreed with this position and voted to discontinue the practice.

The use of prisoners in Iowa has been described by Hodges and Bean [214]. In the beginning, there were no political difficulties. Finally, the state's attorney general was asked to rule on the use of prisoners in medical experimentation; in his judgment, such use was illegal. For a two-year period prisoners were not employed. During this time, the following law was enacted: "The board of control may send to the hospital of the medical college of the state university inmates of the Iowa state penitentiary and the men's reformatory for medical research at the hospital. Before any inmate is sent to the medical college, he must volunteer his services in writing. An inmate may withdraw his consent at any time." Hodges and Bean [214] have observed: "One of the chief advantages of this arrangement is that it permits selection of men of any given age, height, and weight. By screening, the investigator can select persons who have a specific disorder, such as diabetes mellitus or hypertension. He can select subjects with any characteristic that might commonly be found within a prison population. These subjects can then be hospitalized in the metabolic ward under combined prison and research discipline or in the clinical research center under similar supervision for the time necessary to complete an experiment."

REWARDS

In examining the motives for volunteering, Hodges and Bean conclude that relief from monotony is a strong influence. The inmates are paid a dollar a day, about the same as they would earn in prison work. No reduction in sentence is involved, and no specific promise of parole is offered. A letter of commendation is sent to the warden at the end of a given experiment; it is possible that this letter in the prisoner's file could have a favorable effect on the parole board. A resolution adopted by the House of Delegates of the American Medical Association in 1952 asserts that elsewhere prisoners "have in some instances been granted parole much sooner than would otherwise have occurred, including several individuals convicted of murder and sentenced to life imprisonment . . ." Prisoners prefer to receive visits from their children in the hospital rather than in the prison. Altruism may play a part. A few—10 of 224—have used the hospital as an escape hatch. Some undoubtedly hope for future favorable treatment. Feminine proximity, even though limited, is a consideration.

The work of Hodges and Bean with the 224 prisoners[7] led to the publication of more than 80 scientific articles, work carried out under ideal circumstances, a matter of pride to investigators and prisoners alike.

[7] Fox [165], quoting Shuster in the *New York Times,* April 13, 1958, estimated in 1960 that as many as 20,000 federal prisoners were collaborating as volunteers in medical experiments. This may have been a misreading of Shuster's article: he said only that 20,000 federal prisoners composed one of the largest sources of potential volunteers.

While many strong statements can be found to the effect that little or no reward is involved and that commutation of sentence or parole are not offered, the facts are often to the contrary. Leopold and the 441 other prisoners at Stateville Penitentiary in Illinois who volunteered for the malaria project were, in most cases, granted either a commutation of sentence or parole as a direct reward for their services to science [165, 275].

CONDEMNED PERSONS

Kevorkian suggests that prisoners condemned to death be allowed to submit by their own free choice to medical experimentation as a form of execution under complete anesthesia, at the time set for administering the penalty, in place of the methods now prescribed by law [247]. He would allow the condemned man time to deliberate on such a choice and would allow him appropriate guidance from consultants. It is not clear that such a practice would have any great usefulness. It is very clear that such a system, contrary as it is to the ancient and honorable traditions of medicine, could have a demoralizing effect on the physicians involved; the physician is not an executioner. The use of a layman to administer the final *coup de grace,* as he suggests, does not really alter the situation. Freund [170] has this to say on the subject: "The great objection to this proposal is the possible feedback effect it would have on the death penalty itself, making that penalty seem more tolerable, reducing the chances of clemency by the jury or commutation by the executive and perhaps even forestalling the movement that exists in many quarters to abolish the death penalty entirely."

The exigencies of national peril may excuse the careful use of prisoners[8] in medical experimentation, as may other pressing

[8] It is most unusual for normal healthy young males to allow their testicles to be injected and incised, but this was done in recent prison work [205], supported in part by the National Institutes of Health of the United States Public Health Service. The purpose was to study the spermatogenic process in man. The subjects were inmates of a state penitentiary; their ages varied from 20 to 42 years. Bilateral testicular biopsies were made under local anesthesia. The scrotal skin and tunica were incised "and the testicular tissue was separated from the tunica by lateral undercuts . . . Due to internal pressure, the underlying seminiferous tubules protruded above the

needs. The ice is thin. In weighing the pros and cons of such use, one must face the fact that the *bonum communum* was precisely the rationalization claimed by the Nazis.

PRISONERS OF WAR

Prisoners of war are never suitable subjects for medical experimentation. This can be stated categorically.

OTHER CAPTIVE GROUPS

Captive groups *in general* do not present a good source of "volunteers." The reason is plain. One can exert coercion without always realizing it. Where possibilities for coercion exist, however subtle they may be, the use of members of such a group may violate the requirements for valid consent. Such volunteers must be suspect, whether they are one's laboratory personnel, military personnel, medical students, civil or military prisoners, or one's ward patients. Their atypical characteristics have been described above. The use of medical students as subjects for research has been accepted for a long time, but no instructor should permit *his* students to be used in *his* own investigations.

These groups are often considered legitimate subjects by the eager but impoverished investigator, and certainly tradition has accepted their use. To the writer, at least, such groups are, generally speaking, not a good choice for two reasons: (1) These are captive groups, not as prisoners of war are, but nonetheless subject to certain kinds of subtle coercion. A volunteer should be just that, not one who may be subject to fear of the consequences if he does not cooperate. The more domineering the investigator, and thus the more valid the point made, the more likely is this possibility to be disclaimed. Denied or not, the situation does exist; it is better to avoid it in most cases. (2) In quantitative studies of subjective re-

---

tunica and were severed by a stroke of a razor blade." In one phase of the study, radioactive thymidine-H^3 was injected into the testicles and the sites marked with a black thread "so that the exact area could be relocated for subsequent biopsies." Eight previously vasectomized inmates volunteered for this procedure.

sponses over many years, it has become clear to the writer that in this field, at least, subjects must not be in communication with each other. If they are, certain false syndromes are established, presumably through conditioning. Some startling examples of this could be given if space permitted. The hazard to sound conclusion of such action is nowhere more amusingly evident than in the reports of some of those who have studied the psychotomimetic drugs in their own personnel.

Mackintosh [289] expresses a sound and considerate point of view concerning the use of laboratory personnel:

> On the difficult question of laboratory personnel, we had certain decisions to make in the London School of Hygiene. In the study of malarial parasites "resting" in the human liver we had offers from a skilled technician to submit himself to infection and then to have a small liver section taken. In this case the technician was a senior man who was fully aware of the risks involved. His offer was gratefully accepted, but at the same time a regulation was passed that in the future no human experiment should be allowed without a full report being made in advance to the School Council (which is the professional body) and to the Board of Management, which has a considerable representation of scientists, and also lay members. The crux of the decision was whether the volunteer had the training and skill to appreciate the whole situation, although not necessarily the details of the procedure. It was evident that there might be subjective matters of study which the volunteer ought not to know beforehand, so as to avoid vitiating the experiment. The additional point of the decision was to make sure that the volunteer gave his consent freely, or, better still, offered his service in writing. In such cases no fee or reward, apart from any out-of-pocket expenses, should be offered.

3
The Investigator

The physician and the investigator have different immediate aims and divergent long-range purposes. To paraphrase Ladimer, the physician *accepts* patients and is concerned mainly with their welfare; the investigator *selects* subjects—problems as well as individuals—and, while responsive to the patient's interest, is more concerned with solving the scientific problem [256]. While there are some investigators whose standard of ethics is limited to not being caught, these are surely in the minority. Among all safeguards, the *responsible* investigator is the most important to the subject. One hears a great deal about responsible investigators; responsible subjects also are needed.

All of the so-called codes for human experimentation emphasize the requirement that the experimenter be well trained and scientifically competent to undertake the study proposed. Medical research that involves treatment or any but the simplest physical procedures requires that the investigator or his close associate be a qualified physician. No profession other than medicine enjoys such prerogatives, and probably no other profession exhibits such a generally high level of unselfishness and compassion. Of these two qualities, unselfishness is the more important for subject and project alike. Imagination, objectivity, and the power to generalize soundly are all essential.

RESPONSIBILITIES AND SAFEGUARDS

PRELIMINARY RESPONSIBILITIES

The investigator is obligated to fulfill certain responsibilities prior to undertaking an experiment. He must be fully cognizant of the relevant animal data. He must be fully informed on the medical literature applicable to his proposed study. He must be particularly alert to all the possible hazards of his planned procedure. When patients are involved, the investigation must be organized to adduce the maximum information without minimizing the best possible treatment. If valuable long-range goals suggest the need for any deviation from this standard, it can be undertaken only with the full understanding and concurrence of the patient. It is impossible to overemphasize the importance of the well-planned clinical trial focused on the given problem and its solution.

No investigator can expect to be relieved of responsibility for the welfare of his patient as long as the patient is in his charge. In this connection, some writers have advanced the disquieting thought that "no investigator can be successful who allows, or is forced by circumstance to allow, solicitude for his patient to preoccupy his mind." Once again, it is necessary to answer this argument. Science is not the highest value to which all other values must be subjugated.

GENERAL RESPONSIBILITIES

Claude Bernard clearly stated [13] the responsibilities of the investigator:

As far as direct applicability to medical practice is concerned, it is quite certain that experiments made on man are always the most conclusive. No one has ever denied it . . . First, have we a right to perform experiments and vivisections on man? Physicians make therapeutic experiments daily on their patients, and surgeons perform vivisections daily on their subjects. Experiments, then, may be performed on man, but within what limits? It is our duty and our right to perform an experiment on man whenever it can save his life, cure him, or gain him some personal benefit. The principle of medical and surgical morality, therefore, consists in never performing on man an experiment which might be harmful to him to any extent, even though the result might be highly advantageous to science, i.e., to the health of others. But performing experiments and operations exclusively from the point of view of the patient's own advantage does not prevent their turning out profitably to science.

One can take exception to the injunction that one must never perform on man "an experiment which might be harmful to him." Strict adherence to this rule would eliminate all procedures that entail discernible risks. To be contrary, risk *is* permissible under certain circumstances.

In the case of patently nonhazardous experimentation, there is no obligation on the investigator to subject himself first to the experimental procedures. However, when there is doubt as to safety, it is incumbent on the investigator to be *willing* to subject himself initially to the possible hazards involved, although actually doing so may be impracticable in some situations. When it is not known whether a given treatment is likely to be effective, the investigator is entitled to withhold it—as he is not when its effectiveness is assured, except with the consent of the patient—where new and more promising therapy waits trial. In this connection, Green [191] has cogently observed that "where the value of a treatment new or old, is doubtful, there may be a higher moral obligation to test it critically than to continue to prescribe the old remedy year-in-year-out with the support merely of custom or wishful thinking." McCance [293] reinforces this view with the contention that "the medical profession has a responsibility not only for the cure of the sick and for the prevention of disease but for the advancement of knowledge upon which both depend. This . . . responsibility can only be met by investigation and experiment . . ."

The many differences between the practice of medicine and human experimentation have been the subject of repeated comment in this book. Clearly, useful research goes beyond the requirements of the community's standards; there are, nonetheless, certain parallels that can usefully be drawn in examining the investigator's position of responsibility. In questions of malpractice, it is legitimate to ask whether the actions of the physician comported with generally accepted community standards in the given case. So, too, a similar question can be appropriately raised concerning experimentation, as Ladimer [256] has done:

> In research, standards must relate to how the investigator proceeded and how he checked himself. The means by which research of high quality has been managed and the safeguards employed to protect the subject can be generalized into a set of precepts similar to that governing malpractice, to serve as a guide. Thus, willful or negligent deviation, resulting in injury, would constitute a basis for liability. On the other hand, observance of all known precautions, even in the event of an untoward result, would protect the honest, qualified investigator. Neither he nor the physician is a guarantor of success, but each has a responsibility to his own law and credo.

The responsibilities devolving on those who undertake experimentation in man are so great that whenever even remote hazard is a possibility group decision supported by a proper consultative body should be employed. Shimkin [431] contends that self-experimentation "without such collaboration and consultation seems as indefensible as similar experimentation on another individual." In this connection, Ladimer [256] observes: "At the Clinical Center of the National Institutes of Health, for instance, projects involving deviation from accepted medical practice or unusual hazard are presented in writing to a Clinical Research Committee. Consent is obtained from subjects and final approval from the Center's Medical Board and the Director of the National Institutes of Health."

Hill [208] quotes the British Medical Research Council:

> In any particular case—so specialized has medical knowledge become—only a small group of experienced investigators, who have devoted themselves to this branch of medicine, are likely to be competent to pass an opinion on the advisability of undertaking any particular investigation. But in every branch of medicine such a group of investigators exists. It is upon them, and the specialized scientific societies to which they belong, that the medical profession must mainly rely for the creation of the body of precedents and the climate of opinion which shall guide investigators in clinical research . . . it is incumbent upon the medical scientific societies to accept this responsibility and, by en-

couraging critical discussion on the communications presented to them, help to resolve doubts and to form a body of opinion of what is necessary, desirable and justifiable to guide investigators in their field.

Wiggers has expressed a similar view [425].

In 1949, the Department of Hospitals, City of New York, issued the following order:

1. That proposed clinical or laboratory investigations in any hospital or institution of the Department, whether or not under the auspices of affiliated medical schools, be submitted for review and approval by the Executive Committee of the Medical Board of the hospital concerned.

2. That unless it is specifically designed to benefit the patient involved—no research using a patient as a subject is permitted in any hospital or institution of the Department.

The responsibilities of the investigator are heightened when his subject is under the influence of sedatives, hypnotics, analgesics, ego depressants, anesthetics, or even severe fatigue. The partial or complete loss of control of the subject under these circumstances places an increased burden and restraint on the investigator, since he can no longer be assisted by the subject's wishes.

Finally, in this brief discussion of responsibilities, it is clear that the knife must cut both ways: the investigator clearly has grave responsibilities, but society bears a parallel responsibility to ensure that the physician and scientist are not irresponsibly hampered in carrying on studies that will both protect and benefit mankind.

RELATIONSHIPS OF INVESTIGATOR AND SUBJECT

These relationships are very often identical with those of patient and physician. There is good reason to examine this facet of the human experimentation problem. Whenever the physician tries out a new drug or a new technique—not necessarily new in any absolute sense, but perhaps new only for a particular patient—he is experimenting in his effort to relieve or cure the individual involved [293, 425]. To withhold new methods could often be condemned. In principle, such "experimentation" is relatively uncomplicated. Very great complications arise, however, when experimentation on one patient is not expected to benefit him directly, but is designed to help patients in general. The recent increase in this type of experimentation requires consideration, for it involves the most basic elements in the patient-physician relationship, as well as the attitude toward life and its responsibilities harbored by both patient and physician. As Guttentag [196] puts it, "not all experiments performed on men will ever be of value to these particular men. And it is with these breathing men that we are concerned as physicians." Only physicians can legally take the final serious responsibility for human medical experimentation. Occasionally, in certain experiments without discernible risk, others—psychologists or sociologists, for example—may be best qualified to assume responsibility.

Only physicians are well equipped to carry out work "to confirm or disprove a biological generalization with regard to man . . . the profession that is trained more completely than any other in comprehending the somatic and psychological aspects of human life, be it healthy or diseased" [196]. Guttentag [196] points out an additional reason, related to the original patient-physician relationship: "Here *both* the healthy and the sick persons are . . . fellow-companions, partners to conquer a common enemy . . ." He calls it "mutual obligations of equals"; to use von Weizsaecker's term, it is "solidarity." Guttentag regards the physician-experimenter and the physician-friend as representing two distinct aspects of the doctor's activities. In the best situations, a colleague-like intimacy grows between investigator and subject.

Against the background of the two roles played by the physician, Guttentag considers three currently evolving developments. First, there is the use of force, as exercised in Hitler's Germany. It seems unlikely that this will, except for extremely rare local abuses or in the hands of careless or thoughtless investigators, be of importance in the United States, for ". . . the overwhelming majority of physician-experimenters, if not thoroughly aware of the nature of the original patient-physician relationship, are so deeply rooted in the democratic spirit that they agree, and will continue to agree, that the use of force is not justified."

Second, there is the use of the "hopelessly incurable" as experimental subjects. The writer has already stated the reasons for his deep conviction that those who are in imminent danger of death should not ordinarily be subjected to experimentation, except as part of a therapeutic effort to save their lives. An exception to this can be found in the irreversibly comatose individual who may be used as an organ donor under certain rigid circumstances (see Appendix B). Occasionally one encounters reports wherein the term *hopelessly incurable* seems to be used to justify dangerous experimentation. It is not the physician's prerogative to make or to profit from such dubious judgments. According to Guttentag [196], the use of such subjects is

> meant to be noble in the democratic spirit, yet it unconsciously challenges this spirit more subtly but no less than the use of force, because it violates the concept of equality or brotherhood in violating the principle of the original patient-physician relationship. From the experimenter's point of view, the description "hopelessly incurable" is not germane to his purpose. The designation is inadequate, because it does not specify the time element—hopeless within hours, days, months, years? And if months or years are concerned, do all experts agree on the status of their respective sciences and deny the possibility of discovering effective agents within such a period? The term is also unnecessary.

From the standpoint of the physician-friend, the assertion is not germane to his purpose, either. To him it is an expression of detachment between physician and patient, the announcement of a scale of partnership versus domination quite contrary to its original spirit.

Third, one may cite the "increased technicalities of many problems and procedures." To Guttentag this suggests that for the protection of the subject the physician-friend and the physician-experimenter should be two persons, lest selfishness decide the issue. This view should be compared with those of Bean [13, 14]. The physician-friend would play the part of attorney for the defense, while the physician-experimenter would be the prosecuting attorney. Practically, the physician-friend and the physician-experimenter must sometimes be and often are the same person. Nevertheless, it is necessary that the two attitudes be recognized and pondered.

In discussing the role of the clinical investigator *vis-à-vis* that of the patient's physician, Bean comments that Sir Thomas Lewis held to the view that the intense mental excitement of the clinical investigator unfitted him for the personal care of the patient who was the subject of his experiments [14]. On the other hand, Bean and others espouse the opposite view: namely, that unless the clinical investigator *is* the patient's personal physician during the experimentation, his keen quest may unwittingly cause him to jeopardize his patient's welfare and rights. This, of course, is precisely what Guttentag [196] had in mind when he stressed the need for two people, the physician-investigator and the physician-friend. "The moral history of mankind is more important than the scientific."

THE MEDICAL INVESTIGATOR AS SCIENTIST

The investigator of the medical problems of mankind strives to discover, extend, improve, correct, and apply information concerning man. Insofar as his activities are concerned with the discovery and establishment of new concepts, as pointed out in Chap. 2, the investigator is a "basic" scientist and takes equal rank with basic scientists in any field, as described in the section, "The Sick Man and Basic Science" (Chap. 2). The writer has for years marveled at the arrogance of those who, working in laboratories, have claimed that *they* were the true scientists and that anything learned at the bedside of a sick man was applied science, if it were science at all, and certainly downstream intellectually from the high purposes of those confined to the laboratory. With the growth of biologic knowledge, this limited view is less tenable than ever. This matter has also been referred to in the Preface.

The purposes of the physician-scientist are directed mainly toward the discovery and accumulation of biologic and medical knowledge and the testing of this by its application to the prevention, treatment, and eradication of disease.

THE PHYSICIAN-INVESTIGATOR AS HUMANITARIAN

Three individual writers of recent years stand out particularly in their concern for the physician as a humanitarian in a milieu where advancement of medical knowledge is an important goal. These writers are, in the order of their principal writings on the subject: von Weizsaecker [415], Bean [13], and Guttentag [196]. Bean and Guttentag have continued to write occasionally on this or closely related subjects. To this writer, Guttentag's dichotomy is sensible and appealing. It has of necessity been referred to earlier, but requires emphasis here from the point of view of present considerations. There is the physician-experimenter, the scientist, and the physician-friend.

The importance of the dichotomy emerges clearly when one considers some of the current attitudes toward the "hopelessly incurable" patient. Examination of his plight magnifies, but need not exaggerate, the issues; they become clearer here than in less conclusive situations. The experimenter's choice of the hopelessly incurable as subjects may have as one goal to give evidence to others of his thoughtful "conservatism." Such a choice, however, is an exhibition of the use of force, unless the subject is capable of understanding and of truly volunteering. It is conceivable that permission might be granted, when the doomed subject is still in full possession of his faculties, for later study of the mechanism of death, provided such study neither prolongs nor hastens the final process and provided no suffering is attributable to such study.

Characterization of the patient as hopelessly incurable is offensive to the physician-friend relationship. According to Guttentag [196], the use of a patient so characterized for experimental purposes can lead to the paradox that "the healthier the patient, the more he should be the concern of his physician; the sicker, the less." The physician-friend's concern is to restore his patient; if this is not possible, he must attempt to comfort the end.

Von Weizsaecker [415] presents another dichotomy, also useful in considering the hopelessly sick: there are the aspects of pity and of sacrifice. Pity as such does not illuminate the spirit of solidarity between patient and investigator: the patient wants help, not pity. "Selfish motivation, entirely unconscious, may enter in the guise of pity; and, on the other hand, conscious selfishness—for instance, the physician's greed for money—may help a patient more than the physician's pity." Under some circumstances the patient, aware of his hopeless illness, may wish to offer himself for experimentation, in a sense to sacrifice himself. The physician-friend may accept this, under certain circumstances, if he is certain of his patient's lucidity and knowledge, but only with the full understanding that true equality of purpose no longer exists. In this situation, the physician-friend must guard against his own selfish interests. There is, in Fletcher's phrase [161a], a need for the principle of *"mutuality between persons."*

THE DOCTOR-PATIENT RELATIONSHIP IN PATIENT CARE VERSUS SCIENCE

In discussing the doctor-patient relationship, Wolfle makes the point that research not designed to benefit the subject cannot be limited by the doctor-patient relationship [429]. It is not clear just what he conceives the doctor-patient relationship to be. Nearly all therapy involves some experimentation for the good of the patient, and very often this experimentation is extended by the same two individuals beyond the needs of the patient, with his agreement. When this occurs, there has not necessarily been some great or subtle change in the doctor-patient relationship. In any case, one is led to inquire into the exact nature of this much-publicized relationship.

The doctor-patient relationship is an association between two individuals, one skilled in medicine, the other usually not, where the physician tries to be of service in preventing, diagnosing, alleviating, or curing the patient's ailments, and in this relationship the physician may make new discoveries. Does it really make a difference in the relationship whether the beneficiary is a man or the beneficiary science in general? The physician's qualities and qualifications of probity, discretion, honesty, skill, knowledge, and insight, which are the bedrock of the doctor-patient relationship, have not altered as he proceeds from directly benefiting his patient to generally benefiting science. Wolfle [429] says: "Clearly the differences are too great to allow using the precedents of the physician-patient relationship as a total guide in handling the problems of the experimenter-subject relationship." Is this view defensible?

Wolfle argues that a change necessarily occurs when, as in his own experience, he contributed to his physician both time and his person to medical follow-up studies not for his own benefit. He also cites, in support of his view, the much publicized case of the investigators who injected live cancer cells into the patients of another institution without their knowledge. Granted that an ideal doctor-patient relationship did not hold in the latter case, how does this support Wolfle's argument that there is necessarily a change in the doctor-patient relationship when the goal is the advancement of science rather than the welfare of the immediate patient? This case proves nothing more than the fact that an acceptable doctor-patient relationship is sometimes violated. Indeed, the latter case seems to argue against Wolfle's view. If Southam and Levine had followed an acceptable doctor-patient relationship where consideration for their subjects came first, they would have avoided the criticism and official censure they received. Furthermore, if adherence to an acceptable doctor-patient relationship made their experiment impossible, one can only conclude with Pius XII that science is not the highest value. There are and must be limits to human experimentation. Surely a warning of the approach, or the presence, of such limits can be found in situations that require the violation of acceptable doctor-patient relationships as these have been defined over the years.

The doctor-patient relationship is many things, but it includes the understanding that the doctor will act in the interest of the patient's welfare. Any exception to this can be made only with the full understanding and consent of the patient. At one extreme one can visualize a situation where the patient's welfare was the only outcome of the relationship, but the pure case is probably nonexistent and presupposes that the doctor is an idiot, incapable of learning. Every individual case educates the thoughtful doctor; there is no single outcome of the relationship. The real question is not whether this relationship should have one outcome or whether, in addition to providing for the patient's welfare, the outcome should advance education or science. The point at issue is that the patient's welfare must not take second place to education and the advancement of knowledge. The doctor-investigator cannot be any more neglectful of the interest of a group of individuals under his responsibility in the laboratory, for the sake of science, than he is of one patient in his consulting room who comes for therapy. This is emphasized by the American Medical Association in *Ethical Guidelines,* 1966, Rule 2.

Wolfle has no more interest in quibbling over small details than the writer has. It seems, however, that some serious ethical errors recently exposed are attributable to failure to maintain a responsible doctor-patient relationship even when the beneficiary is not a single patient, but science in general. One can envisage even more serious dangers in parting from the spirit of the doctor-patient relationship in human experimentation. Many have already been demonstrated.

"STANDARD" TREATMENT WITHHELD BY THE INVESTIGATOR

Until the Food and Drug Administration called a halt in 1962, it was not uncommon for proposed remedies to be released from the laboratory before adequate animal work had been completed and certainly before well-designed tests in groups of human subjects had substantiated the claims made. Responsibility for such precipitate action must often be divided among the manufacturers; the detail men who make unwarranted claims; the uncritical physician sometimes honestly seeking better patient care, but also sometimes seeking acclaim for "introducing" a new and possibly valuable agent; and finally the public for its acceptance of blatant advertising.

It would be difficult at this late date to unravel the chain of events that led, for example, to the widespread use of meperidine (Demerol). This agent was introduced and promulgated, among other claims, on the basis of three nonexistent qualities. It was said to be nonaddicting; it is now known to be viciously addicting. It was said to be an effective morphine substitute that did not depress the respiration as morphine does; it is now known to depress the respiration as much as morphine in equianalgesic doses. It was said not to cause smooth muscle spasm, as morphine does; in the only place it has been carefully tested in man, on the sphincter of Oddi, it produces a spastic effect equal to that of morphine. This is not to deny that meperidine is a powerful agent and truly useful in situations where patients are sensitive to morphine. For generations morphine has represented the standard treatment for severe pain. Was it a mistake to study other agents in seeking for a better analgesic? Certainly not. To freeze any treatment, however "standard" it has become, and to forbid a search for better agents is to block advance in medicine.

Under what circumstances can a new treatment be tried out? If there is no standard treatment, the ethical problems are comparatively few. If animal work has been completely reassuring, and this has been confirmed in early tests in man based on valid consent, then, in the view of the writer, when no discernible risk is involved it is not necessary to discuss the use of the new agent with patients who have come, let us say, for relief of pain. Comparison of such an agent with a placebo can be carried out. Better still, it can be compared with the standard morphine. It is possible that discussion of this could lead to distortion of the results obtained. This is unlikely if the patients are told in advance that they may be receiving a new agent or a placebo, but they will not be told if or when this may occur. It is necessary to point out that the Food and Drug

Administration does not concur with all details of the above policy.

In desperate situations where there is no standard treatment, it may be proper to try dangerous and doubtful remedies. Each case must be appraised independently. The procedure should be discussed with the patient if he is capable of understanding the situation; if not, it should be submitted to the responsible next-of-kin. In such situations, also, it is prudent to obtain the group support of one's peers. In less serious situations it is often important, if one is to go beyond an accepted, standard treatment, to strive for the informed consent of the patient, and the support of one's peers. Common sense need not be abandoned here. In this connection, one can remember that when a sick man comes to a physician for relief he gives, in the act of coming, consent to *reasonable* efforts to relieve him.

"Standard" treatment is a relative phrase, far from absolute. A number of examples come to mind to suggest the need for a healthy skepticism as to how really established a standard may be: a case in point is the report of Thulborne and Young [408]. It is common practice in some clinics to give penicillin prophylactically before and after surgery to patients with chronic chest disease or to patients who are believed to be especially susceptible to postoperative chest infection. In this study, 65 such patients were given penicillin, and 70 controls were not. The agent neither cut down the incidence of postoperative pulmonary infection nor reduced the severity. Hill [209] poses this question: "Was it more ethical to continue to use unquestioningly a powerful antibiotic, day in, day out, with no measure of its benefit than deliberately to withhold it from a specific group of patients in an attempt to find out?" The controlled clinical trial is no occasion for discarding common sense in the search for accuracy and effectiveness. "Here we have an instance—and by no means unique—of the wheel turning full circle. At the start of the trial was it ethical to withhold the treatment? At its end, was it ethical to give it? It is very easy to be wise (and critical) *after* the event; the problem is to be wise (and ethical) *before* the event."

Lay pressures can be very strong. Mainland describes the early efforts to determine the effects of oxygen on premature babies [290]. The suspicion had grown that oxygen in high tension was a possible cause of retrolental fibroplasia and subsequent blindness. A controlled comparison of two levels of oxygen was planned. The nurses present were indignant that half the premature infants would be denied the high oxygen. As the trial continued and the suspicion was strengthened that high oxygen was a factor in the disease, the nurses switched sides completely and believed it was criminal to place any babies in a high-oxygen atmosphere.

Another example may be given. Despite some conflicting information, there was "striking" evidence that anticoagulants were of value in treating cerebrovascular disease. Hill, Marshall, and Shaw, evidently with some misgivings at denying this therapy to half of a considerable (142 patients) group, decided that a controlled clinical trial was necessary to settle the matter [210]. Judging from the favorable reports available when the trial was set up, it could have been agreed that it was unethical to withhold the treatment from half of the patients. However, by the time five fatalities from hemorrhage had occurred in the treated group and none in the untreated group—not completely significant at the 5 percent level—the investigators decided to terminate the experiment earlier than planned; others had found comparable results. Thus, it was questionably ethical at the beginning of this study to withhold the anticoagulant; at the end, the evidence tended to indicate that it was unethical to administer the anticoagulant, an opposite attitude.

Numerous other examples of the breakdown of too hastily presumed standard treatment can be found: cortisone *versus* aspirin in rheumatoid arthritis; cortisone *versus* placebo in status asthmaticus; and, less conclusively, the recent trials of anticoagulants in acute myocardial infarction, not yet quite completed by the Medical Research Council, as reported by Pickering [342].

There can be a problem in leaving human controls untreated, although this can be exaggerated. (1) The question is not a serious one when the disease is mild and improvement may be expected in a few days. A well-planned trial is much to be preferred to the casual and uncertain use of a drug. (2) A new and potent drug is not likely to be available in quantity; it may also have powerful undesirable side effects. For both of these reasons, it needs to be compared with untreated cases. It is essential to obtain the maximum information from the available material. The only circumstances in which alternative treatment of an ailment is permissible, according to the British Medical Research Council, is when doubt exists as to which of two approaches is better. If doctors were certain of the benefits of penicillin, for example, yet did not use it, their decision could be construed as running counter to the basic rule of the physician, *primum non nocere*—above all, do no harm.

In experimentation one is uncertain of the outcome. In this sense, all or nearly all therapy is experimental. One takes an aspirin for a headache; it may or may not relieve the headache. One recommends a resection of the stomach for ulcer; it may or may not be successful. Perhaps a legitimate distinction between frankly experimental therapy and standard therapy is simply this: in experimental therapy one primarily seeks information whereas, in standard therapy, treatment and cure of the patient is the goal.

THE INVASION OF PRIVACY

One aspect of the investigator's activities so far has been given too little attention: his sometimes offhand invasion of the privacy of his subject. All of the signs indicate that this matter is to be thoroughly examined in the immediate future. This area is of such importance in human experimentation that it requires a rather extensive presentation. As a basic principle, intrusion into a human body or mind under any circumstances is no more permissible than casual search and seizure in a home.

Looking backward for a moment, it is evident that the modern origins of an interest in privacy stem from the historic study of the subject by Charles Warren and the young Louis Brandeis. This was published in 1890; the word privacy thus appeared in legal literature for the first time. Nothing is said about privacy in the United States Constitution. Ernst and Schwartz [147] refer to the

Warren and Brandeis study as "a spurt of legal imagination which takes us far beyond what at the time were considered by many to be immutable principles of law and logic. Here are Warren and Brandeis in 1890, ambushing from the previous . . . cases the perhaps unspoken elements that bound them all together at that time, and moulding these elements into a new legal principle that deftly expresses what all the inadequate fumblings of the past had not been able or inclined to do."

Sometimes epoch-making events have their origins in trivial situations, as was the case here. The Warrens were active in the Boston Back Bay social life of the late nineteenth century and gave frequent dinner parties. The press went to unusual lengths to learn the identity of the prospective guests. This attempted invasion of his privacy annoyed Warren and occasioned his persistent interest in the subject. He sought the collaboration of young Brandeis, and American law has not been the same since.

A recent stimulus to interest in privacy was the remarkably fine paper by Ruebhausen and Brim [368], published in 1965. In 1967 a government panel report on *Privacy and Behavioral Research* was published. The panel's concern was based on questions as to the propriety of certain procedures in behavioral research raised by the Congress, by officials in the several agencies of the government, by university officials, by the scientific community generally, and by leading members of the professional societies that serve the behavioral sciences.

The invasion of privacy by the investigator takes many forms. There are the countless questionnaires with their sometimes impertinent questions, beginning at the grade-school level and continuing through applications for jobs and licenses, married life, and on through senescence. Those who are supported by public welfare funds can expect official invasion of their privacy; so also can the entire population during the collection of data for the government census. Although the original aims of such studies may be justified, there is always the danger that the accumulated data may eventually be used for unintended purposes. Men are spied on, recorded, reported on, and harassed by a whole gamut of persons and devices ranging from the simple-minded Peeping Tom to the devilishly complex and effective electronic surveillance techniques. Some of this is motivated by competition in business or by domestic tangles; some of it is for criminal purposes; some of it for law enforcement; but much of this is for "research," and hence comment on it is appropriate in the present consideration.

When the collection of data is mandatory, as in certain governmental procedures, in industry, in welfare situations, there is a great burden on the sponsoring agency to protect the subject against disclosure unless this is specifically sanctioned by the individuals concerned or by statute. Sometimes proper regulations must be observed, as in the case of the physician, who is required by law to report venereal disease. Only a small proportion of the population may currently be exposed to serious invasions of privacy; however, as the report of the Committee on Privacy and Behavioral Research (1967) points out [119], there is enough of such action against the minority to "risk eroding the quality of life for the majority."

The extent of the invasion of privacy can hardly be surprising to those who are familiar with behavioral research, for all social science, political science, economics, anthropology, sociology, and psychology are concerned with the behavior of individuals, of groups, and of communities. In 1966, some 35,000 behavioral scientists were engaged in such research in the United States, and 2,100 new Ph.D.s pour forth each year; 40,000 students are presently seeking advanced degrees in the behavioral sciences. In 1966, the Federal government contributed 300 million dollars to behavioral research.

The individual's right to be let alone conflicts with the advancement of society through scientific research, since the purposes of behavioral studies are directed to the assessment and measurement of many qualities of man's mind, feelings, and actions [119]. Clearly, there is conflict between the individual's right to seclusion and the right of the public to be informed in many areas. So also is there conflict between the right to privacy and the guarantee of free speech and a free press. The violation of privacy is an indignity to the individual. The concern for privacy arises from concern for the individual. In a totalitarian state, only the dictator is allowed privacy.

When studies are made without the consent of the subject, they constitute an invasion of privacy that can be serious. At the same time, however, it must be recognized that prior discussion of the work planned can distort the results; thus, the honest investigator faces a dilemma not easily resolved. In the end, most scientists in the field accept something short of the ideal: a situation in which a state of mutual trust exists between scientist and subject whereby the latter's dignity and anonymity are preserved.

In his inquiry into the autonomy of the individual, Shils [382] recognized that respect for privacy is a rather recent addition to the values of modern liberalism, that the value of privacy is derived from our belief in "the sacredness of individuality." This must be respected by the investigator. Deception is contrary to such respect. Margaret Mead has commented on the subject [298]. Privacy can be suspended only by the deliberate decision of the subject involved, except where sanctioned by statute, as in the required reporting of venereal disease.

The Committee on Privacy and Behavioral Research concluded: "Neither the principle of privacy nor the need to discover new knowledge can supervene universally." As with other conflicts in our society, according to the committee, there is need for adjustment and compromise in determining which value is to govern in a given situation. The cost in privacy is balanced against the gain in knowledge, which leaves one with a feeling of uneasiness and the fear that the individual will be sacrificed. The following quotation from the report has the same effect: "Furthermore, the investigator is first and foremost a scientist in search of new knowledge, and it would not be in accord with our understanding of human motivation to expect him always to be as vigilant for his subject's welfare as he is for the productiveness of his own research." Neither is one reassured by the committee's conclusion: "If intrusion on privacy proves essential to the research, he (the investigator) should not proceed with his proposed experiment until he and his colleagues have considered all of the relevant facts and he has determined, with support from them, that the benefits outweigh the costs." André Gide has well stated: "Everything has been said, but it is necessary to say it again because some have not listened." In that spirit, one must reiterate one's contention that ends do not always justify means. Unfortunately, also, the committee report's concluding remarks evince no awareness of the fact that some experiments simply cannot be carried out; again, science is not always the highest good.

A number of factors have coalesced to produce emphasis on the rights of the individual in our society. There are, of course, the common law and the Bill of Rights, giving assurance that an individual will be safe in his person, but they have been on the books for a long time. Important as they were and are, they alone are not responsible for the recent upsurge of social consciousness. Some causative factors are evident: there is the continuing reaction to the Nazi outrages of recent memory; the present struggle for equal civil rights for all men; and the publicity given to unethical medical experimentation, to mention a few. While the last factor is, in comparison with the others, of small extent, it has nevertheless received wide publicity; the extent of this sudden publicity is perhaps a barometer of the temper of the public. No doubt other less clear causes are at work. One can see some evidence for them in the influence of the labor movement, in the anti-trust laws, in the dispersal of money through taxation, coupled with anti-poverty legislation. The last three are personal and corporate attacks on "accumulations of power." This complexity of society gives the individual a feeling of bewilderment.

The development of science requires reasonable freedom for the investigator; at the same time for the sake of the individual, a healthy society imposes restraints. Thus, tensions exist between society and science. "This tension between society and science extends to all disciplines in the social, physical and life sciences. It affects the practitioner as well as the research investigator." There is also the "conflict of science and scientific research with the right, not of private property, but of private personality" [368], which will now be considered.

Complex as is the individual's right to a private personality, this is nowhere nearly as secure in law as the right to private property, as Ruebhausen and Brim point out [368]. There are, nonetheless, two major aspects: there is the "right to be let alone," so movingly espoused by Cooley [111], and there is Lerner's "right to share and to communicate" [276]. There is also the need to share and the need to withhold.

While the individual strives always to protect his privacy, the collection of individuals and institutions called society invariably tends to invade the individual's privacy. Serious or not as this may be, the test of importance is this: is the threat or the invasion by the investigator unreasonable or intolerable [368]?

New threats, new techniques are made possible by science [368]:

> Modern acoustics, optics, medicine and electronics have exploded most of our normal assumptions as to the circumstances under which our speech, beliefs and behavior are safe from disclosure, and these developments seem to have outflanked the concepts of property and physical intrusion, and presumed consent—concepts which have been relied on by the law to maintain the balance between the private personality and the public need. The miniaturized microphone and tape recorder, the one-way mirror, the sophisticated personality test, the computer with its enormous capacity for the storage and retrieval of information about individuals and groups, the behavior-controlling drugs, the miniature camera, the polygraph, the directional microphone (the "big-ear"), hypnosis, infra-red photography—all of these, and more exist today.

This threat is not new, for Warren and Brandeis long ago [417] spoke of the same thing: "Recent inventions and business methods call attention to the next step which must be taken for the protection of the person, and for securing to the individual . . . the right 'to be let alone.' Instantaneous photographs and newspaper enterprise have invaded the sacred precincts of private and domestic life; and numerous mechanical devices threaten to make good the prediction that 'what is whispered in the closet shall be proclaimed from the house-tops.' "

The President's Crime Commission in 1967 considered electronic surveillance, which includes wiretapping and bugging. These consist in the secret installation of mechanical devices for the purpose of receiving and transmitting conversation. Law enforcement officials almost unanimously agree that the evidence required to bring criminal sanctions against the upper levels of organized crime will not and cannot be obtained without these modern electronic techniques. They contend that they are indispensable in developing adequate strategic intelligence concerning organized crime, to arrange specific investigations, to develop witnesses, to corroborate their testimony, and in the end to serve as substitutes for witnesses. These instruments and techniques have been developed in response to the operational methods employed by organized crime. It must be admitted that these instruments have created unique problems for both law-enforcement officers and scientific investigators.

It is proper to ask, who has the right to overhear and for what purpose? If such eavesdropping is permitted, how is it to be limited or controlled [279]? Former Vice President Humphrey [219] observed, "We act differently if we believe we are being observed. If we can never be sure whether or not we are being watched and listened to, all our actions will be altered and our very character will change." Associate Justice William Brennan has spoken [44] of another aspect of this dark subject: "Electronic aids add a wholly new dimension to eavesdropping. They make it more penetrating, more indiscriminate, more truly obnoxious to a free society. Electronic surveillance, in fact, makes the police omniscient; and police omniscience is one of the most effective tools of tyranny."

THE THREAT TO PRIVACY

One dare not overlook the threat to individual privacy inherent in the field of electronic surveillance. Privacy of communication is essential among citizens. Fear or suspicion that one's activities or speech are being supervised by a stranger has a seriously inhibiting effect upon a willingness to present critical and constructive ideas. In this connection, the President's Crime Commission in 1967 observed: "When dissent from the popular view is discouraged, intellectual controversy is smothered, the process for testing new concepts and ideas is hindered and desirable change is slowed. External restraints, of which electronic surveillance is but one possibility, are thus repugnant to citizens of such a society."

The development of these electronic surveillance techniques in recent years has been remarkable; the electronic cocktail olive is only one illustration. Parabolic microphones can pick up conversations held in the open hundreds of feet distant. These devices can be purchased commercially. Laser beams have shown promise in picking up conversations within a room by focusing on a window pane. Further progress has led to the production of equipment of extremely small size. Bugging can detect and provide for a record of what is said anywhere. It is not dependent upon the telephone; it poses a universal threat to privacy.

Just how widespread such surveillance activities really are is not known. Many who employ these techniques, fearful that their conduct may be declared unlawful, are unwilling to report their activities. This applies to scientific investigators, as well as to others. Individuals familiar with the field believe that electronic surveillance is widespread and its use rapidly increasing. The threat to privacy becomes wider.

PRESENT LAW AND PRACTICE

The United States Supreme Court in 1928 decided that evidence obtained through tapping a defendant's telephone *outside* the defendant's premises was permissible in a federal criminal prosecution. The point to be noticed is that the Court found no unconstitutional search and seizure under the Fourth Amendment. The Federal Communications Act of 1934, Section 605, forbids interception and disclosure of wire communications. The interpretation placed on this by the Department of Justice permits interception as long as no disclosure of the material is made outside the Department. Wiretapping by a federal agent is thus facilitated, but the results must not be used in court. Disclosure of such information is a violation of federal law.

In recent times, law-enforcement experience with bugging has been more limited than with the use of traditional wiretapping. Curiously, the legal situation concerning bugging is also different. Regulation of the national telephone communication network falls within clearly recognized national powers. Any future legislation that attempts to authorize the placement of electronic surveillance equipment would break new and uncharted ground, according to the President's Crime Commission. It was determined by the Supreme Court in 1961 that the use of bugging equipment that involves unauthorized physical entry into a constitutionally protected private area is in violation of the Fourth Amendment and that evidence obtained in this way is inadmissible. Eavesdropping that does not involve such trespass or that is undertaken with the consent of one of the parties recorded presently encounters no such prohibition. In a decision announced in December, 1967, the Supreme Court made it clear that the Constitution does not forbid electronic bugging by law enforcement officers if they first obtain warrants authorizing the procedure. The Court also extended the scope of the Fourth Amendment by requiring enforcement officers to obtain such warrants even when they plan to eavesdrop on persons in such semipublic places as telephone booths. A good deal of confusion has arisen between state and federal law enforcement agencies, based on the fear that information obtained in one investigation "will legally pollute another."

As indicated above, one very serious consequence of the present state of the law is that private parties, and even some law-enforcement officers, are invading the privacy of many citizens without court sanction and without reasonable legislative standards. The President's Crime Commission concluded: "The present status of the law with respect to wiretapping and bugging is intolerable. It serves the interests neither of privacy nor of law enforcement. One way or the other, the present controversy with respect to electronic surveillance must be resolved."

RECOMMENDATIONS CONCERNING NEEDED LEGISLATION DEALING SPECIFICALLY WITH WIRETAPPING AND BUGGING

All members of the President's Commission agreed on the difficulty of maintaining a balance between the law-enforcement benefits that arise from the use of electronic surveillance and the threat to privacy such use may involve. If such a balance is to be struck, important constitutional decisions must be made by the Supreme Court [cf. 412, U.S. Supreme Court, *People v. Berger*]. Further, there was agreement among the members of the commission that if authority to utilize these techniques is granted it must be accompanied by stringent limitations. The members of the commission believe that all private use of electronic instruments for surveillance should either be placed under rigid control or outlawed. Such action would affect investigators in the special areas of sociology and psychology. Some members of the commission seriously doubt the desirability of such control and believe that short of a searching inquiry, such as a Congressional consideration of electronic surveillance, there is insufficient basis to strike a balance in favor of the interests of private individuals. It should be noted that matters concerning the national security not involving criminal prosecution did not come within the commission's mandate.

We have entered the electronic age, with its manifold possibilities for the invasion of privacy. As late as 1967, no legislation had been enacted by the Congress to control the situation. Until its December 1967 decision, the Supreme Court had done little to settle these matters. It would appear that insofar as one can depend on news reports (see *Boston Herald-Traveler* Dec. 19, 1967, "Wiretapping Legal with Warrant," Supreme Court decision Dec. 18, 1967) the new rulings should help a good deal to clarify those areas where eavesdropping is permissible and to lessen what has been called, "a moral and legal vacuum, within which the partisans of stiff law enforcement and those who fear our liberties are being ignored snipe away at each other."

As mentioned, most of the President's Crime Commission members want a law giving carefully circumscribed surveillance powers to law officers. Various suggestions have been made, including the view that electronic supervision be permitted only in cases involving national security or on direct court order. Professor Alan Westin of Columbia University would allow specified state and federal authorities to use electronic surveillance, but under narrowly prescribed conditions [424]. This same proposal would make it a crime for private individuals or organizations to use such devices. Unless modified, this proposal could severely limit legitimate scientific enquiry.

The tools just mentioned facilitate the scientific invasion of privacy, but one must not lose sight of the fact that a serious invasion of privacy is the use of subjects in experimentation without their knowledge or specific consent.

OTHER TYPES OF INVASION OF PRIVACY

Modell makes the point that, in earlier years when drugs were evaluated on an empirical basis, the disasters that followed this method were not very apparent; now, however, with carefully planned evaluation of drugs, great attention is being drawn to the scientist's activities, with the result that he is sometimes "pilloried for his meticulousness" [305]. The overall result is that the medical scientist is wrongfully placed on the defensive.

Modern sciences and technologies have given rise to major health hazards that lead to an invasion of the private person without his knowledge or consent; as with early medicine, when no attempt was made to estimate the hazard, these modern sciences and technologies have remained free to expose masses of people without limit. As examples, Modell cites the contamination of air, soil, watersheds, and water by industrial wastes, only recently a matter of organized concern, applied especially to automobile exhausts in the air and detergents in the soil [305]. Since no careful experiments were carried out to determine the extent of these hazards, they were not labeled inhumane.

Inconsistencies abound in degrees of regulation, as was stated by Modell [305]: "The Food and Drug Administration does not require the application of any of the ethical safeguards for human subjects exposed to insecticides in experiments that it requires for medicinal drugs, even though the former are by their very nature toxic. The Government participated with the airplane industry in an experiment to determine the effects on mind and body of repeated frequent sonic booms involving all the inhabitants of Oklahoma City without anyone's permission.[1] And, of course, we are all subjects of a still unfinished long-term chronic experiment on the effects of ionization to which no one willingly or knowingly gave consent." Experimentation without consent is not uncommon in government circles. In this same context, Cahn [56] has said, "I wish to suggest that, in the areas of scientific interest which impinge on government and law, there are limits to the permissibility of experimentation, that the limits are imposed by institutional factors on one hand and moral factors on the other, and that they require much more attention and respect than lawyers, ethicists, or experimental scientists have been giving them."

It would seem only reasonable that the same ethical consideration should apply to all controllable exposures, not to the medical alone [305]. ". . . we are obligated to discover the size of the hazard by preliminary trial or experiment in man; and that a meaningful ethical basis for their operation will be developed only when all the influences of scientific and technologic progress on man's health are, as with drugs, examined in disciplined experiments before mass exposure. This is the primary ethical decision" [305].

Over a period of many years, Modell has very properly supported these views [305]. The fact that responsible public figures have for one reason or another not had Modell's insight—or if they had it, have not acted on it—does not alter the fact that improvements are needed in all areas, including the medical. There is need

[1] A *New York Times* editorial, June 8, 1968, discusses the "cruel irony in the sonic boom" that shattered 200 windows at the Air Force Academy. A dozen persons were injured by flying glass, in addition to the large numbers subjected to the other unpleasant effects of the boom." The editorial concludes, "The convenience of the few does not justify this imposition on the many."

for specialists to give attention to all of these areas, which so clearly demonstrate invasion of the private person and the private personality.

When diagnosis or therapy for the benefit of the given individual is at stake, such invasion of his privacy or his body can be proper, for the individual has, in the act of coming to the physician for relief, already given consent to reasonable efforts to relieve him. But when such invasion takes place without the knowledge or consent of the individual involved and not for his benefit, a powerful and hostile public reaction is provoked when the matter is exposed, however well motivated the perpetrators considered themselves to be. Take, for example, the injection of live cancer cells into unconsenting, unknowing individuals or the withholding of effective penicillin in hundreds of unknowing, unconsenting young airmen with streptococcal throat infections, resulting in more than a score of rheumatic fever cases [28]. These physical transgressions are simple to find and to identify. More subtle invasions of the private personality are more difficult to single out. The public reaction against such acts has been and is likely to be violent, and this violence inevitably leads to harsh and arbitrary restrictions.

While not dangerous to life as might be the injection of live cancer cells or the withholding of penicillin, a well-known invasion of privacy[2] was carried out by the University of Chicago with the support of the Ford Foundation [68]. In this case, in the course of behavioral research, "bugging" of a jury was done with the consent of the court and of the counsel for both sides. The jurors were subjected to surveillance. Revelation of this invasion of institutional privacy was roundly condemned and was followed immediately by restrictive legislation.

The scientist recognizes the need for straightening out his own

[2] In five civil cases in the Wichita, Kansas, Federal District Court, the jury room was bugged with the consent of the trial judge and counsel, but without the knowledge of the jurors, partly in order to learn whether post-trial interviews with jurors would permit reconstruction of the events in the jury room. When this was disclosed, a national scandal ensued, with public censure by the Attorney General of the United States (1955). Following this report, there was enactment of statutes in some 30 jurisdictions prohibiting jury tapping [236].

house, something he has attempted to do through the establishment of guiding codes. In most cases these are both unrealistic and unsatisfactory. These problems and shortcomings are discussed elsewhere (page 215). The thoughtful scientist recognizes that, unless he is more successful in the future than he has been in the past in his police efforts, he faces seriously restrictive and coercive legislation. Indeed, this situation is exemplified by some of the rulings of various governmental agencies, notably those of the Food and Drug Administration (page 299).

While the questionnaire is a legitimate instrument of record, public sensitivities are rather easily aroused when attention is brought to imprudent invasion of privacy through this means. Restraints are necessary, but these usually cannot be applied routinely. Conrad has listed eight questions and describes them as basic criteria for consideration in the evaluation of questionnaires [109]. They are as follows:

1. Does the item deal with an area which—either through custom or through Constitutional or statutory protection—is generally regarded as highly personal or optionally private?

2. Does the item (or series of items, taken as a whole) seem likely to have an adverse psychological effect upon a significant number of susceptible respondents?

3. Does the item call for self-incriminating or self-demeaning admission or confession? (This criterion obviously overlaps No. 1.)

4. Does the item seem excessively "psychiatric"; i.e., does it refer to extremely abnormal or discreditable behavior, attitudes, feelings, impulses, etc.? (This obviously overlaps No. 1 and No. 3 above; it may also overlap No. 2.)

5. Does the item seem to countenance (or give unduly neutral recognition to) behavior or views which are generally considered highly reprehensible, immoral, contrary to public policy, etc.—if not actually illegal?

6. Does the item request highly personal or confidential information *about someone other than the respondent himself* (without permission of the other person)?

7. Does the item seem to favor, or is it likely to be interpreted as "propaganda" for or against, one side or another of a highly controversial, emotionally charged issue?

8. Does the item enter a domain which is politically sensitive, from the viewpoint of the individuals who may be affected?

It would be most unfortunate if the social scientist became identified in the public mind with violations of privacy, with snooping. Shils [382] observes: "The respect for privacy rests on the appreciation of human dignity, with its high evaluation of individual self-determination. . . . This value of privacy is derived from our belief in the sacredness of individuality." It is unthinkable to accept progress in medicine founded on deceit, on a subject defrauded of his privacy or his physical safety. Such procedure runs counter to all that medicine stands for.

THE INVESTIGATOR'S USE OF PERSONALITY TESTS

In the past decade there has been considerable resentment of personality testing [see reference 274 for a series of references substantiating this]. The abuse of personality tests has been the subject of discussion before the Senate Subcommittee on Constitutional Rights (1965), as well as before the House Special Subcommittee on Invasion of Privacy of the Committee on Government Operations. Unless psychologists voluntarily restrict their activities in this area, it seems probable that they will be subjected to legal restrictions. Indeed such a bill has already been introduced into the House of Representatives (1966). The psychologists' response that their potential troubles are attributable to (1) public ignorance or (2) political extremism misses the point. Lovell, who represents an authoritative view, has said [284]:

> In my opinion, the protests we have heard, however ill informed and inarticulate they have been, are directed at misuses of psychology which are quite real and very serious, to which our vested interests have blinded us.
>
> Fundamentally, I think the issue is one of reconciling three divergent interests: (a) the public's right to privacy; (b) the social scientist's freedom of inquiry; and (c) the personnel worker's right to determine fitness for employment. Solutions, insofar as they have been proposed,

have usually taken the direction of *restricting test content*. I do not think this tack can ever lead to any resolution of the basic conflicts involved.

While most of the objectionable invasions of privacy concern information on sex, politics, or religion, there remains considerable probing of private thoughts. These matters are at times of concern in research, but probably occur more often in the determination of job fitness. In testing for research, serious situations arise when the subjects are subjected to coercion, deception, or to revelation of the material obtained, the breaking of confidence, or, of course, when subjects are unaware of their participation in an investigation, conceivably acceptable, depending on circumstances. The ethical standards of the American Psychological Association (1963) state in Principle 7d:

> The psychologist who asks that an individual reveal personal information in the course of interviewing, testing, or evaluation, or who allows such information to be divulged to him, does so only after making certain that the responsible person is fully aware of the purpose of the interview, testing or evaluation and of the ways in which the information may be used.

This is analogous to the legal principle which demands that the accused be informed that anything he says may be held against him, but the analogy is not carried out consistently. The accused may not decline to testify against himself. His psychological interrogator need obtain no search warrant in order to examine his psyche.

THE STUDY OF TOXIC SUBSTANCES

As commented elsewhere, disease presents us with an opportunity to study the deranged body, the body under stress, ready for comparison with the normal subject. The field of toxicology presents the same opportunity in two general circumstances: first, the acute situation where accidental ingestion of a toxic substance or a useful drug made toxic by a large dose occurs; second, where more or less prolonged exposure occurs in commerce, as to food additives, to fruit sprays, pesticides, and the like. Toxic effects emerge, and the subjects are ready for study. Happenstance has readied the material; the alert investigator can take advantage of the situation to the profit of all.

The deliberate introduction of "functional chemicals" into our environment and into foodstuffs represents further gigantic human experiments by invasions of the body, where the public has no control. The public has a right to expect that those responsible for this will ensure the determination of what are safe levels and then ensure their maintenance. Animal studies are essential, but of themselves quite inadequate to guarantee safety. While various findings in animals may be accurate, that does not answer the question of whether they are relevant to man. Studies in man are required.

Coulston [115] has said: "It is granted that much of the human toxicology would be done on a relatively small number of individuals and may not have a total transfer to the general population. Nevertheless, it would seem that data derived from even relatively few numbers of human subjects are better than none. In this way, very important protection could be accomplished for the nation as a whole." It is difficult to understand how "very important protection could be accomplished for the nation as a whole" from "even relatively few numbers of human subjects" when one takes into account the hazards and difficulties inherent in studies of this kind. Coulston's view is at best a risky one. One wonders, too, how he could say, "Certainly, not all food additives, advertent or inadvertent, need to be studied in man."

In various studies—for example, those of food chemicals—certain risks cannot be studied experimentally in man. Other examples are cancer risk, the stunting of growth, or irreversible pathologic change. Such effects can sometimes be studied in cause-and-effect-situations, for example, the relationship among cigarette smoking and chronic bronchitis, pulmonary fibrosis, emphysema, lung cancer, and arterial and myocardial disease.

There are certain inherent limitations in human studies of toxic substances. These have been considered by Frazer [167] in a comparison of animal and human studies. (1) *The nature of the ac-*

ceptable risk. Here, animal studies up to and including death are useful, for such studies cannot be done in man. (2) *Permissible dosage range.* Here again, dosage can be extended to the production of severe toxic effects or even death in animals, but in man the dosage range cannot be extended beyond that which produces minor and reversible effects. (3) *Possible experimental situations* that aid in interpreting chemical effects can be created in animals; this is rarely ethical in human volunteers. (4) *Methods of assessment of biologic effects.* Detailed study in animals is easy; survival is not required. Post-mortem examination can be carried out at once after death; this may be more useful than biopsy studies. In man, the detailed study of effects may be greatly limited. (5) *Numbers available for experiment.* Differentiation between two groups of treated subjects may require large numbers, easier with animals than man, if statistical significance is to be achieved. (6) *Human time scale.* Animals with their usually shorter life span, their greater metabolic rate, and more rapid growth and development are sometimes more valuable than man, with his longer life span. Some long-term toxic effects may appear in man only after, say, 25 years. Until earlier effects are recognized, human studies may have no predictive value. (7) *Effect of ethical considerations and veto.* While certain ethical considerations are present in animal studies, these are more complex and difficult in man. The human subject must always have the power to veto participation or to terminate a study if he chooses to do so. This leads to potential restrictions not present with animals. From the foregoing, it is evident that in terms of quantity the biologic information derived from man will be less than that from animals, but the *quality* of that obtained from man usually supersedes the value of animal data.

There is increasing evidence that species differences are in many cases attributable to differences in absorption, distribution, metabolism, and elimination of the substance studied. As Frazer has pointed out, the question involves the access of an adequate amount of active metabolites at the site of action [167]. When these biochemical matters are better understood, it should be possible to make a better choice of animal material to precede human experimentation. Some reactions may, of course, be limited to man. For instance, hypersensitivity reactions are sometimes difficult to produce in animals. Toxic effects owing to inborn genetic faults are not likely to be found in animals. For that matter, normal human volunteers are just as unlikely to predict such effects. Some planning of human studies may be of help, as in the choice of allergy-prone subjects or the choice of those with inborn errors of metabolism. The requirement of such subjects greatly limits work in this area. Some forms of arsenic are said to be carcinogenic in man alone.

DECEPTION BY THE INVESTIGATOR IN HUMAN EXPERIMENTATION

Deception in human experimentation can take various forms, some of which are legitimate, if hedged about with certain restrictions and requirements, some of which are not legitimate. Worst of all is the risk of patients' health or life without their knowledge and consent. It will be helpful to take a look at the several kinds of deception.

PLACEBOS

These provide good examples of the point just made: some deception is defensible, and some is not. The defensible requires restatement of one or two points made elsewhere. When a patient comes to a doctor for relief, he gives, in the act of coming, his consent to reasonable efforts to relieve him. The physician may very properly wish to pit a drug the patient has been receiving against a placebo, to see if the drug has any specific value. This is in the patient's interest. The information cannot be obtained in any other way, and the temporary deceit is acceptable.

As another example, a placebo is not "nothing." It is a powerful therapeutic tool [see Lasagna and Beecher, 269, and Beecher, 18], on the average about one-half to two-thirds as powerful as morphine in the usual dose in relieving severe pain. In the presence of stress, under special circumstances the placebo may be more than three-quarters as effective as morphine in relieving pain [19, 25]. There is no requirement that the physician must always use the most powerful therapeutic agent in treatment. The more powerful the agent is, usually the more powerful its accompanying undesirable side effects will be. Thus, the deception inherent in the use of a placebo in some therapeutic situations can be legitimate.

The above two examples emerge from therapy. When placebos are used in experimental work in volunteers, the situation changes. Some will argue that, if no discernible risk is involved, the secret use of placebos is legitimate, provided disclosure of their presence would vitiate the information sought. The argument is a dubious one at best. In most cases, if not in all, a statement to the volunteers that they *may* get a placebo suffices; however, it must be explained that they will not know if or when this will be. The subjects thus have the right to accept or reject the situation. If they accept it, the deception they will experience is legitimate. This of course applies to other kinds of deception, as well as to placebos.

"STOOGES"

Instead of the unpleasant term *deception,* sometimes the more felicitous but tricky term, *unannounced observations,* is used. However it is put, an unfavorable picture emerges. One wonders why so little is said about it by the President's Panel on Privacy and Behavioral Research. Without approving or disapproving comment, the panel seems to accept the existence of deception in research, and thus gives approval of a sort. One study is mentioned where all subjects present in a room, except one, are stooges. The point of interest is how the one's judgment may be affected by the deliberately misleading influence of the stooges. Following the deception, the subject is told the purpose of the study and its results. "It is clear that an experiment of this sort may put a subject under stress and raise self-doubts." An admonition is given to the investigator to bear in mind the possibly adverse effects of the deceit, but what to do about this is not made clear. While one could wish for a stronger statement by the President's panel concerning the use of stooges in experimentation, this detail should not obscure the value of this thoughtful examination of the existence and consequences of the invasion of privacy in behavioral research.

With characteristic eloquence and forthrightness, Margaret Mead [296] has taken sharp issue with the use of stooges:

> Is it scientifically and ethically permissible to deceive the subjects of research by disguising oneself as a "participant observer," or by introducing stooges into an experiment, or by making use of long-distance television or hidden microphones or other devices for concealed observation? When a human being is introduced who is consciously distorting his position, the material of the research is inevitably jeopardized, and the results always are put in question as the "participant" —introduced as a "psychotic" into a mental ward or as a "fanatic" into a flying-saucer cult group—gives his subjects false clues of a non-verbal nature and produces distortions which cannot be traced in his results. Concealed instruments of observation may not distort the subjects' course of action, but the subsequent revelation of their presence—as in the jury room that was tapped for sociological purposes—damages the trust both of the original participants and of all others who come to know about it. The deception violates the conventions of privacy and human dignity and casts scientists in the role of spies, intelligence agents, Peeping Toms, and versions of Big Brother. Furthermore, it damages science by cutting short attempts to construct methods of research that would responsibly enhance, rather than destroy, human trust.

It must, of course, be accepted that threats to the security of the nation may require the use of deceit. Such acts are not to be confused with science and its advancement.

In a further discussion of this problem several years later, Mead points out [297] that the "primary consideration is whether the human beings who are involved shall either be lied to or asked to lie to others, i.e., to function as stooges." She does not deal here with issues involving drugs or physical harm of any sort. First, she considers the effect of such activities on the subject; second, the effect on the investigator; third, the effect on the validity of the experiment itself; and fourth, "the effect upon the whole culture of the presence of methods of observation and experimentation in which human dignity is violated as contrasted with methods in which human beings are fully respected and protected, or in which human beings are asked knowingly to sacrifice their own safety or privacy for the benefit of others or later generations."

Her arguments in these four categories can be summarized. If one fails to acquaint the experimental subject with what is happening within reasonable limits, this reduces his stature as a human being where he is not permitted to judge for himself. All problems are not solved by "debriefing" the man. He is told he has been tricked, deluded, spied upon, and lied to. Acceptance of such information requires that the subject identify himself with the lying investigator or "the decision that social science is a bunch of confidence tricks and now he also knows a few." If the subject cannot use such self-satisfying rationalizations, he can consider himself abused, or he may decide that being lied to is merely the price he must pay for some other advantage sought, such as education or preferment. And all of this can lead to a cynical attitude toward such experimentation. Deceit can, in some situations, have a more serious effect on the investigator than on the deceived subject.

The tricky investigator becomes accustomed to deceiving and manipulating other human beings. Even though this is explained after the fact to the subject, it still carries the implication that manipulation of people is acceptable. Contempt for others grows out of this. The investigator becomes omnipotent. The end result is a threat to the integrity of his own scientific work.

It must be acknowledged that deceit may be necessary; if, as mentioned earlier, the subject is aware of this possibility and accepts it, even though he is temporarily demeaned as a human being, it must sometimes be accepted. For example, the fabricated situations and the use of stooges to test the strength and resilience of astronauts come to mind; so also does the choice of candidates for dangerous secret activities, as in warfare or in explorations. Even here, the important question is whether the deception is absolutely necessary in an experiment that is itself required.

As for the effect of deception on the experiment, the first question is, does the experimental design absolutely require deception of the subject? Next, is an experiment which incorporates deception ever a *valid* experiment? One must accept the well-demonstrated fact that many individuals are able to pick up cues that other individuals are not aware of giving, so that one or more of the subjects may realize that the investigator is lying. It is not possible to control this element, and the validity of the experiment is thereby jeopardized. It may be possible to avoid the unconscious delivery of cues by the use of mechanical guides or mechanical instructors that can, if cleverly and imaginatively arranged, spare the subject from the feeling of deception by the experimenter. Mead observes, "If the potential invalidity of all experiments where lying occurs is recognized, this will stimulate the use of other kinds of experiments."

TRUST

Science becomes more and more significant in the modern world; it is absolutely essential that this be a *trusted* activity. Mead emphasizes [279] the point: "The image of the scientist as someone who is trustworthy and humane is impaired every time that there are accounts of research which have disregarded basic human rights of consent, as in revelations about medical experiments on unconsenting patients, or scientists using lying, deceit, disguises and spying in the collection of data, or misquoting or suppressing evidence in the discussion of public policy . . . Trust in the responsible use of power is essential for an ordered society. Trust in the responsible use of knowledge, which increasingly gives overweaning power, is crucial today."

Margaret Mead's opening comment at the 1968 American Academy of Arts and Sciences Conference on Human Experimentation epitomizes the requirement for most such work. She said that although her field of anthropological research does not have subjects, *"We work with informants in an atmosphere of trust and mutual respect."* This is as broad as the Golden Rule; it is the basic requirement for ethical experimentation in man. I should like to refer to several more of her points in the material immediately following.

There is responsibility to the subjects that they not be exposed to ridicule, legal sanctions, or danger without their informed concurrence. Thoughtless invasion of privacy is not to be tolerated. The trustworthy investigator will not overlook his obligation to his own discipline, as well as to the public image of scientific work. "The more powerless the subject is, per se, the more the question of ethics—and power—is raised. It is assumed that trust will follow status, and therefore more precautions must be taken to see that the trust is not abused."

Any careless or reckless downgrading of the status of human experimentation, any denigration of human rights, any exposure of unethical procedures, submission to unnecessary hazards, deceit, and wiretapping not only arouse fear, but destroy trust. Whenever advantage is taken of the helplessness or unprotected state of the subject, whenever deceit is involved, trust is impaired. This rules out the use of stooges or other disguised participants. On the other hand, the heroic acts of a Walter Reed not only support, but advance, the status and dignity of human research. A most important obligation is that the scientist, supported as he is by society, maintain the trust given to him.

THE DEFENSIVE INVESTIGATOR AND A POSITIVE APPROACH

Several factors have placed the medical scientist on the defensive; for years the antivivisectionists have haunted his activities. One must recognize that careless, thoughtless, and sometimes even cruel investigators have, through their wrongful acts and publications, provided material for these groups to use. At the same time, the antivivisectionists constitute a crippling threat to sound medical studies in animals. The inconsiderate, careless, thoughtless, risky, sometimes dangerous use of human beings, as exemplified in Chap. 4, has also added to the investigator's unfavorable image.

Consequently, even conscientious, responsible investigators sometimes adopt a defensive attitude. It is high time that the latter, largely the majority of individuals, admit, as they usually do, the fact of their past errors and evince a determination to avoid them in the future. (Very few of us have been without fault.) This will be easier than it has been in the past, for in recent years the issues and the sources of error have been clarified.

It is time for a positive approach, time for frank encouragement of research in man, time for the public to be informed of the reasons for and the fruitful consequences of human experimentation. It is time for professional men to think, not defensively, but affirmatively about these matters. It is time for the medical schools to recognize the need for teaching the rights and the wrongs, the freedoms and the limitations, the compelling reasons for experimentation in man.

The public also requires education. The education of the public can be effected along several lines; a volunteer corps has already been described (page 62). The role of the great teaching hospitals in the advancement of medical knowledge can be forcefully but discreetly presented to the public. Man's spirit of adventure can be channeled in this direction as effectively as in climbing Mt. Everest or in exploring space.

4
Questionable Ethics in Experimentation

> It is not admissible to do a great right by doing a little wrong . . . It is not sufficient to do justice by obtaining a proper result by irregular or improper means.
>
> MIRANDA V. STATE OF ARIZONA, 384 U.S. 436, 447 (1966)

Medicine has achieved greater advances in the last 50 years than ever before; they must continue. In this half century, medicine has become "scientific"; that is to say, the traditional methods of medicine have been joined with the methods of science. Observation has been subjected to analysis, and new procedures have evolved through study of the sick and the well. Complexities abound; these entail, not only scientific, but moral, ethical, and sometimes legal problems. The confidence of the public in those who engage in such experimental pursuits is indispensable. Only if the public can be assured that self-discipline and ethical study are the rule will the necessary confidence be maintained. Careless or misunderstood investigations can do incalculable harm to medical progress. It is our collective obligation as a profession to see that this does not take place.

On an earlier occasion, the writer [28] published in the *New England Journal of Medicine* twenty-two examples of what he believed were unethical or questionably ethical studies. These were chosen by the editor from fifty examples submitted. The prevalence of such material and the ease of finding it have been discussed earlier in this book (pages 15 and 17). Thoughtful investigators without bias can easily verify these statements.

These examples were not cited for the condemnation of individuals. They were recorded to call attention to a variety of ethical problems found in experimental medicine. It has been and is the writer's hope that calling attention to these studies will help to correct any existing abuses. Some evidence that this is so can be seen in the remarkable decrease in "problem" applications made to the National Institutes of Health from 1966 to 1968 (page 15). During many years of study of these matters, it has become apparent that thoughtlessness and carelessness, not a willful disregard of the patient's rights, account for most of the difficulties encountered. Nonetheless, it is evident that in some of the examples presented the investigators have risked the health or the lives of their subjects. Evidence is also at hand that many of the patients in the examples referred to never had risk satisfactorily explained to them, and it is clear that further hundreds have not known that they were the subjects of an experiment [28], although they suffered grave consequences as a direct result of the work described. These are troubling charges. They have grown out of troubling practices. They can be documented by examples from leading medical schools, university hospitals, private hospitals, the Army, the Navy, and the Air Force, the National Institutes of Health, Veterans Administration hospitals, and industry. The basis for the statements is a broad one.[1]

American medicine is sound, and most progress in it is soundly attained. There is, however, a reason for concern in certain areas; the type of activities to be mentioned will do great harm to medicine unless soon corrected. It will certainly be charged that any mention of these matters does a disservice to medicine, but not so great, one believes, as a continuation of the practices to be cited.

One often hears the remark, "Why bring up these cases?" Ques-

[1] At the Brook Lodge Conference (1965) on "Problems and Complexities of Clinical Research," the writer commented that "what seem to be breaches of ethical conduct in experimentation are by no means rare, but are almost, one fears, universal." It seemed obvious that by "universal" he referred to the fact that examples could easily be found in *all* categories where research in man takes place to any significant extent. Judging by press comments, that was not obvious; hence, this note.

tions have to be raised; problems have to be identified before they can be resolved. Santayana's conviction is relevant. (See page 5.)

Curiously, some critics have implied that only an expert on liver function could reasonably object to the deliberate infection of 250 mentally defective children with hepatitis virus; that only an expert cardiologist or epidemiologist could object to withholding penicillin in the treatment of streptococcus throat infection after the investigators' own data had demonstrated its spectacular effectiveness in preventing rheumatic fever; that only an expert in the area could object to the use of hundreds of military personnel in the just-mentioned study of rheumatic fever without their knowledge; that only an expert immunologist could object to thymectomy in young children to determine if this would facilitate the "take" of a homologous skin graft! It is doubtful that most reasonable investigators hold such views.

It has seemed better not to give references, for, as Professor Richard Field of the Harvard Law School has pointed out, some of the principal investigators who are responsible for these studies might be subjected to criminal charges. Certainly, the writer has no such purpose. On the other hand, there could always exist in the minds of some the thought that the writer might have distorted or exaggerated the material presented. One way around this dilemma is to confine the case material to that presented in the *New England Journal of Medicine* [28]. This material was thoroughly checked by its greatly respected editor, Dr. Joseph Garland, and two of his associates, who themselves inserted into the manuscript the statement that all examples were "documented to the satisfaction of the editors." They agreed wholeheartedly with the writer that anonymity of reference should be preserved in that publication, a policy also followed by Blumgart in a recent paper [39].

De Bakey [133] makes a stirring appeal for the application of the Golden Rule in human studies; he believes that it has been "largely overlooked or undervalued." This seems to have been the case in some hundreds of examples cited by the writer, where the health and the life of the subjects were put in jeopardy without their consent or even the knowledge that they were being experimented on [28].

It has seemed to the writer that recapitulation of the cases published in the readily available *New England Journal of Medicine* [28] would serve no useful purpose, with one exception [253a], the Willowbrook case.[2] This example is no longer anonymous, since it has repeatedly been identified in the press. It is referred to here, for further pertinent material has become available since it was first discussed.

In several of the examples presented in the 1966 paper, there is room for argument by men of experience and good will. Indeed this is also true of the Willowbrook case. For example, one can find the present editor of the *New England Journal of Medicine,* Dr. Franz J. Ingelfinger, commenting with regard to that case [225a].

> How much better to have a patient with hepatitis, accidentally or deliberately acquired, under the guidance of a Krugman than under the care of a zealot who would exercise intuitive management, blind to the fact that his one-track efforts to protect the rights of the individual are in fact depriving that individual of his right to good medical care.

Whether or not this severe statement, with its remarkable conclusion, takes into account certain important principles such as concurrence or rejection of experimentation in children below the age of consent, it seems unlikely that the British Medical Research Council [49] would have agreed, for they say,

> The situation in respect of minors and mentally subnormal or mentally disordered persons is of particular difficulty. In the strict view of the law parents and guardians of minors cannot give consent on their behalf to any procedures which are of no particular benefit to them and which may carry some risk of harm.

[2] In an effort to be fair to Dr. Krugman and to avoid inaccuracy, my comments on this significant case were sent to him October 1, 1968. He replied by telephone on October 24, 1968, and agreed to send a written discussion to me by December 25, 1968. It is now more than a year later (November, 1969). He has not replied, and the material will, regrettably, have to go to press without his comments.

Nor would the World Medical Association have agreed. Their statement is as follows:

> Under no circumstances is a doctor permitted to do anything which would weaken the physical or mental resistance of a human being except from strictly therapeutic or prophylactic indications imposed in the interest of the patient.

Professor R. A. McCance of Cambridge University speaks out as strongly as Ingelfinger but with an opposite view [293]. Both men are distinguished.

Thus it appears evident that there is room for disagreement with Ingelfinger, from the viewpoint of other individuals as well as of the responsible organizations quoted.

This study was directed toward determining the period of infectivity of infectious hepatitis. Artificial induction of hepatitis was carried out in an institution for mentally defective children (many of whom were 5 to 8 years old) in which a mild form of hepatitis was endemic. The parents gave consent for the intramuscular injection or oral administration of the virus, but little is said as to whether they were informed of the hazards involved.

The authors give references to two earlier papers where their "justification" is presented. It is repeated here and is as follows: "It was inevitable that most of the newly admitted susceptible mentally retarded children would acquire the infection . . . [the disease] was especially mild at [Willowbrook] . . . facilities were available to provide optimum medical and nursing care . . . and [*post hoc*] observations on more than 50 (now 250) patients who acquired artificially induced hepatitis at [Willowbrook] reveal that the average experimental disease observed was even milder than the observed natural infection" [253a].

Comment. A death rate of 1 or 2 patients per 1,000 is not negligible. There is no assurance that the sequelae in the years to come will be innocuous.

Several other problems are presented by this case. First, there is the question of legality. As one understands it, a strict interpretation of English law forbids experimentation on children, even with parental consent, unless it is done for the direct benefit of the child. While much of American law is derived from English law, the issue is not so clear in the United States. (See page 63 for further comment on the use of children in experimentation.)

There has been reason to believe gamma globulin is useful in reducing or ameliorating infectious hepatitis ever since the pioneer work of Stokes in 1945, nine years before the study under discussion was started [253a]. Krugman's own work supports this: "The efficacy of gamma globulin in the control of infectious hepatitis with jaundice has been clearly established in studies by Stokes and Neefe [1945], Havens and Paul [1945], Gellis and coworkers [1945] . . ." In the present study (1960), Krugman and colleagues say, "In the second trial the dose of gamma globulin was increased to 0.06 ml per pound of body weight. A tenfold reduction in incidence of overt hepatitis followed this larger dose." During a third trial, the same dose resulted in "a thirtyfold decrease in incidence of hepatitis with jaundice [and] was observed for a five month period following inoculation." (See also [348].)

Admittedly the situation is complex and perhaps it is not practical to try to protect the children at Willowbrook prior to admission; but since gamma globulin is known to be useful it seems surprising that discussions of this possibility have not been reported by the Willowbrook team. In terms of principle, Bradford Hill (1963) has raised questions as to whether an established new treatment can be ethically withheld from any patients in the doctor's care [209].

According to the *Medical Tribune* of February 20, 1967, Dr. Saul Krugman said that it is "inevitable that most newly admitted children will become infected [with hepatitis] at Willowbrook, in the first 6 to 12 months after entering the institution." The nearly universal infection described by Dr. Krugman compares oddly with the statement of Dr. A. D. Miller, Commissioner of the State Department of Mental Hygiene, who said, according to the *Medical Tribune* of February 15, 1967, that the 11-year-old hepatitis immunization research program had resulted in an "80 to 85 percent reduction of this disease at Willowbrook for both patients and employees." Which statement is correct?

In the *Medical Tribune's* account of Dr. Joan Giles's comments to the parents, it was not clear whether any or all parents were told that hepatitis sometimes progresses to fatal liver destruction or that there is a possibility that cirrhosis developing later in life may have had its origin in earlier hepatitis.

The preliminary survey that led to the present Willowbrook study began 13 years ago; the specific investigation was initiated 11 years ago following presentation, it is said, of the proposal to New York University's Committee on Human Experimentation and its approval. Most universities did not have such committees until recently. This pioneer group should be acclaimed, if it had any such committee so long ago. (Assurance has been given that it did not have such a committee at that time.)

Let us consider another seeming discrepancy. According to the *Medical Tribune,* Dr. Krugman said that he was "certain from the outset" that there would be criticism of the program. "We set it up very carefully . . . and in accordance with the World Medical Association's Draft Code of Ethics on Human Experimentation." [3] How he reconciles his statement with what that code actually says is not clear. The code says, "Any act or advice which could weaken physical or mental resistance of a human being may be used only in his interest."

Whether the studies at Willowbrook have been useful is beside the immediate point. If a study is unethical, it does not become ethical because it produces useful results.

In a further study of infectious hepatitis, Krugman, Giles, and Hammond [253] emphasize that "during the course of the experiment the subject of it should be free to withdraw from it at any time [the subjects were 3 to 10 years of age] . . . that the investigator or investigating committee . . . should be free to discontinue the experiment if in his or their judgment it may, if continued, be harmful to the subject of the experiment."

This sounds very well until one considers the situation: once the

[3] One wonders how this was possible, since Dr. Krugman's study began in 1954, whereas the World Medical Association's Code was not set down until 8 years later (1962).

infection has occurred, what good would be withdrawal from the experiment? As a matter of fact, it could be undesirable, for they say the patients on the study received better care than the others. Finally, they say, ". . . any risk to which the subject of an experiment may be exposed should be carefully assessed in terms of direct benefit to himself." Is one to conclude, then, that infectious hepatitis is a good thing?

The administrator at Willowbrook, Dr. Jack Hammond, according to the *Medical Tribune,* said the "biggest fuss" arose over a "complete misinterpretation." Parents were informed that admission to Willowbrook was closed in late 1964, owing to overcrowding. Shortly after this notice had gone out, in some cases as soon as a week after the first notice, a second letter was sent out, advising the parents that there were some vacancies in the hepatitis unit and that if parents would volunteer their children for that study they could be admitted. As reported, Dr. Hammond seemed surprised at the ensuing uproar when those involved were charged with a "high pressure method of obtaining consent from parents desperate to institutionalize their child."

In discussing the deliberate infection of a human being with hepatitis virus, the distinguished Professor of Experimental Medicine, R. A. McCance of Cambridge University, made [293] a pertinent comment concerning the general problem of hepatitis (prior to the Krugman study):

> To inoculate someone with icterogenic serum is a risk that I personally would never take, nor would I ever have cared to take it even before the risks were so well known, for once the inoculation had been made, I would have lost control. Everyone working experimentally with normal human subjects or with patients must remember not only his responsibility to the subject or patient but also his responsibility to the discipline of experimental medicine. One irresponsible experimenter can do great harm to medical science.

SUMMARY

1. There is an unresolved question of legality, even with parental consent, to carry out experimentation in children not for their direct benefit.

2. Dr. Krugman has asserted that it was "inevitable that most newly admitted children would become infected [with hepatitis] at Willowbrook." Commissioner Miller said the 11-year-old hepatitis immunization research program had resulted in an "80 to 85 percent reduction of this disease at Willowbrook for both patients and employees." Which statement is correct?

3. The statement of Dr. Krugman that his study was approved by New York University's Committee on Human Experimentation before the 11-year-old study was started is not in accord with the facts, as stated by an official of that university, who admitted that no such committee then existed. If it had, it would have been a great pioneer, for most such committees are of recent origin.

4. Despite Dr. Krugman's statement that the program was set up in accord with the World Medical Association's Draft Code of Ethics on Human Experimentation, this clearly is not the case.

5. The suspension of admissions, with a following letter to the parents that their children could be admitted if they agreed to participate in the hepatitis study, is startling.

SOME ESTIMATED DEATH RATES

In the examples referred to [28], a number of procedures, some with demonstrated death rates, were carried out. The following data were provided by three distinguished investigators in the field and represent widely held views.

CARDIAC CATHETERIZATION

Right side of the heart, about 1 death per 1,000 patients; left side, 5 deaths per 1,000 patients, "probably considerably higher in some places, depending on the portal of entry." (One investigator had 15 deaths in his first 150 patients.) It is possible that catheterization of a hepatic vein or the renal vein would have a lower death rate than that of catheterization of the right side of the heart, for, if it is properly carried out, only the atrium is entered en route to the liver or the kidney, not the right ventricle, which, if entered, can lead to serious cardiac irregularities. There is always the possibility, however, that the ventricle will be entered inadvertently. This occurs in at least half the cases, according to one expert, "but if properly done is too transient to be of importance."

Blumgart states, in the case of the ill, that about 3 percent show serious irregularities that can be successfully terminated; approximately 1 percent suffer acute myocardial infarction; and about 1 in 200 dies as a consequence of cardiac catheterization [38].

LIVER BIOPSY

The death rate here is estimated at 2 to 3 per 1,000 patients, depending in considerable part on the condition of the subject.

ANESTHESIA

The general anesthesia death rate can be placed at about 1 death per 2,000 patients.

5
Ethical Problems in Transplantation

It is evident that the transplantation of tissues or organs is not purely a medical problem. Perplexing questions abound; some are medical or partly medical, and some are not. The Ciba Foundation symposium (1966) was interested primarily in transplantation, but it considered as pertinent subjects as diverse as how and when a potential donor can be considered free of undue influence [430]. How long should "life" be maintained in a patient with irrevocable brain damage? When does death occur in an unconscious patient maintained only by artificial aids to the circulation and the respiration? Are there ever circumstances under which death may be mercifully advanced? Can a parent rightly refuse necessary treatment of his child? How does one protect minors, the ignorant, and prisoners in the transplant situation? When may pregnancy be terminated? Is it legal to mutilate a donor for the sake of another person? What protection from society do medical men need in the development of new life-saving techniques? What is the community's financial responsibility in developing and maintaining life-supporting measures? Clearly, the problems arising in transplantation are wide-ranging.

Since nearly all cases of transplantation involving homografts imply experimentation for the benefit of the ailing subject, the ethical problems encountered are usually relatively straightforward. The donor, with reasonable explanatory effort on the part of the physician, cannot avoid knowing that he is to participate in a therapeutic experiment. There are instances of transplantation, however, where the above situations are not present, where transplantation has been carried out in an experiment not for the benefit of the subject. Beecher has referred to the matter [28] where skin homografts were carried out in children who had been subjected to thymectomy, to determine whether thymectomy provided a better "take."

When Woodruff set about organizing a skin bank in Scotland, he discovered that it was illegal to proceed under the Anatomy Act of 1832. The act had been passed as a consequence of the activities of the Edinburgh murderers, Burke and Hare. The need for a skin bank was finally appreciated, and the situation was set right by the passage in 1961 of the Human Tissue Act. Here murder first led to restrictive legislation, a sequence one can often observe when ethical violations less final than murder occur. One can take some comfort in knowing that when need for revision was demonstrated, correction of the law followed, however belatedly.

Another example of the crippling power of the courts was demonstrated in the 1932 case of the rich man who bought a testicle from a young Neapolitan. A surgeon transplanted it, with the result that article 5 of the Italian common code of civil rights was promulgated in 1940. This forbade the donation of organs or other parts of the body that could produce a *permanent* deficiency in the donor. According to Cortesini, blood transfusion or skin grafts were thus not made illegal [112]. A more enlightened bill is currently before the Italian Parliament for final approval.

Unlike Oliver Wendell Holmes's "Wonderful One-Hoss Shay" which disintegrated

> All at once and nothing first
> Just as bubbles do when they burst

human beings are likely to fail in a given part; hence the interest in transplanting a particular tissue or organ. Sometimes, of course, the ailing organ can be compensated for by the administration of its missing secretion: cortisone in Addison's disease or insulin in diabetes. Sometimes a mechanical device such as a heart valve will do, but at other times nothing less than a transplanted organ gives hope of prolonging life.

Murray believes that the lung is a likely organ to be successfully transplanted and that of the nonpaired organs, the liver is the most promising [317]. Remarkable progress has already been made in liver transplantation. Transplantation of the endocrine organs is being studied. In the material to follow, transplantation of blood, cornea, kidney, and heart will be especially discussed in terms of the problems they present that are germane to transplantation in general.

According to Couch, if there were no legal or logistical problems, there would be available each year an estimated 10,000 cadaver kidneys in the United States and 6,000 livers for 4,000 potential liver recipients [114]. These data are based on "neurologic" deaths, when the tissues to be transplanted would be satisfactory. Merrill has sharply criticised the use of organs of primates in man as premature. He estimates the hazard to life of the kidney donor as about the same as that of traffic death attending a male United States inhabitant who drives less than 8,000 miles each year [300].

Some generalizations can be supplied as useful guides in the transplantation field [363]. These have been emphasized for years by responsible investigators in the area. It may be helpful to summarize them. Before transplantation is undertaken, there must be a reasonable chance of clinical success. An acceptable therapeutic goal must be in view. Adrenal or pancreatic transplants violate this "rule," since acceptable replacement secretions can be obtained. The risks and uncertainties must be presented to the families of the donor and the recipient, as well as to the two principals. The protocol for each transplantation must be devised so as to gain and preserve the maximum information. There must be probing evaluation of the results by independent observers. Careful, accurate, and conservative information is to be disseminated through legitimate channels, both medical and lay, in order that cruel hopes will not needlessly be raised. The field of transplantation carries great hope for the future; this should not be discredited in the present by unscientific practice or proclamations.

BLOOD TRANSFUSION

In 1668, a pamphlet of 80 pages on blood transfusion was published at Bologna, Italy. According to Keynes, it is fair to call this the first textbook on this subject [248]. Thus, for three centuries the possibility of the transfusion of blood had been in man's mind, although its widespread and successful practice really dates from about the time of World War II. Between these two periods, 1668 and World War II, there was considerable animal and human experimentation, some of it indefensible. Blood transfusion has interest and relevance to the present consideration: it represents the greatest and most successful transplantation of tissue. The considerable seventeenth-century interest in blood transfusion was succeeded by a minimum of interest in the eighteenth century, a sequence one often encounters in the history of science: men turn away from unsolvable problems, only to return to them when some event or discovery gives renewed hope that they can be solved. In the nineteenth century, several books on the subject published in Europe stimulated interest in the field, an expanding interest that has continued to the present.

From the earliest times, blood has been considered to have an almost mystic importance, doubtless because of the evident fact that much loss of blood promptly leads to loss of life. It was believed that the weak could be made strong by drinking the blood of the latter; thus, the blood of bulls and gladiators became a popular beverage. Keynes describes the attempt toward the end of the fifteenth century to rejuvenate the aged Pope Innocent VIII, by giving him a drink prepared from the blood of three young boys, who thus died in vain [248]. The history of blood transfusion follows a common pattern of science. First, there was the concept of introducing various materials into the circulation of an animal; then this was extended to blood. Animal experiments were carried out. Finally, these were applied to man.

Very often before the eruption of a great new advance in science, there is created a *climate* wherein many men have similar ideas and it becomes impossible to be certain who first had the new concept. Certain it is, however, that that busy man, Dr. Wren (later Sir Christopher), must be given the credit for first experiments, in 1657, of intravenous injection of foreign substances into animal veins. Then, toward the end of February 1666, Richard Lower first demonstrated to a distinguished company at Oxford that a bled-out dog could be revived at once by the blood from a donor dog. When his blood was restored, the recipient "promptly jumped down from the table, and, apparently oblivious of its hurts, soon began to fondle its master, and to roll in the grass to clean itself of blood." This was the first public demonstration of a successful dog-to-dog transfusion. Lower's priority was challenged by one Jean Denys of France, who managed to have *his* claim translated into English and even published in the *Transactions* of the Royal Society for June 22, 1667, without the knowledge of the Secretary, Henry Oldenburg, who unfortunately at the moment was confined in the Tower of London. He was released just in time to have Denys's letter suppressed, although some copies still exist, according to Keynes [248].

In experiments in 1667, Denys succeeded for the first time in transfusing animal blood into man, first into a sick boy who was made miraculously well by a little lamb's blood and then in an experiment in a *well* man, without ill effects. Similar experiments were carried out in England until, inevitably, disaster struck in 1668: a patient died and the widow sued Denys. Denys lost, with the injunction that no further transfusions be made unless approved by a member of the Faculty of Medicine at Paris. Opposition there led to discontinuance of the procedure.

Samuel Pepys recorded in his *Diary* on November 14, 1666, comments on an animal-to-animal transfusion and, nimble-witted man that he was, suggested that it would be interesting to inject the blood of a Quaker into an Archbishop. The next year Pepys wrote, November 21, 1667, of a "poor and debauched man, that the College have hired for 20s. to have some of the blood of sheep let into his body." There were no apparent ill effects, although considerable uncertainty as to the outcome had been expressed before the fact. This "poor and debauched" man may have been the first *paid* experimental subject, at least in England. There is some evidence that the French had preceded the English in this experiment.

In 1794, Erasmus Darwin proposed *hiring* a donor so that frequent transfusions could be made into a sick man. The potential recipient "now found himself near the house of death"; he felt it useless to proceed with the experiment, and it was not carried out. The world had to wait until December 22, 1818, for Blundell's account of the first successful man-to-man transfusion.

Many lesser but still important milestones must be passed over, such as the attempts by Braxton Hicks to prevent clotting [207]. In 1914 Agote [3] first used citrated blood, and in 1821 Prévost and Dumas first used defibrinated blood. Landsteiner discovered blood groups in Vienna, 1899–1902; Jansky in 1907 [231] identified four blood groups and transfusion was well on its way to becoming a standardized technique. The use of a subject paid to participate in an experiment 300 years ago and E. Darwin's suggestion 175 years ago that a donor be hired indicate that some of our modern practices have ancient origins.

Robertson [362] established the possibility of storing blood in World War I, a practice widely followed in World War II, first by British and then by United States forces, but only after a tragic error made in Washington was overcome: the American Forces entered North Africa without adequate blood-transfusing equipment and without plans for the use of blood in quantity. Here was fatal human experimentation on a massive scale. This incredible mistake came as a result of believing that the newly developed blood plasma, wet or dried, would suffice.[1] It soon became apparent that the infusion of plasma would indeed restore the blood pressure to a level where bleeding would be resumed in those already

[1] I am indebted to Col. Edward D. Churchill, Surgical Consultant to the North African Theater of Operations (later Mediterranean Theater), for the information to follow. A complete account will be presented in his book now nearing completion.

nearly exsanguinated and much of the remaining essential hemoglobin washed out [16].

This is not to deny the value of plasma in certain situations, but its range of usefulness had not been adequately determined before it was shipped to North Africa. Plasma's limits of usefulness could easily have been tested under the direction of the well-established National Research Council. Unfortunately, however, that body had wholeheartedly adopted the view that shock was different from hemorrhage and that shock was associated with hemoconcentration (National Research Council's *Manual on Shock,* 1943).

Any second-year medical student could have been expected to understand why plasma was not an adequate remedy for hemorrhage. There were in Washington at the Walter Reed Army Hospital, in the Surgeon General's office, and elsewhere able men who recognized the need for whole blood in the treatment of hemorrhage. So did doctors who were caring for battlefield casualties in North Africa. For various reasons, these men were not influential in correcting the error, most probably because Surgeon-General Kirk, on the advice of the National Research Council, had decided that plasma and electrolytes would fulfill battlefield needs. Later, that honest and forthright man took full responsibility for the decision.

One man, and one alone, must be credited with marshalling the evidence for the need for whole blood, Colonel Edward D. Churchill. He tried earnestly to overcome the erroneous views concerning plasma and, having failed, with great courage defied the military and the National Research Council establishment and "leaked" an account of the situation to a reporter. The information was published in the *New York Times* of August 27, 1943. The anticipated explosion occurred, but thereafter whole blood for the wounded became increasingly available. Colonel Churchill was vindicated, and one of the most irresponsible experiments in the history of medicine was terminated, but not until many lives had been needlessly lost.

The first blood bank for civilians was established as part of a military effort in Barcelona in 1936. The following year, Fantus in

Chicago founded the first completely civilian blood bank [153]. Blood substitutes, ranging from milk in the 1870s to modified fluid gelatine during and after World War II, have been disappointing. Fractionating blood into its components has made it possible to satisfy a patient's needs more accurately than formerly.

Wolstenholme has taken a look at those who give and those who receive blood [430]. He estimates that some 7 million transfusion units are at present administered in the United States each year. The number is not accurately known. Blumgart estimates 4.5 million, with 30,000 cases of hepatitis [39]. The donors are usually 18 to 65 years of age, from whom 500 ml is drawn without ill effect. The use of cadaver blood was suggested by Rubin in 1914 [366] and had for a time a considerable vogue in Russia in the 1930s. Such a practice is limited by infection developing after death and by the difficulties in obtaining an adequate history to rule out infectious hepatitis, malaria, and syphilis in its early stage. It has been estimated that blood transfusion in the United States is annually responsible for 30,000 cases of hepatitis, of which 3,000 are fatal. Sometimes blood is taken over a period of weeks and stored for reinfusion into the donor at the time of operation.

Even when infection-free and compatible blood is available, it is not always welcomed. Wolstenholme tells of a press report during World War II of a fanatic Nazi soldier captured at Tobruk who killed himself as soon as he realized he was being given British blood. Some Britishers had a similar aversion. In North Africa a British general ordered the destruction of 100 blood transfusion units derived from German prisoners of war rather than to have any of it used to save the lives of British wounded. One learns with relief that, as soon as the general's back was turned, the order was ignored. Arkansas has introduced legislation to control or to prevent the administration of "racially different" blood.[2]

[2] Arkansas Statutes 1947 Annotated, 1960 Replacement, vol. 7A, chap. 16, "Blood Transfusions." "82–1601. Blood labeled as to race.—All human blood used or proposed to be used in the State of Arkansas for transfusions of blood, except such units of blood which will have been transported across the State line into Arkansas, shall be labeled with the word 'Caucasian,' 'Negroid,' 'Mongoloid' or some suitable designation so as to clearly indicate the race of the donor of such blood. No human

Aside from these bizarre cases, Jehovah's Witnesses provide a greater and more serious difficulty, one that bristles with ethical problems. One eminent chief of service at a Harvard hospital decided, on the advice of counsel and with trustee support, to overrule the wishes of an adult Witness. She was transfused. If one can ignore or overcome such blood prejudice, can one also force a kidney transplant? What are the limits of coercive therapy? What is to be the end of this complex decision? The rather large group of Jehovah's Witnesses would prefer to lose their lives than contravene what they believe to be God's instruction (Leviticus XVII: 13, 14): "You shall eat the blood of no manner of flesh for the life of all flesh is the blood thereof." (The Bible also says "Thou shalt not kill.") It is customary to accede to such prejudice, but not always. A great ethical problem arises in the case of the children of Jehovah's Witnesses or in the case of a Witness too ill to make a rational decision. If the emergency is not great, legal advice can be sought; when the situation is critical, some physicians desist and others do not. The law as yet offers no guide in this area.

It is unquestionably true that blood transfusion is too often too lightly undertaken. One distinguished authority in the field has argued vehemently in the past that blood transfusion should not be carried out during surgery under general anesthesia lest a previously undetected incompatibility or a frank error in matching go unnoticed. To accept as decisive this remote possibility against the undoubted lifesaving power of blood transfusion during surgery is sadly unrealistic. When contemplating overuse, one must always remember the possibilities and hazards of sensitization. Wolstenholme estimates [430] the overall mortality rate for transfusion to be "not higher than 3 in 10,000."

In offering extra pay to persons who engage in hazardous pur-

---

blood not labeled in accordance with the provisions of this act [82–1601—2–1605] shall be used for transfusions in the State of Arkansas." [Acts 1959, No. 482, 2, p. 1923.]

"82–1602. Notice when blood of different race to be used in transfusion.—Any person about to receive a blood transfusion or a parent of said person, or the next of kin of said person shall be informed of the race of the donor of the blood proposed to be used if blood from a person of a different racial classification is to be used." [Acts 1959, No. 482, 2, p. 1923.] Certain emergency provisions are also spelled out.

suits, society has accepted the view that risk is reimbursable. One wonders if the question whether the sale of major organs, with the risk this entails, will eventually find the same acceptance as the sale of blood for transfusion. When the immunologic problem is solved, this could become a pressing question. Legislation now pending in Italy would make illegal any payment for an organ.

CORNEAL TRANSPLANTATION

In reviewing the history of corneal transplantation, Rycroft concluded that credit must go to Pellier de Quengsy for attempting in 1789 to stitch a glass disc into the cornea after removing a scarred patch of that tissue [372]. He does not record the outcome. A few years later, in 1796, Erasmus Darwin in London wondered whether a "small piece of cornea" could not be trephined out. Such ideas led to the first graft of corneal tissue on a human cornea by Reisinger in 1817. He derived the idea from watching Astley Cooper place a skin graft on the stump of an amputated limb at Guy's Hospital. The first successful human corneal graft was achieved by Zirm in 1905. The donor in this case was a small boy whose eye was removed because of an intraocular foreign body. Later the Russian, Filatov, demonstrated that donor material from cadavers could be used after storage at low temperatures.

Corneal grafts involve avascular tissue, unlike other material whose grafting has been attempted, and this undoubtedly accounts for the early and continued success. Since the material can be obtained from cadavers or surgical sources and stored, most of the harassing ethical problems surrounding other tissues or organs are not present here. Prior to World War II, donor material was difficult to find and came mainly from eyes containing tumors. After World War II, when the demand for donor material greatly increased, surgeons turned to cadaver material. Once again, the Anatomy Act of 1832 hindered this approach in Britain and one was forced to depend on the occasional permission of relatives of the deceased. This situation was improved by the 1952 Corneal Grafting Act, which was later incorporated in the Human Tissue Act of 1961.

The Queen Victoria Hospital's Eye Bank at East Grinstead received in 1965, about 15 years after its founding, over 400 eyes. International donor services are now provided. These widespread activities are made possible by public education through lectures, the press, radio, and television. Such ethical success can perhaps be extended to more complicated transplantation problems by similar educational efforts.

The law concerning what can and cannot be removed from a body and under what circumstances varies with the country or state involved. Much of it is unclear or ambiguous.

INTERMITTENT HEMODIALYSIS

While intermittent hemodialysis does not of course involve the transplantation of tissues or organs, it very often is a means of maintaining life while awaiting the availability of a suitable kidney for transplantation; it therefore seems not unreasonable to consider the matter in this chapter on transplantation. It also is required to support the patient when a graft fails.

Hemodialysis is a promising example of an experimental-practical procedure enveloped in problems both mundane and ethical. De Wardener has discussed the ethical and economic problems of keeping human beings alive with hemodialysis [137]. The main function here, of course, is to adjust the electrolyte and water content of the body so as to maintain them within constant limits and make certain that wastes derived from protein metabolism are eliminated. If the kidneys cannot do this, the subject will die; however, life can be maintained even in the absence of kidney function by circulating the blood through an artificial kidney. This process is called hemodialysis. It requires that the patient be placed on the artificial kidney some 12 to 14 hours twice weekly. It is customary to carry out this procedure at night in order to interfere as little as possible with normal activities. The patient's liberty is severely limited. The site of the arterial and venous connections must be kept absolutely clean; it cannot be put into a bath, nor can the subject swim. Vigorous exercise is unwise. The site must be protected from injury. Strict dietary limitations are necessary. In most cases the procedure must be carried out, at the present time at least, in a hospital.

If the procedure is carried out correctly, the mortality is low. For example, Pendras and Erickson [334] at Seattle have treated 23 patients for over 40 patient-years with only 3 deaths. De Wardener [137] reports that he at Charing Cross and Shaldon at the Royal Free Hospital have treated 35 patients for a period of 43 patient-years, with 1 death owing to a technical accident. Eight of Shaldon's patients are on home dialysis. Combining the data from the three centers gives a total of 58 patients treated for 83 patient-years with only 4 deaths.

In England, the initial cost of the equipment is $4,200 (1966) per bed. For dialysis carried out for 3 patients six nights a week, the capital cost per patient is thus $1,400. This does not include the cost of housing. Maintenance cost, nursing staff, technicians, and disposable items come to $84 per patient per week [137].

In the United States, Pendras at Seattle estimates the in-hospital cost at $5,000 to $10,000 per patient per year [333]. He believes that present facilities can accommodate only about 10 percent of those in need. He estimates that with a cumulative patient load after five years of some 15,000 to 25,000 patients, 75 to 250 million dollars for therapy would be required. At present, hemodialysis can be offered only on a limited basis.

In 1962 de Wardener estimated that in England 2,230 patients would have been acceptable and would have profited from dialysis. Aside from initial capital expenditure, the cost of treating this number in a hospital would be 9.8 million dollars for one year. He provides other interesting estimates of cost over a period of years. He estimates the need ultimately for care of 11,000 patients, whose annual cost would be equivalent to that of two 800-bed district hospitals [137]. Clearly, dilemmas persist.

Rusk estimates that each year kidney disease kills 6,000 Americans who could be saved if sufficient dialysis resources were available [370]. A special committee recommended to the President in November 1967 that the federal government spend about 1 billion dollars over the next 6 years to save these lives. In 1968 it was estimated that there were about 7,000 terminal uremic patients who could benefit from dialysis, but that facilities were available for only about 1,000. Some 25,000 lives could be saved over the next 6 years if the recommendations are carried out. In the meantime the Public Health Service, the Veterans Administration, New York State, and other agencies are struggling with the problem, seriously aggravated by economy drives in governments.

Rusk presently estimates hospital costs for dialysis at about $14,000 per patient per year, an estimate at variance with that of Pendras. Home dialysis costs $3,000 to $4,000 per year. Unless substantial government help becomes available for the 6,000 patients presently unprovided for, new laboratory facilities cannot be made available to them, and ability to pay will be a substantial consideration in determining who lives and who dies.

The United States Department of Health, Education, and Welfare has established 12 units in a Kidney Disease Control Program to determine the feasibility of prolonged home dialysis in different settings with different population groups and equipment. It is expected that from 800 to 1,000 patients in this program will be on home dialysis by 1973.

It is generally believed that kidney transplantation is the preferred treatment. By 1968, some 2,000 kidney transplants had taken place, with about a 75 percent chance for function lasting more than a year. The chances are lessened if the kidney is obtained from a nonrelative or a cadaver. There is some evidence to show that the patient who receives a transplant can expect to live twice as long as a patient on dialysis. Nevertheless, it is to be remembered that transplant patients require on the average 3 months of preoperative dialysis and, if the graft fails, indefinite dialysis.

With these elementary considerations in mind, we may turn to the ethical problems, the questions that must be faced, and in this it will be well to follow de Wardener's thoughtful comments [137].

Have we the right to prolong life in this way? Despite the limitations imposed, life can still be pleasant and productive; the answer to the general question must be a positive one.

Granted that the procedure is justified, who shall be treated? It has been the practice of the initial center to broaden responsibility by committee action, as at Seattle, where the committee includes both lay and medical members. De Wardener doubts that the results of sharing responsibility are any better than decisions made by one or two individuals [137]. Schreiner also argues against committee decision as to which candidate will be placed on dialysis [375]. Committee decision involving laymen ultimately requires organization and presentation of medical data to the lay group, and here the physicians' biases can be expressed. However, many aspects of society must be considered in the decision as to who will and who will not be accepted in a dialysis program, areas in which the physician is as incompetent to make decisions as the layman is to decide on medical issues. Pendras seems to be on firm ground [333]. His group considers two bases for selecting patients: (1) the medical-psychological and (2) the social-moral, rehabilitation aspect. In essence, the Seattle screening is done by two committees in which laymen as well as physicians participate. In choosing candidates, they consider "worth to the community." For example, a 32-year-old man with a stable history of employment and responsibility and a family of six to support was chosen over a 45-year-old widow whose children were grown up and had left home. Pendras is a strong advocate of the group decision.

In de Wardener's program, decision is required only when a place becomes available. The first obligation is to patients already under treatment. A new patient is not accepted until the last one has been well launched, for experience has shown that most difficulties occur in the early weeks of treatment. Moreover, a new patient is not accepted when any staff shortage exists. The subject to be chosen is one who must be showing signs of deterioration notwithstanding a low-protein diet. Since hemodialysis facilities are in short supply, a choice must be made among needy candidates.

Usually such a choice is made from patients between puberty and menopause, subjects who are clear mentally and cooperative and not suffering from some other disease that dialysis will not control. Often patients who have young children are chosen.

A definition of suitability for dialysis depends on a number of factors, some arbitrary, some empiric. For instance, children are not treated because, if dialysis is started before adolescence, puberty is unlikely to develop. The subject chosen should have the possibility of a prolonged survival. It seems reasonable during the period of establishment of a new technique to choose in the early years those subjects who will probably do best.

Who ought to pay? Few individuals can afford the cost of dialysis, although in some countries only those who can pay are accepted; in other countries, the state pays. In still other countries, no hemodialysis is available.

The cost is such that few can pay for the procedure without reducing their standard of living and without jeopardizing their children's futures. Thus, such a patient must choose between his family's comfort and dying. Some call this a form of suicide, a charge hotly denied by others. The sad fact is that a patient may feel obliged to make such a choice when his judgment may be clouded by his disease. Once the treatment has begun, a drastic step by the patient is required to stop the procedure and spare the family further financial distress; this has been accomplished, for example, by such a deliberate dietary indiscretion as choosing a high-potassium diet, or by tearing out the tubes to bring on death by hemorrhage. It is unquestionably true that financial hardship preys on the minds of many confronted with these problems.

In the face of such tragic decisions, it is good to know that the United States is financing programs from both government and charitable funds. These are still in short supply, but the trend is hopeful. In Great Britain, if the Health Service is to be truly comprehensive, it is the responsibility of the Ministry of Health to provide for intermittent hemodialysis. The Minister of Health accepted this responsibility in 1965.

Is it right for such large sums to be directed to hemodialysis? The size of the financial commitment has discouraged some. De Wardener [137] takes the creditable view that this is nothing new for, as Lord Platt has pointed out, in earlier years vast sums were spent on tuberculosis patients without questioning the cost. Indeed, de Wardener has recently found that the cost per week of sanitarium care of a patient with tuberculosis is the same as that of maintaining a patient on intermittent hemodialysis in a hospital. Few tuberculosis patients confined to a sanitarium can lead productive lives, whereas those on intermittent hemodialysis can do so. This is a sound argument in favor of extending the availability of intermittent hemodialysis. Others may argue that placing the tuberculosis patient in a sanitarium removes a threat to the health of those who might otherwise come into contact with him and that it is less urgent to treat the man with renal failure because he will not infect those about him—a specious argument.

De Wardener presents interesting comparisons of the cost of treating or housing patients with mental disease and those with renal failure. As he says, if patients with mental disease are not treated or confined, they will roam the streets and prod one's conscience. In contrast, a patient with failing kidney function will die and leave us in peace. The treatment of those with hemodialysis is not as radical an economic venture in the treatment of disease as some have supposed.

A further ethical question to be considered is whether the considerable number of skilled individuals involved in hemodialysis should be employed in this way, taking into account, for example, the shortage of nurses. In some hospitals, wards are closed because of this shortage. De Wardener estimates for England that if the present nurse-to-patient ratios hold in 1980, some 4,000 nurses will be engaged in this activity. Automation and the employment of less skilled personnel may help with staffing problems. However, legal problems can arise when care of patients is delegated to an unqualified staff. Although the doctors involved are fewer in number than the nurses, too few nephrologists are willing to take on the time-consuming demands involved in maintaining a hemodialysis program.

Schreiner has raised the question as to whether the physician might not possibly better be occupied with trying to discover how the streptococcus produces glomerular nephritis than to spend his time treating the consequences of this infection [375]. This is really not very relevant; many physicians are competent to supervise a dialysis program, but few are endowed with native research ability to discover the cause of the kidney failure. It is the old problem of research versus patient care. A more basic problem is the availability of the necessary kinds of talent.

The cost of hemodialysis in money and in manpower cannot be overlooked. Any serious examination of the subject must necessarily raise the question of whether this cost may threaten the success of such other desperately needed programs as education, urban renewal, or prevention of disease. This seems most unlikely in a country as rich as the United States.

KIDNEY TRANSPLANTATION

The general, although not unanimous, view is that an individual with two healthy kidneys can ethically give one, providing the gift is truly voluntary and is given with the full knowledge of the risks he runs, including the possibility that his sacrifice may turn out to be useless. One must face the fact that family pressures are often so great that it becomes difficult or impossible to determine whether the donor is truly a volunteer. Attempts to ensure this have sometimes led to standardized psychological examinations by which the examiner attempts to determine whether the potential donor is "stable, well-balanced and rationally motivated." Another purpose of such an examination is to uncover possible family pressure. The donor is told that if he does not want to give a kidney no one will know, for the physician will state that the donor is unsuitable. In these circumstances, about three of five donors are found to be genuine volunteers. A major purpose is to prevent external pressure on the prospective donor. There is the recurrent question as to whether one is justified on ethical grounds in refusing to transplant a kidney from a relative who would then feel that he had, in the refusal, failed to save the life of a loved one. One can raise the question whether it is really ever possible with truly free will to exercise free choice in a situation where the inherent pressures are as strong as they are in family situations. Family pressures can lead to choice of a donor on the basis of his presumed expendability. As Daube [131] puts it, family pressure is nevertheless "consonant with the dignity and responsibility of free life." There are also subtle and strong internal pressures within each possible donor. These pressures are rooted in traditional religious and social education concerning the propriety of self-sacrifice. It is difficult to see how any individual or any panel of experts can be absolutely certain that free and uninhibited consent exists when the prospective donor is aware that he is making a life-or-death decision and that the decision is under scrutiny. The potential anguish of such a situation could be most acute for the identical twin, who is a unique donor, but in view of the excellent results after other intrafamilial transplantations, it is not limited to twin cases [394]. Excepting identical twins or other close relatives, the whole issue is clouded by the contemporary brief prognosis, in most cases one or two years [186]. It has been estimated, excluding fraternal twins, that there are probably no more than 15 patients in the world who have survived kidney transplantation for more than three years [394]. It is thus not now possible to know the value of the procedure in terms of a 5- or 10-year prognosis. Even if the benefit proves to be limited to a few years, this is a significant gain for the individual who fills a useful place in society. Starzl [394] asks searching questions as to who is equipped to determine the "usefulness" or "value" of a given individual: "A system of selection based upon such materialistic criteria is founded on the dangerous assumption that a few people are qualified and have the right to adjudicate the value of someone else's years."

Under some circumstances it is not ethical, or perhaps even legal, for a patient to accept an organ. For example, if the patient knows that the donor's spouse strongly disapproves of the donation, it may be unethical for him to accept. If he knows that a prisoner or a lunatic is donating the organ, it might be both unethical and illegal to accept it, for, as Daube [131] says, a "person under restraint cannot be presumed to consent."

Woodruff finds it curious that so much emotional concern is voiced over a kidney donation, while during the Battle of Britain no one saw any moral problem in allowing a man to become a fighter pilot [431]. Most persons would rather give a kidney than engage in such dangerous activity. Bentley objects to such an analogy, for moral theologians make a distinction between direct and indirect effects [34]. For the fighter pilot, the possible maiming is never the means of achieving his objective. The maiming, if it occurs, is an indirect effect, foreseen as possible, but in transplantation the maiming, the loss of a kidney, is the direct means to the end desired. Thus, a moral difference is present. One can speculate on the consequences of a breach in the present immunologic barrier: the transplantation of skin can be life-saving in the severely burned. In another area, with the present population of the United States at 200 million, one can estimate the need for 10,000 kidney transplants each year [317].

A difficult early period in any specific experimental work is likely to be the time when success is rare. Platt believes [346] that the ethical position of removing a kidney from a healthy person when the chances of its survival as a transplant for a long time is 5 percent is different from what it would be if the success rate were 90 percent [346]. "Rarity of success" is a real and complicating factor not usually discussed. In such a situation, whether to continue or to call a halt is a troubling decision. If an acceptable success rate is to be achieved, experimentation must continue. This problem is not limited to organ transplantation; it is common in the development of most complex diagnostic and therapeutic procedures.

Platt [346] takes the view that in certain rare and dangerous developmental procedures not yet ready for general use but nevertheless *for the patient's welfare,* "There is a slight ethical danger here, in that one is selecting patients for such procedures partly because they may benefit other people in the future and not wholly because of possible benefit to the present patient." As long as the purpose of the procedure is truly diagnostic or therapeutic, there can be little ground for complaint, if at the same time it adds to knowledge or is of benefit to others. It seems likely that the only questionable situation would grow out of deception of the subject or oneself when there was no true expectation of helping the patient. Platt is of the opinion that too little thought is given to whether the proposed experiment is really a *sound* experiment [346]. Beecher has emphasized for years that the improperly designed experiment, one that cannot give useful data, is an unethical experiment, regardless of whether it is "harmless" [27]. There is the requirement in all human experimentation that the ends sought not be trivial.

The next few years may show that kidney transplantation has a better chance of success than has resection of the esophagus for cancer: 15 percent five-year cures for the lower one-third; 5 percent for the middle third; no five-year cures for the upper third [427]. Esophageal surgery would not ordinarily be called experimental, yet kidney transplantation is usually so designated. One may not fairly equate experimental procedures with procedures that have a low success rate. It must be borne in mind that for some diseases as, for example, cancer of the esophagus, there is no real alternative to surgery except palliation, whereas there is an alternative to kidney transplantation: intermittent hemodialysis.

Murray has made the point that an operation on the donor is not a medical procedure at all: it is not making a sick person well, but a well person sick. Any maiming of a patient should be for his benefit [317]. The principle of totality covers this: a part of the body may be sacrificed for the good of the whole. The donor loses a kidney, but has spiritual gain in his sacrifice.

Questions involve both donor and recipient: whether a kidney transplant, for example, will do any good and, if so, to whom. If the transplant lives, the recipient is obviously benefited. Whether the transplant lives or dies, the donor can be benefited psychologically and spiritually. This was affirmed by the Supreme Judicial

Court of Massachusetts in the case of the first identical twin transplant.

Giertz has proposed that a considerable number of persons might agree, when healthy and fully conscious, that a kidney might be taken if certain conditions ensue later in life; a second solution might stem from a reevaluation of widely accepted moral principles, with alteration of legislation [177].

HEART TRANSPLANTATION

Transplantation of the heart represents a desperate effort to save a desperate situation. It is a therapeutic effort that will be widely practiced, once the rejection phenomenon is overcome.

Barnard's first heart transplant focused attention on a great need. The excitement and the educational effect resulting from it will in all probability lead to the availability of funds and the stimulation of investigation, so that transplant problems, not only of hearts but of other organs as well, will be solved sooner than would otherwise be the case.

A considerable debate is at present under way involving whether further heart transplants should be attempted until the rejection phenomenon is better understood and better controlled. Another imponderable in the heart transplant situation is that it is difficult to judge with accuracy the prognosis in survival time of the prospective recipient without transplantation. Certainly, a heart transplant would not be contemplated if widespread crippling atherosclerosis or other major disease were present.

An especially difficult problem with single organ transplants, such as the heart or liver, is that this is, at least so far, a once-and-only procedure, whereas with the kidney as many as three transplants in a single patient have been carried out. Then, too, in the case of renal disease there is the fact that the man with no kidney function can often be kept alive and functioning for years with intermittent hemodialysis. There are, clearly, basic differences in the problems surrounding the several organs.

A further restriction pointed out by the Board on Medicine of the National Academy of Sciences (Walsh McDermott [294]; see the full statement, page 306) is that the number of surgeons with the knowledge and skill to perform the actual transplantation of the heart is greater than the number who have available the full capability to conduct the total study in terms of all relevant scientific observations. The Board would restrict cardiac transplantation to institutions in which there exists, not only surgical expertise, but also a thorough understanding of the biologic processes that lead to rejection and its control. In this hazardous field, it is especially important that careful planning be established prior to the event; that systematic observations be recorded; and that all findings, good and bad, be communicated to the few others engaged in such activity. Rigid safeguards must be established to cover the rights of donor and recipient.

LEGAL PROBLEMS IN THE FIELD OF TRANSPLANTATION

A considerable dilemma is to be encountered in this area. The rights of donors, alive or cadaver, insofar as the latter can be said to have "rights," and the rights of recipients have not been spelled out in law. At the same time, history indicates that it is very often undesirable to bring legal decision into a situation that is in a state of rapid change.

The use of live donors who have been properly informed, who understand the risks involved and the uncertainty of success, and who have agreed in writing, has not yet led to serious legal problems. The use of a minor twin has been discussed (page 122). Cadaver donors are in another category. In the first place, true emergency planning is involved so that the kidneys or other organs can be removed and perfused in an hour or less. In such a case, good hope for success is justified.

For those who, like Alexandre [4], insist that the removal of organs is proper after the brain is dead, although the heart still beats (page 155), the philosophy is simpler than for those who do not agree. (See report of the Harvard *ad hoc* Committee on a Definition of Irreversible Coma, Appendix B.) There is a difference, of course, when one of paired organs is removed and when a single organ such as the liver or the heart is taken. Such a view falls into the category of "statistical morality" (page 206), for all major surgical procedures have their own mortality rates and, when a sufficient number of operations is carried out, even the removal of one of a pair will lead to death.

Since the transplant must sometimes be effected in minutes,[3] not hours, what legal procedure can be prepared ahead of time? Eventually, as Giertz has suggested, it may be possible to persuade large numbers of individuals to agree, when still healthy, to organ removal if brain death later occurs [177]. This could, if extensive enough, make a real impact on the situation. Alternatively, legislation might be passed to ensure—unless the individual or his family explicitly objected or it was contrary to his religion—that tissues might be taken legally after death without further arrangement. The situation might also be handled by legally authorizing a previously designated person to give consent to tissue or organ removal after death. The "definition of death" is discussed later (page 311).

Under present legal restrictions, a living person has limited powers to dispose of his body or its parts after death, although some states permit such disposal by will, as in California, and more recently in Massachusetts. The law has not kept pace with science; as suggested above, this may be fortunate until many situations and problems are better clarified. (For further discussion of this field, see the scholarly review by Wasmuth and Stewart [419].)

ETHICAL PROBLEMS CREATED BY THE HOPELESSLY UNCONSCIOUS PATIENT

> Vex not his ghost: O, let him pass! he hates him
> That would upon the rack of this tough world
> Stretch him out longer.
>
> KING LEAR, V. iii

These remarks will be limited to the single situation of the *unconscious* and irretrievably injured man who is kept "alive" only

[3] Not so in the cases of prolonged irreversible coma, considered in Appendix B.

by extraordinary means. Four very different kinds of questions arise from this situation [29a]:

1. Under what circumstances, if ever, shall extraordinary means of support be terminated, with death to follow?
2. From the earliest times the moment of death has been recognized as the time the heartbeat ceased. Is there now adequate evidence to support the thesis that the moment of death should be advanced to coincide with brain death while the heart continues to beat?
3. When, if ever, and under what circumstances is it permissible or proper to use for transplantation the tissues and organs of a hopelessly unconscious patient?
4. Is it right to discard the tissues and organs of the hopelessly unconscious patient when they could be used to restore the otherwise hopelessly ill but still salvageable individual?

This matter is pertinent to the theme of our common interest, for the ever-broadening experimentation in the transplantation of tissues and organs has already led to the use of organs of hopelessly unconscious patients while their hearts were still beating. The ethics of this procedure have been questioned. We are therefore under the compulsion to face up to these problems.

In Judge Cooley's memorable phrase [111], there is "the right to be let alone." Implicit in this is the right to live and the right to die; there is also the opposite right, to communicate. The individual's right[4] to be let alone conflicts with society's right to use scientific research for the advancement of all. These thoughts and others to be discussed are relevant to this presentation because of current pressures to use the hopelessly unconscious patient's tissues and organs in an attempt to help the otherwise hopelessly ill but still salvageable patient in certain experimental procedures.

COMMENT ON DEFINITION OF DEATH

The moment of death can have legal importance,[5] but the criteria by which death is established must depend upon medical evi-

[4] These matters have been more fully discussed in Chaps. 2 and 3.

[5] *And theological, as well.* Pope Pius [344] has said: "Extreme Unction would certainly not be valid [after death], for the recipient would certainly not be a man any more," an indispensable condition for receiving the sacraments.

dence. Granted that there may be a time when it is good—that is, appropriate—to die, when does that moment arrive? What are its criteria?

Starzl has spoken of "the declining curve of life," implying that as the end approaches there is lessening life in the individual, that there is present a quantitative factor, a sort of death by inches [394]. At the same time, one can share Schreiner's [375] discontent and insist that "a coordinating vital principle exists which is either there or not there." This vital principle comes into being when the sperm fertilizes the ovum and persists until life departs. The moment of death can only be approximated; it is an imprecise term. That is the principal reason why the Harvard Commmittee chose to give a definition of irreversible coma (Appendix B), rather than to attempt a definition of death.

From ancient times to the recent past, it was perfectly clear that when the respiration and heart stopped, the brain would die in a few minutes; thus, the obvious criterion of a heart in standstill as synonymous with death was sufficiently accurate. This is no longer the case when modern resuscitative and supportive measures are involved. These improved activities can now restore and maintain "life" as judged by the traditional standards of persistent respiration and continuing heartbeat. This can be the case even when there is not the remotest possibility that an individual will recover consciousness following massive brain damage. In other situations, "life" can be maintained only by means of artificial respiration and electric stimulation of the heartbeat; in temporarily bypassing the heart; or, in conjunction with these procedures, reducing the body's oxygen requirement by cooling.

All organ and nerve centers do not become irreversibly damaged simultaneously. Consciousness as a brain function is often irretrievably destroyed months before the respiratory and vasomotor centers fail. Death occurs at several levels. Civilizations die, yet many of the component societies live on. Societies disintegrate, while the individuals involved survive. Individuals die legally, spiritually, or physiologically, but many of their cells continue to metabolize. Cells are destroyed, but their enzymes still function.

Which of these states are we to call death? The answer must necessarily be arbitrary. Medawar [299] surveys all of this, and one can almost hear him sigh as he concludes: "But legally, I suppose, a man is dead when he has undergone irreversible changes of a type that make it impossible for him to seek to litigate."

However it is phrased, our basic concern is with the presence or absence of physiologic, especially neurologic, life. The lack of an accepted definition of death handicaps many of the activities within the hospital, as, for example, the cadaver transplant problem. This is a medicolegal problem; it is also a sociolegal problem that arises in the difficulties of handling a corpse.

It is interesting that we are forced to ask the *series* of questions: When is death, what is death, what is life? It is self-evident that there is no simple answer to the first of these questions. Quoting the fictional Dr. Zhivago as saying that we live solely in others, one can submit that life is the ability to communicate with others. If this ability is lost in permanent unconsciousness, the future will surely confirm that a man is dead. One can make a considerable case that if a physician judges that his patient's ability to communicate is lost beyond retrieval through permanent unconsciousness, he not only may, but *must,* declare the man dead. He can doubt only his judgment, not the criteria.

When is death? The traditional compulsive urge to know and record the moment of death is usually not very important. The moment of death is important, however, in the transplant situation and sometimes for legal purposes. What often matters is, not the time of death, but the time when a physician undertook to declare the patient dead. So much for general comments; the "specifics" are spelled out in Appendix B.

In Belgium, Alexandre has in nine cases used unconscious patients with head injuries, whose hearts had not stopped, as kidney donors for transplantation [4]. "Five conditions were always met in these nine cases: (1) complete bilateral mydriasis; (2) complete absence of reflexes, both natural and in response to profound pain; (3) complete absence of spontaneous respiration, five minutes after mechanical respiration had been stopped; (4) falling blood pressure, necessitating increasing amounts of vasopressive drugs; (5) a flat E.E.G." Some have spoken of taking organs from a dying person. "I would like to make it clear [says Alexandre] that, in my opinion, there has never been and never will be any question of taking organs from a dying person who has 'no reasonable chance of getting better or resuming consciousness.' The question is of taking organs from a dead person, and the point is that I do not accept the cessation of heart beats as the indication of death." Certainly, such individuals have lost their ability to communicate. The question is, have they also lost their right to be let alone?

Calne [59] states bluntly that Alexandre was "in fact removing kidneys from live donors." He believes that "any modification of the means of diagnosing death to facilitate transplantation will cause the whole procedure to fall in disrepute with the entire profession."

Alexandre and Calne agree that two separate teams should be involved in deciding these matters: one concerned with resuscitating the patient and the other with an interest in donor possibilities, if such become apparent [4, 59]. Schreiner [375] differs; he does not "believe that mechanical separation of two teams and the problems of the surgeon's disrepute are really germane to the philosophical problem . . . The moral problem can't be settled on the basis of what might happen to a reputation . . . This question of deciding death transcends the problems of transplantation." He contends that if cadaver transplants become available by "updating" death and do as well or nearly as well as organs from live donors, then we must question the morality of continuing to use transplants from live unrelated donors.

These matters have been presented in some detail to show the differences of opinion and uncertainty among experts who have given much thought to the as yet unresolved question of what constitutes true death.

Woodruff and Louisell speak of the need, in view of current medical realities, for a conference of nonmedical and medical participants to focus directly on a redefinition of the moment of death [283, 431]. This will require the collaborative and precise thinking of physicians, lawyers, theologians, and philosophers. It seems clear that, in view of the differences among the experts who have given much thought to the matter, any updating of the moment of death would be a *legal* impossibility at this time, however theologically and scientifically sound it might be. This is not to argue against updating; it is to suggest the propriety of caution. There are encouraging signs. Consider the following celebrated case [144, 283, 306]:

An inquest was held in Newcastle on a man who, on being struck, fell backward onto his head. Respiration failed 14 hours after hospital admission, and he was placed on a respirator. A day later, with his wife's consent, a kidney was removed for transplantation. Following the nephrectomy, the respirator was turned off. There was no spontaneous respiration. A medical witness declared that the man had virtually died at the time he was put on the respirator, although it was legally correct to say that death occurred following the interruption of artificial respiration. The surgeon, described as an assailant, was charged by a jury with manslaughter. He was then committed for trial by the coroner. The coroner had consented to the nephrectomy in accordance with the Human Tissue Act of 1961; the jury found that the nephrectomy *had not contributed to death*. In the discussion following, it was proposed that the moment of death be defined as the moment when a spontaneous heartbeat cannot be restored. Louisell and others [283] raise the question whether the moment of death might not best be defined as "the moment at which irreversible destruction of brain matter, with no possibility of regaining consciousness, is conclusively determined."

Louisell, who is Boalt Professor of Law at the University of California, has given much thought to these matters. He concludes, "In the present state of the law I could only advise a client that he would incur the danger of a possible charge of homicide if by removal of an organ he causes death, if life still continues in the conventional sense"; that is, if there is still a heartbeat.

It is our hope that the Harvard *ad hoc* committee's "Definition of Irreversible Coma," which is presented in full in Appendix B, will be accepted and will clarify and solve many of the problems mentioned above.

DEATH AND THE CHURCH

In an address, "The Prolongation of Life," Pope Pius XII raised many questions [344]; some conclusions stand out. (1) In a deeply unconscious individual whose vital functions are maintained over a prolonged period only by extraordinary means, "the soul may already have left the body." As mentioned, verification of the moment of death can be definitely determined, if at all, only by a physician. It is not "within the competence of the Church" to decide this. The assumption is that life is present as long as vital functions persist spontaneously or even with some help from artificial processes. (2) It is incumbent on the physician to take all reasonable ordinary means of restoring the spontaneous vital functions and consciousness and to employ such extraordinary means as are available to him to achieve this end. It is not obligatory, however, to continue to use extraordinary means indefinitely in hopeless cases. "But normally one is held to use only ordinary means—according to circumstances of persons, places, times, and cultures—that is to say, means that do not involve any grave burden for oneself or another." There comes a time when resuscitative efforts should stop and death be unopposed.

VESTED INTERESTS

Vested interests impinge on most moral choices. Here, this situation is no different. It will be best to consider the source of these pressures. Their presence calls for caution.

Let us first consider the *patient's* point of view. If conscious, he is not obliged to avail himself of extraordinary means of survival. A good case in point is the use of intermittent hemodialysis for the man with kidney failure. At a recent symposium [430], considerable discussion was devoted to the question of whether a man commits suicide when he has the opportunity to avail himself of intermittent hemodialysis and rejects it. The answer is surely in the negative: the subject has the right to withdraw. It is an extraordinary process for maintaining life and therefore not obligatory.

It must be recognized that when the patient is in full possession of his mental faculties, the situation is not comparable to turning off the respirator of an unconscious patient with irreversible brain damage. The patient who has the opportunity to reject hemodialysis must weigh, not only the financial and emotional cost to his family, but also the cost to the society to which he belongs. Medical resources in this field are limited: utilization by one deprives another, and rejection by one benefits another.

The unconscious patient with overwhelming brain damage can be maintained only by extraordinary means. When it becomes evident that the brain is dead, there is an obligation to discontinue extraordinary supports, but one must remember that the termination of extraordinary care, even for just reasons, with death to ensue, can have a shocking effect on observers. Conversely, the patient's relatives and family very often wish to terminate their agonizing death watch and often urge a discontinuance of extraordinary measures. Some of those who have an interest in organ transplantation demand a new appraisal of what constitutes death so the organ sought may be taken while circulation continues. Hospitals and society in general have a vested interest in terminating the appalling cost of useless procedures in hopeless cases. Occupancy of a bed in such circumstances jeopardizes the salvageable.

The presence of vested interests, however correct may be their point of view, raises the possibility of selfish rationalization and is a warning of the need for caution. Then, too, a new definition of death, when there are those who have a vested interest in it, could lead to public questioning and doubt and an unfortunate blurring of the line between the permission sought and euthanasia. These are simply points to be considered; they do not preclude a new definition of death. It would be a grave mistake to underrate the attitude of the public as to the inviolability of the body. In many cases, this is based upon religious beliefs concerning the resurrection of the body. While Roman Catholics and Orthodox Jews oppose cremation, this refusal to violate the body is prevalent also in some atheistic countries. Perhaps the theologian, with his distinction between ordinary and extraordinary means of sustaining human life, will also say (ironically or not) with Arthur Hugh Clough:

> Thou shalt not kill; but need'st not strive
> Officiously to keep alive.

A MAJOR PROBLEM

These situations and these possibilities pose a serious problem for hospitals. Inevitably, with increasingly bold, venturesome, and commendable attempts to rescue the dying, there will be an accumulation of individuals in hospitals who can be kept "alive" only by extraordinary means despite the fact that there is no hope of recovery of consciousness, let alone recovery to a functioning, pleasurable existence—all of this at an individual cost of $25,000 to $30,000 per year. Burdensome as this expense may be, it is the lesser of two expenses. If the average hospital stay is two weeks, the irretrievably unconscious patient then occupies space that could have been used by 26 other patients in a year's time, a cost beyond measure. There are today great delays in hospital admissions, even of patients with cancer, because of bed shortages. A life may often be lost owing to delay in getting definitive hospital care because a bed is occupied by a hopeless case.[6]

It seems clear that the time has come to reexamine this situation. Money *is* human life; so are available hospital beds. The money spent to maintain unconscious and hopelessly damaged individuals could be used to restore those who are salvageable. What are our privileges and responsibilities in this confusing situation? [7] What decision must we make about this "striving officiously to keep alive"? It must be borne in mind that "hopeless," when established by a killing disease, is often not the same thing as "hopeless" result-

[6] If ever a legal precedent is established by a successful suit involving failure to place a patient on a respirator or for turning off a respirator, then one can expect an increase in numbers of the irretrievably injured and unconscious requiring hospital care. Doctors will be fearful to use their best judgment.

[7] The *London Times*, 16 July 1964, reported the death in Montreal of a woman aged 21 who had been in a coma since a traffic accident twelve years before.

ing from a recent accident. Astonishing recoveries have occurred in the latter case.[8]

A child submerged for 22 minutes would have been considered dead, unquestionably so; but new techniques made it possible to resuscitate such a child in Norway. Leicester asks [274], "Was he, in fact 'alive' or 'dead'? What meaning do those words carry in this context?"

It must be remembered that such advanced techniques as were employed in this case are sometimes the result of intensive, even desperate efforts to alleviate the hopelessly ill. There *is* profit for mankind sometimes in the prolongation of dying, justified as it can

[8] A 5-year-old boy, for example, was submerged for 22 minutes in a Norwegian river at a temperature of $-10°$ C [254]. Before he went under, he was seen in the water clinging to the ice. Doubtless his body temperature rapidly fell during this period, and the resulting hypothermic state probably accounts for his survival. Although the boy seemed to be dead, with blue-white skin and widely dilated pupils, he was given mouth-to-mouth insufflation. The mouth and pharynx were filled with vomitus. This was partially cleared. No pulse was felt. The trachea was intubated, the airway aspirated, artificial respiration instituted, and external heart compression started at once and continued on the way to the hospital. On arrival, there was some evidence of peripheral circulation. The ear lobes became pink. The heart was pricked with a needle and epinephrine and procaine were administered, without apparent result. Blood was withdrawn for typing and for determining the extent of hemolysis. Two and one-half hours after submersion, the heart started to contract spontaneously. Chlorpromazine was administered in an effort to improve the peripheral circulation. Gasping breaths now followed and soon became normal, but in an hour pulmonary edema appeared. Lanatoside and theophyllamine and morphine were given to control it. Three more pulmonary edema episodes ensued. An exchange transfusion was given to eliminate the free hemoglobin and potassium. Respiratory failure occurred five times in the next 24 hours. Hydrocortisone, antibiotics, heparin, and chlorpromazine were given. He was transfused. Examination two days after the accident showed no pupillary or corneal reflexes and no reaction to painful stimuli. On the fifth day, these signs returned. In a week, the boy began to swallow and to cough. On the tenth day he could obey simple commands, recognize his mother, and say "Yes," or "No." The next day he began to shriek and became restless and unconscious. Except for the brief period mentioned, he was unconscious for about six weeks. The agitated period lasted 14 days. He seemed to be decerebrated. Gradual improvement followed, but he appeared to be blind. Six weeks after the accident his mental condition improved. He began to speak, but still seemed to be blind. A week later, his vision began to return. On discharge, two-and-a-half months after the accident, he behaved like a normal child, except for a little ataxia. Six months after the accident, his mental condition was almost normal for his age, although he was still clumsy, and peripheral vision was reduced. Neurologic examination, including an electroencephalogram, was normal. By the usual clinical standards, he behaved as a normal child.

be by concern for the specific sick man. The rights of the individual and the rights of society are interrelated.

This is no place to deal with the complex matter of euthanasia. Present concerns are in no way related to it. However, while we are considering the subject of advances made in the care of the sick, it can be observed that one frequently stated reason, so-called justification for euthanasia, has been to terminate the patient's agony. Nowadays physical agony is almost always controllable with drugs; consequently, as Leicester [274] says, the "justification . . . for killing the patient . . . would now have to be stated less in terms of mercy to the patient and more in terms of consideration for those who grieve for or rebel against his condition. Such a justification would be correspondingly harder to maintain."

With the developments of recent years, there has been an extraordinary increase in the power of the doctor, and from this increase new and unexpected dilemmas and moral choices emerge. They require decision and action. A major difficulty lies in having to choose among values that are not really measurable or of clearly comparable moral weight. With progress in medicine, technical decisions become easier, whereas moral problems become increasingly significant and difficult.

SUMMARY

Many physicians today would take the view that the moment of death arrives when consciousness is permanently lost, when it has passed the point of no return, and when the brain is destroyed. Its criteria, maintained for at least 24 hours, are a failure to respond in any way to intense stimulation over a prolonged period, no breathing, no reflexes (except for rare spinal reflexes), and no movement. If an electroencephalograph is available, the cessation of electric activity in the brain provides useful confirmatory evidence, provided no central nervous system depressants are present and provided also that the patient's temperature is above 90°F. These matters are dealt with in detail in Appendix B. Justice Holmes defined the obverse of this when he said, "To live is to function; that is all there is to living."

As with all things in medicine, judgment enters decision, for example, as to what is "consciousness permanently lost" or what is a "hopelessly damaged brain." To take a nihilistic view and say that these are incredibly difficult questions impossible to answer can be as immoral as to treat these matters lightly. *To fail to act, to fail to decide, can have a desperately radical result.* The curable, the salvageable can thus be sacrificed to the hopelessly damaged and unconscious who consume time and occupy space better devoted to those who could be helped. To pretend that no such alternative exists is nonsense; one is inevitably deprived of what the other receives.

Two yardsticks must be recognized: the one measuring the welfare of the individual, the other the welfare of science, which is to say, in the best sense, the welfare of society. Since these two areas are essentially interrelated, the one dependent on the other, then surely it must be granted that on occasion the brief prolongation of dying may be justified. One can and should place the welfare of the individual first. There are often circumstances that justify prolongation, for example, in trying out an uncertain, new therapeutic procedure of remote but still possible benefit to the patient. There is the frequent situation where young doctors or nurses or paramedical personnel may, for compassionate but ignorant reasons, misunderstand the reasons for and the right to terminate extraordinary means of therapy for the hopelessly unconscious man. In such a situation, the prolongation of dying may be utilized to educate these groups, to the elimination of bitter recriminations and unfortunate gossip.

We have already stated the reasons for caution in updating the time for discontinuing extraordinary therapeutic efforts when vested interests exist. At the same time, the rule of double effect can operate in the experimental situation involving organ transplantation. It would perhaps be unwise to make categorical statements about this at this time. When decisions are as difficult to make and as various as they are at present, one suspects that there is need for more information and more education.

CONCLUSIONS

1. Advances in resuscitative and supportive measures are enabling us to make bold, venturesome, and commendable attempts to rescue the dying. Inevitably, at times these efforts succeed only partially, with the result that individuals who can be maintained "alive" only by extraordinary means accumulate in hospitals. Resources devoted to such individuals jeopardize the salvageable.

2. Earlier criteria of death, such as absent heartbeat, are often no longer adequate. Brain death seems to be an important relatively new concept (Appendix B).

3. The position of the Roman Catholic Church is that when deep unconsciousness is judged to be permanent, extraordinary means to maintain life are not obligatory. These means can be terminated and the patient allowed to "die."

4. Certain vested interests would like to advance the criteria of irreversible brain damage to make a new definition of death. Such pressures indicate the need for caution; however, criteria of brain death, based upon a large mass of carefully studied material, appears to be sound and to constitute a justifiable new standard of death, but one not yet accepted as legal death.

5. It would be a mistake, probably, to invoke legal action *at this time* in the present unclear and rapidly changing situations and attitudes concerning the use of the tissues or organs of hopelessly unconscious individuals. Any such decisions would almost certainly be restrictive.

6. Problems must be recognized and questions stated before they can be answered. One great question stands out here, in addition to questions of ultimate legality. Is it morally right or wrong to use the tissues and organs of hopelessly unconscious patients with continuing circulation; if right, under what circumstances is it right? Granted that a time comes when resuscitative measures must stop and death be unopposed. In the hopelessly unconscious individual, the question is whether the *body* must be left untouched. The principal question is thus posed; to do this is our major purpose here. We believe that Appendix B contains an answer.

7. One can distill from the foregoing two major conclusions: (a) It is clear beyond question that a time comes when it is no longer appropriate to continue extraordinary means of support for the hopelessly unconscious patient. (b) A strong case can be made that mankind can ill afford to discard the tissues and organs of hopelessly unconscious patients so greatly needed for study and trial to help those who can be salvaged. This can come about only with the prior concurrence of the individuals involved, the agreement of society and, finally, approval in law.

The Uniform Anatomical Gift Act is an example of how wise and dedicated men can smooth out legal difficulties that go back as far as the seventeenth century. The Act is concerned with the procurement of human tissue from both living and dead persons and thus is especially relevant to the newly arising problems of organ transplantation. The final draft was endorsed by the American Bar Association, August 7, 1968. As of September, 1969, some 37 states had approved it. Credit for this major achievement goes to a remarkable trio, Alfred M. Sadler, Blair L. Sadler, and E. Blyth Stason [372a].

6
The Law and Human Experimentation

While human experimentation has accompanied the practice of medicine from times of antiquity, the current concept of planned medical research has not really been presented as such to the courts. As the courts have understood it, human experimentation has not been, nor is it now, *legally* recognized as a legitimate part of the physician's activities except as this may be necessary in treating a patient, with his consent, or in preparing for his treatment as required, for example, by the Food and Drug Administration's drug testing program. Beecher has stated that the universal and long-standing recognition that human research is essential to the advancement of medical science and the newer recognition that some aspects of even basic science cannot advance without it, have led to a correct, although still in most cases, extralegal, expansion of human experimentation [24]. Curiously, when well conceived and soundly conducted, such work is everywhere recognized as being properly within the ethical and moral concepts of our time, but is not yet broadly recognized in law. It would be unrealistic and a mistake for medicine to wait for guidance from the law. We have attempted to lead in advancing the concept of brain death in our definition of irreversible coma [Appendix B]. It is our hope that eventually the law will find our point of view useful in its formulation of legal attitudes. It is also our hope that pertinent law will not be established in this changing area for a long time to come, until the issues involved are much clearer than is presently the case.

We may grant that little current law deals explicitly with human experimentation. Jaffe points out that the common law, the law devised and administered by the courts, has developed and continues to develop doctrines that are applicable [229, 230]. The physical touching of an individual without his consent may be actionable even when no physical injury results. Manipulation of an individual by deceit may be actionable as fraud. Carelessness in experimentation may be actionable as negligence if it leads to injury.

The legal considerations, such as they are, surrounding human experimentation have been reviewed and documented by several writers [55, 122, 123, 255, 256]. Presently appropriate is a statement of the circumstances, the basic assumptions, the general principles involved, and the conclusions reached. It may or may not be true that "most legal problems which arise in connection with clinical investigations do not have . . . criminal implications," as Ladimer and Newman editorially assert [263]. Very few such cases ever come to the attention of the courts.

BACKGROUND

The practice of medicine has been hedged about with innumerable oaths, precedents, customs, rules, orders, and laws for the protection of the patient. Certain rules indirectly concerning human experimentation have been formulated by early writers—Aristotle and St. Thomas Aquinas, for example—as well as in Roman law. Curran [123] points out that the natural law concept of jurisprudence is at the foundation of international legal theory: "Under this system, laws are tested on the basis of 'right reason' as being in conformity or in conflict with the 'rational and social nature of man.' In other words, *man* is the central value: the society exists to serve man. Man has certain basic rights which cannot be taken from him by the state." This view may be compared with that of Grotius [175].

As ancient as common law is the principle that the individual shall be protected in his person and in his property. Starting from this, Warren and Brandeis [417] long ago recognized that "political, social and economic changes entail the recognition of new rights, and the common law, in its eternal youth, grows to meet the demands of society . . . Later there came a recognition of man's spiritual nature, of his feelings and his intellect. Gradually the scope of these legal rights broadened; and now the right to life has come to mean the right to enjoy life,—the right to be let alone." Thus, nearly 80 years ago there was recognition by legal scholars of the value of sensations, "feelings," and enjoyment. Warren and Brandeis also point out that, as concepts of the "right to life" expanded, so also the legal view of property broadened:

> From corporeal property arose the incorporeal rights issuing out of it; and then there opened the wide realm of intangible property, in the products and processes of the mind . . . The intense intellectual and emotional life, and the heightening of sensations which came with the advance of civilization, made it clear to men that only a part of the pain, pleasure, and profit of life lay in physical things. Thoughts, emotions, and sensations demanded legal recognition, and the beautiful capacity for growth which characterizes the common law enabled the judges to afford the requisite protection, without the interposition of the legislature.

There is ". . . the right to privacy, as a part of the more general right to the immunity of the person—the right to one's personality." The right to privacy was established in the law of France a century ago. The current invasions of privacy carried out as a part of human experimentation are of such importance that a separate section is devoted to it (page 94).

While this background may seem remote from the principal concern of this book, it gives encouraging evidence of the growth of the law. One can hope that the time is not distant when the law will embrace protection not now present, both for research subject and for investigator (page 36).

The Food and Drug Administration regulations are enforceable as law, and the rulings of the National Institutes of Health have the force of law. These requirements are new in the field of experimentation in man. These two bodies have approached their responsibilities in different ways. The Food and Drug Administration has established its own standards and rules in Washington, whereas the National Institutes of Health have set up a system of self-regulation at each research center through review by local peer groups.

Quasi legal decisions were made at Nuremberg; when specific laws are formulated, these "precedents" will doubtless be taken into consideration. Medical research, like all activities, is covered by common law principles of general applicability. "The law" governing this activity remains somewhat uncertain or, more precisely, undeveloped [263; see also the Declaration of Helsinki, Appendix A].

SOME SPECIAL CASES AND PARTICULAR SITUATIONS

The legal precedents and interpretations have to do mainly with the comparatively simple situation of experimentation designed to benefit the immediate patient. The important but much more difficult situation remains and is scarcely mentioned in legal discussion: that is, the situation where the research is not designed to benefit the immediate patient, but patients in general. To the writer, this is an instance where the law and its interpretation are very far removed from actual practices and very far away from current universally accepted ethical and moral concepts of Western civilization.

As mentioned, until recent times there have been no true legal precedents, no laws specifically covering experimentation in man. There is the somewhat early example of the Nuremberg Military Tribunal in the Medical Case of the War Crimes Trials [96]. According to Ladimer and Newman [263], this judicial summary of expert testimony against the Nazi doctors establishes two precedents: ". . . first, that improper human experimentation can constitute a crime against humanity; and second, that the propriety of experimentation may be judged according to expert testimony as to practices and standards professionally recognized at the time of the alleged offenses." The so-called Nuremberg Code, derived from these deliberations, holds that certain basic principles must be observed in order to satisfy moral, ethical, and legal concepts. This is not the place to determine whether the Nuremberg Code represents a true precedent in the legal sense. At any rate, violation of its principles was considered sufficient basis for imposing nine prison terms and seven death sentences.

A number of judicial decisions and laws impinge on or at least are relevant to the area of human experimentation; Jaffe [229] has discussed these problems. These decisions will be reviewed with the hope that when the inevitable accident occurs in the course of human experimentation and the matter is brought to court, it will then for the first time be examined and decided on its true basis as experimentation, not as heretofore always the case, on the basis of whether what was attempted was done in accordance with the medical standards of the community, that is, precedents derived from medical malpractice litigation. Useful experimentation cannot be judged against such a yardstick, for it is new; it is different; it goes beyond the old. Perhaps the somewhat gloomy conclusion of Swetlow and Florman is not entirely warranted [404]. There is a hopeful view to be found in a careful examination of the precedents that underlie the common law. The writer is indebted to Crawford Morris [311] for his discussion of present trends extrapolated from the past:

Public policy is determined by both the legislatures and the courts, and the latter usually pay lip service to the statement that public policy is best determined by the legislature, although this is very often not the case.

There is a clear legislative intent that favors human testing or experimentation. The recent Federal Food, Drug and Cosmetic Act not only authorizes, but *requires,* human study of all new drugs destined for use in man.

In the area of the common law, no court in the United States has been asked to decide a controversy between two citizens or between a state and a citizen as to the propriety of human experimentation. Legal precedent in this area is lacking. Nevertheless, that great pioneer of the law, Justice Brandeis, once had this to say: "Yet the advances in the exact sciences and the achievements in invention remind us that the seemingly impossible sometimes happens. There are many men now living who were in the habit of using the age-old expression: 'It is as impossible as flying.' The discoveries in physical science, the triumphs in invention, attest the value of the process of trial and error. *In large measure, these advances have been due to experimentation.*"

In *Fortner v. Koch* a Michigan court, in ruling [164] on a medical malpractice case, remarked: "We recognize the fact that, if the general practice of medicine and surgery is to progress, there must be a certain amount of experimentation carried on. . . ." In *Brinkley v. Hassig* the court [47] remarked, "It is true, as counsel argue, that the great advances in medical science have come about by the courage of pioneers, whose efforts often met with ridicule from their professional brethren." In the *Board of Medical Registration and Examination v. Kaadt* the court [41] said, ". . . a physician is not limited to the most generally used of several approved modes of treatment and the use of another mode known and approved by the profession is proper, but every new method of treatment should pass through an experimental stage in its development and a physician is not authorized in trying untested experiments on patients. . . ." While this seems to reaffirm the old saw that nothing shall ever be done for the first time, it does at the same time recognize the need for experimentation.

The judgment of the Nuremberg Military Tribunals in 1949 (Codes, page 227) set down ten basic principles that "must be observed in order to satisfy moral, ethical and legal concepts" in human experimentation. Thus, the tribunals clearly approved of human experimentation under the conditions they laid down.

In the recent case of *Hyman v. the Jewish Hospital* [224], it was ruled that Hyman, a member of the hospital's board of directors, had the right to examine the medical records of 22 patients who had participated in a cancer study. The decision of the Regents of the State of New York [322], which grew out of the Hyman case, was that two physicians were guilty of unprofessional conduct, *not in what they did, but in the manner in which they acted;* that is, without informing the subjects fully of what they were doing—injecting live cancer cells—and without consent. There were four reviews of part or all of these matters by New York courts: the Supreme Court, its Appellate Division, the Court of Appeals, and the Board of Regents. The manner of carrying out, but not the propriety, of the basic study was questioned. This is a very important milestone.

In another recent case, *Saron, Admr. v. State of N.Y.*, the appellate division affirmed a judgment for the defendant against the claim that the patient's death was caused by an experimental drug [374]. The experimental nature of the procedure was not frowned on; it was specifically approved. The court found no evidence of negligence in the use of the drug. In the case of *Fiorentino v. Wenger,* the New York appellate division affirmed a verdict for the plaintiff against the surgeons and the hospital when death from exsanguination occurred following an unorthodox procedure [159]. This decision was rendered, not on the basis that the surgeon "experimented at his peril," but rather on the ground that the departure from orthodox procedure required informed consent, which was not obtained.

A legal precedent was established by the first kidney transplant from an identical twin, a minor [122]. (The first transplant of a kidney in adult twins occurred in 1954; since children were not involved, it is not relevant to the issue of experimentation in children, page 63.) The Supreme Judicial Court of Massachusetts in 1957 set a precedent by declaring kidney transplantation proper in the case of 19-year-old twins. The benefit of the proposed transplant to the sick twin was obvious. It was also determined that the well twin would suffer irreparable psychological damage if he were denied the opportunity to donate his kidney to his brother. The consenting parents and twins understood fully the risks and benefits involved. Since the procedure was construed as also beneficial to the well twin it is not, strictly speaking, a new precedent, but it emphasizes that "benefit" need not be physical, but can be psychological. Subsequent to this case there have been other similar litigated transplant cases with like decisions.

In these examples drawn from decisions extending back perhaps 30 years, it is evident that the precedents that form the basis for the common law clearly imply an enlightened view of medical experimentation and its essential nature. These precedents will undoubtedly be considered when a definitive court test of experimentation as such is finally undertaken.

As a step in the direction of protection, the Law-Medicine Institute of Boston University, under the direction of William J. Curran, in 1960 began a long study of self-regulation in clinical investigation. This study made it evident that little self-regulation existed; indeed, it disclosed that many investigators and administrators considered such regulation to be undesirable. In the view that the doctor experiments at his peril one can see conflict with the federal statutes and administrative regulations that *require* the testing of new drugs in man before they are placed on the market.

However valuable for the human race a new procedure appears to be, if disaster occurs, the high-minded purpose of the investigator will give him no legal protection. The *Duke Law Journal* attempts to take a more cheerful view of the matter. While considering the legal implications of psychological research with human subjects, this legal review surprisingly stated: "If a legal action is brought against the scientific experimenter, its result will depend upon the existence of a privilege conferred on the experimenter by society, determined by balancing the risk of possible harm to the subject against the potential returns to society" [139a]. The basis for this sweeping statement is not clear. In any case, here is the view that the ends justify the means.

This approach is echoed by the Chief, Stress and Fatigue Section, Aero Medical Laboratory, Wright-Patterson Air Force Base, Captain George E. Ruff [139a, 369], who says: "We feel that the limited possibilities of danger in our work are more than outweighed by its potential returns. Both the need for data on personality structure and function and on environments important in space flight are more than enough to justify these particular experiments. Such reasons would probably not justify studies where a high percentage of the subjects might be harmed." In the view of this writer, this "statistical morality" leaves much to be desired.

It may be helpful in practical terms to take a look at the statements of a lawyer widely experienced in this area concerning the protection of experimental projects and those involved. Morris's [311, 312] views can be summarized:

1. The approved protocol must be carefully adhered to.

2. Informed consent must be obtained in writing and the known or suspected risks spelled out. If the risks are not known, this, too, is a risk to be faced; especially uncertain are the long-range effects.

3. Adequate insurance programs to protect both investigators and subjects are desirable. Ordinary liability insurance may not protect the investigator. The existing policy with increase in premium, or a new policy should be taken out specifically covering the risks in question.

Protection must include, not only the subject and the investigator, but also the scientific discipline involved. Science in general must be protected from any loss of confidence or any other consequence that might make future scientific work difficult. Concerning loss of confidence, Mead indicates [296] that there is general recognition that the investigator ". . . should not infuriate the local citizenry or outrage the board of trustees of a university by his research methods or the way in which he presents his results."

THE KEFAUVER-HARRIS AMENDMENTS AND THEIR INTERPRETATION

One can find a parallel to the current problem in the activities of the grave robbers, the "resurrectionists," as a result of the fact that there was no legal way to acquire an adequate supply of cadavers for the instruction of medical students. The law did not take notice of the situation until a public outcry, coupled with vigorous measures, forced action. According to Blake, Massachusetts in 1831 passed the first law in the English-speaking world designed to provide a satisfactory supply of cadavers [37]. This was the result of pressure from the Harvard Medical School and the Massachusetts Medical Society. Other states slowly followed suit, but it was not until 1895 that the District of Columbia took legal action to rectify the situation. The parallel with the problems of human experimentation is clear when one views the reaction to unethical or questionably ethical experimentation. A new and restrictive law on the books concerning the use of new drugs is already in effect.

The federal government is deeply involved in medical research, much of it involving man; the Food and Drug Administration is actively regulating the use of experimental drugs in interstate commerce. The former activity is based largely on such rulings as the requirement of the National Institutes of Health that all applications for support must be approved by a committee of the applicant's peers.[1] It is probable that other governmental agencies will adopt this policy. The authority of the Food and Drug Administration is derived from the amendments to the Food and Drug Act of 1962. The Food and Drug Administration first took up problems of manufacturing and distribution and then promulgated regulations as to safety and now efficacy.

As mentioned in Chap. 5, the Kefauver-Harris amendments to the Federal Food, Drug and Cosmetic Act (1962) have legal force, for the first time, directly concerned with human experimentation. These amendments require that the physician inform his patient that he proposes to use a new drug. Before this time, no federal or state laws required that a physician inform his patient that he was using an experimental drug in treatment. At that time, the physician was guided in the use of such a drug by earlier court decisions and by statements made by the Judicial Council of the American Medical Association.

Some attempt was made in both the House of Representatives and the Senate to face up to the thorny problem of consent. Discus-

[1] Based upon the Surgeon General's memorandum of February 8, 1966, amended July 1, 1966.

sion in both houses made it clear that they intended to make exceptions to the requirement of consent in the case of urgent need for treatment of (1) an unconscious person, (2) a child in an emergency when the parents cannot be reached, (3) a mentally incompetent patient with no known representative, and (4) a patient suffering from an incurable disease when the doctor fears that knowledge of the nature of the disease would be against the patient's best interests. Notwithstanding this, the Food and Drug Administration concluded that there was no real basis for exception in the circumstance where the investigator feels that informed consent would interfere with the design of the experiment, as is possible, even likely, in studies of the effects of drugs on subjective responses. Neither would the Administration make exceptions when informed consent might disturb the doctor-patient relationship. Evidently, discussion in the House and Senate is one thing and the law that emerges from such discussion something else, presumably the epitome of what the Congress deemed valid and important and necessary. The *interpretation* by the Food and Drug Administration goes beyond what the law actually says.

The regulations became effective March 8, 1963. They specify other safety conditions that must be met before an experimental drug is tested in man. Oddly, the regulations distinguish between clinical pharmacology and clinical trials. Two forms are available. In Form 1572, the Statement of Investigation with reference to clinical pharmacology says: "The investigator certifies that he will inform any patients or any persons used as controls, or their representatives, that drugs are being used for investigational purposes, and will obtain the consent of the subjects, or their representatives, *except where this is not feasible or in the investigator's professional judgment, is contrary to the best interests of the subjects.*" (Italics added.) Kelsey quotes the law [244], and yet she blandly says, one paragraph later: "However, the law states that consent must be obtained from any 'human being' to whom an investigational drug is administered." The writer is quite unable to reconcile these conflicting statements. Kelsey goes on to say:

The law provides that a human being must be informed if he is to take part in an experiment involving an investigational drug, even though he may only serve as a control in such a study. Such a control could receive either an inactive placebo or a drug of established activity. The law does not require that the subject be informed as to which preparation he receives and thus it would not be necessary for the subject or the physician to have prior knowledge of which agent will be administered. This permits the use of "blind" or "double blind" studies for the controlled evaluation of drugs. There are other legal safeguards to protect the patient in the event that the physician gives an inactive placebo for a life-threatening condition for which either the drug under consideration or another drug is generally recognized to be of therapeutic value.

The concept that placebos are "inactive" indicates a considerable misunderstanding. Placebos are, in general, powerful therapeutic tools, having one-half to two-thirds as much power to relieve pain of pathologic origin as the optimal dose of morphine given at the rate of 10 mg per 70 kg body weight [18].

Evidence that Kelsey's 1963 statements were indeed administration policy and that the Food and Drug Administration had applied its own interpretation to the consent "loophole" is to be found in the following letter of September 24, 1965, to the writer from the then Commissioner, George P. Larrick:

> First, let me say that there are no regulations which undertake an interpretation of the provision of law on patient consent. [But see the contrary statement below in this same letter.] We have left the matter to the words used in the statute itself, because Congress placed the prime responsibility on the investigator to certify that he is familiar with the consent provision and will comply with it.
>
> Second, we read the law to require that each investigator notify all persons involved in investigational drug use, or their representatives, that investigational drugs are being used and obtain their consent.
>
> There is an exception to this which permits investigators not to obtain consent "where they deem it not feasible or, in their professional judgment, contrary to the best interest of such human beings."
>
> To us, this means that the investigator must seek and obtain patient consent or make a professional judgment that he has an exceptional case in which consent is in fact not feasible or would be adverse to the patient's best interest. [So far, so good.]

The "best interest" part of the exception applies only to those physician-patient relationships where the investigator responsible for the patient has reached a professional judgment that informing the patient and obtaining consent would be contrary to that patient's best interest. It does not, as Dr. Kelsey said, apply simply because the investigator may feel that it would interfere with the design of the experiment. It does not apply simply because the physician-patient relationship might be disturbed—the test is whether consent would be contrary to the patient's best interest. [It is difficult to understand how a disturbance of the physician-patient relationship would not be contrary to the patient's best interests.]

The "not feasible" part of the exception is intended to cover the situation where consent is not capable of being obtained. [The basis for this highly restrictive interpretation is not clear; the Commissioner disavowed interpretation in his first paragraph, above!]

There are still other types of problems. After the Food and Drug Administration's legislation was passed, the agency was then obliged, as indicated above, to interpret the meaning of the several provisions. The widely acclaimed Declaration of Helsinki was used as a guide, but this did not solve all problems. The "loophole phrases" made trouble, especially with the concept of informed consent. Here it was determined that consent is "not feasible" where it cannot be obtained "because of inability to communicate with the patient or his representative; for example, where the patient is in a coma or is otherwise incapable of giving informed consent, his representative cannot be reached, and it is imperative to administer the drug without delay." This narrow exception seems to approve experimentation on the very ill, even on unconscious persons. This is certainly questionably ethical, as Curran has pointed out [126].

Another loophole problem arises in the situation described as "contrary to the best interests of such human beings" when obtaining consent might seriously affect the patient's disease status if consent were sought. Again, Curran observes: "This definition seems to sanction experimentation on patients who are either unaware of the nature of their illness (e.g., cancer) or are unaware or are misled about its seriousness . . . Consent is dispensed with because getting . . . *informed* consent would require telling the patient some *truth* which had been kept from him up to that point." The term *physician,* not *investigator,* is used in this patient's case. The physician is exerting therapeutic judgment. "He is assumed to be wearing two hats, one as attending physician to his patient and the other as investigator to his subject. Here he is allowed to base his judgment to eliminate a research requirement upon his therapy role, not his investigator's role." The Food and Drug Administration seems to have made another questionable ethical assumption. It has assumed that such a patient can be used for experimental purposes, but the overriding question is whether such a patient who does not know the facts of his case should be used in experimentation at all. The regulation allowing the investigator to wear two hats can be challenged for, as Curran has pointed out, he is thus able to make judgment about the research requirement while he wears the doctor's hat.

The rulings included this statement: "The degree of risk to be taken should never exceed that determined by the humanitarian importance of the problem to be solved by the experiment." Superficially but not necessarily, this seems to say that ends must justify means. Presumably, what is meant here is that grave risk shall not be undertaken for trivial ends. The Surgeon General or his associates seem to be asking for an impossible balancing of unknowns. A sounder approach would seem to be that serious risk in an experiment should in almost all cases be taken only when the subject promises to profit directly from it; that is, when the need for diagnosis or therapy designed to profit the individual patient, not science in general, is at stake.

SOME GENERALIZATIONS

There is an ancient association of medicine and the law. Cortesini observes that some of the earliest signs appeared in the *jus gentium* of Rome [113], and the union was perfected further in the *corpus juris* of Justinian. A great difficulty has been that legal and medical thinking have been so different that physicians have not been very effective in contributing to the formation or enactment of legal measures. There is considerable evidence that a new day has arrived and we may be allowed to expect that these conflicts will be resolved. The prestige of the medical scientist has risen; at times, he is necessary in framing laws, especially in new aspects of medicine, both experimental and therapeutic. This intervention is necessary because the advances in the medical sciences pose many moral and social problems that must be solved at a legal level. "The legislator must therefore sanction, adjust and frame laws concerning medical improvements as they affect present-day life" [113].

The physician describes the discoveries made in his realm objectively and without prejudice and thus provides the jurist with the data required. Thus, the jurist can examine and evaluate the material from the social and political viewpoint, but always with regard to biologic truth. The integrations of these kinds of data must lead to generalizations that exclude tentative scientific definitions and conclusions that may quickly become obsolete as investigation proceeds. Ill-considered or hasty action here could greatly interfere with the progress of clinical research, as well as with the development of the law. In his review of the subject, Ladimer [255] says:

> The term "experimentation" must be considered objectively (preferably discarded if it retains the connotation of improper medical practice) so that it is recognizable as a legitimate scientific endeavor which can be advanced by the recognized research scientist. The legal issue would then become not experimentation versus accepted practice of the art of medicine but an evaluation of the plan and conduct of research in relation to specific fact situations, that is, whether the research was conducted with due regard to the interests of the subject. The law has a duty to comprehend the scope and elements of diverse human activity and their places in society if it is to assist in making individual judgments and setting or recognizing general values . . . Essentially, medical research on human beings consists in experimentation, that is, deliberately inducing or altering body or mental functions, directly or indirectly, in individuals or in groups primarily for the advancement of health, science and human welfare.

As Curran [123, 126] has put it: "For many years the problem was to balance interests; this was the predominant theory of American law, often attributed to Dean Roscoe Pound of the Harvard Law School and his Sociological Jurisprudence. Opposed to this theory are the natural law or fundamental justice exponents who assert that no end of social justification warrants deprivation of certain basic rights." According to this view, individual rights may be curtailed for the sake of public benefit. Curran goes on to say:

> Thus individuals were required to endure noises or smoke so that factories and railroads could make America grow. But this legal philosophy is not in such good standing today as it was in the expansionist years of America. In earlier times, the courts were the protectors of property and of industrial growth. But the times have changed. The courts are now much more concerned with individual rights than they were . . . Now the more dominant legal philosophy is humanistic with the concepts of the natural law receiving the greatest application . . . The newer courts are not so apt to look kindly on the imposing of substantial risk on human subjects because of the potential benefits to greater numbers coming from the experiments.

Ladimer believes [255] that medical research

> is significantly different from medical practice in such respects as purpose and attitudes, scientific problem or medical hypothesis, study design or treatment, relative obligations of physician-research and patient-subject and general environment including scientific staff, facilities and types of clinical material selected . . . The conduct of medical practice, generally conceived to be diagnosis, treatment and care, is governed by state statute and supporting administrative licensing and regulatory bodies. Medical research on human subjects, except as it is an inherent but not predominant incident of such practice, would appear to be outside the scope of [medical practice]. There is no existing broad police power statute for control of human research although it is, by its nature, subject to the general police power. [Human research] . . . today warrants [legal] recognition as a separate endeavor affected with a public interest as significant as medical practice itself.

In Freund's view [169], the time has not yet arrived when the law can be expected to guide human experimentation in terms of precise answers to ethical problems. Before this can come about, there will have to be a close interchange between law and medicine, with each discipline clarifying the issues of its own field based on its particular experience. Before any such dialogue can take place, an understanding of "certain characteristics of the legal process and the legal mind must be achieved." Freund describes them. First, the law is inherently conservative; there must be continuity with the past; the law is addicted to principle, and it fears setting a bad precedent; the law likes to balance risks; it is "deeply protective of human integrity and life"; the law is dialectic in method. "The adversary system assigns roles to the advocates and to the judge, and it would disrupt the system if anyone attempted to play a role other than his own." Too often, as observed elsewhere, in the field of medicine the same individual attempts to encompass both the role of the patient's physician and the role of the physician investigator. It is clear that experimental medicine can profit from an examination of legal procedure. The law contains built-in safeguards, reciprocity—in effect, a feedback mechanism.

Although conservative, the law is also creative and responsive, as Freund emphasizes. He believes that just as the law has erected the right of privacy for both property and private personality (page 94), so also the law could recognize the right of human experimentation. "Social interests and expectations, if they are in fact justified, can expect eventually to be reflected in the law." Ruebhausen [367] puts it thus: "Law is the ethical conviction of society and the legal process is how these convictions are enforced."

In many fields of activity society accepts risk: the new plane; mountain climbing; the young automobile driver; the construction of buildings, highways, and tunnels; the exploration of space —all carry a significant risk. One seeks safeguards; one seeks to balance gains against risks. In medicine, the first rule is to do no harm; if serious risk is to be taken, however, this can often be limited to the situation where the subject, a patient, promises to profit directly from it, other methods having failed. When serious risk is to be taken for the sake of science alone, the problem is much more complicated; the welfare of the subject is paramount. Ruebhausen believes that human experimentation is of more concern to science than it is to the law, but that legal limitations will almost certainly be forthcoming [367]. When this occurs, the laws must assure that (1) human dignity and the values of society will be upheld; (2) that there will be no infringement of the individual's right to determine the use of his own time and his person; and (3) that experimentation will take into account freedom of choice.

One can generalize. In *therapy,* the patient is an end; he may also secondarily be a means in that what is learned in his treatment may have general scientific value. In *science,* the patient or subject is a means, not an end, to general scientific advancement, when what is done is not for his direct welfare, but for that of science in general. As one moves away from therapy, disclosure and consent assume a new urgency. If risk is considerable, consultation with one's peers also becomes urgent.

Freund [169] has faith that the law on the subject of human experimentation will be worked out "in close reliance on the moral sensibilities of the community." To this end it is important that the medical profession take the public into its confidence, educate it, and avoid the revulsion that inevitably follows when some flagrant secret activity is exposed.

CONCLUSION

Notwithstanding the wealth of both legal and lay confusions in this area, it is evident that there is wide understanding and approval of what human experimentation entails and of its importance, indeed, its necessity. If advancement in the field of medicine is to take place, experimentation in man must proceed with the valid consent of the subjects, insofar as this can truly be obtained, and certainly with the subjects' awareness that they are participants in an experiment in all except the most trivial situations where there is no discernible risk. It must proceed in the presence of adequate precautions against risk of injury. Hatry [204] believes that "The clinical investigator who is guided by his competence, integrity, and conscience has little to fear from our machinery of justice and much still to achieve for humanity." McDermott [294] is convinced that it is most unwise to attempt to extend the principle of "a government of laws and not men" into an area of great ethical subtlety such as that found in human experimentation.

The law allows certain degrees of freedom of action; it also imposes restraints. These freedoms and these restraints are bound to shape the growth of medicine. In giving continuity and stability to society, the law is conservative. Ethical errors evoke restraints and an expanding and sometimes crippling conservatism. This diminishes the law's "suppleness of adaptation to varying conditions" so prized by Justice Cardozo.

Laws change; even the United States Supreme Court reverses itself as society's moral convictions change. The law is really a formulation of these convictions. For example, in 1854 the Supreme Court said, in the Dred Scott case, that Negroes are property; in 1896 it held that separate but equal school facilities are constitutional, but in 1954 it changed this view to hold that separate cannot be equal. Society must reach moral conclusions before the law can be expected to deal with a given situation. There are heated controversies about the invasion of privacy, about human experimentation, and about artificial insemination, to mention a few examples. The latter situation is fraught with awkward questions that the law has not attempted to resolve. Does the sperm donor have any rights to the child? Does the child have inheritance rights? Or is the whole business simply adultery and, if so, who is the adulterer: the donor or the mediating physician? Obviously, these are moral questions, and the law cannot be expected to deal with them in any final sense until society has made some considered decisions. Stumpf [400] puts it very well: "On one side there is medicine creating new problems and raising new questions for the courts, but the courts cannot deal effectively with these problems and questions because, on their side, the source upon which they rely—namely, the moral consensus of society—has not yet taken recognizable shape."

7
Science in Relation to Moral, Ethical, and Religious Issues

Man finds science a prodigal benefactor in ways which virtue had not used to reward him . . . So in the childish tendency to pledge allegiance to what seems the more generous protector, modern man is likely to place all his trust and all his hopes in science, forgetting that well-being may derive from more than one source. Plants flourish from neither rain alone, nor sunlight alone.

ALAN GREGG, 1941

The central factor in the troublesome problems that arise in human experimentation is the moral one. Morals pertain to the distinction between right and wrong and good and evil; they are rules of conduct. Ethics is sometimes called—loosely, one fears—the *science* of morals. At any rate, ethics is concerned with rules of conduct that are recognized in certain limited departments of human existence; at the same time, however, ethics is concerned with human duty to its widest extent, and sometimes also with the good life. While a system of ethics is not a religion, all religions embrace an ethical component, and this component is of fundamental importance in determining the quality of a religion. The existence of a moral element in religion is implicit in Euripides' statement, "If the gods do aught that is shameful, they are no gods." Ethical concepts are the warp and woof of the human aspects of religion; they are indispensable in any particular system of faith and worship. In this sense, religious and moral considerations seem to be inseparable and therefore have been considered together; they are, in the end, issues of conscience. It is interesting parenthetically to observe in a ten-year survey of *Index Medicus* that discussions of medical economics are listed far more often than considerations of medical ethics.

Sometimes one can dismiss troublesome thought as to one's moral responsibilities. It is easy to suppose that standards of medical ethics are self-evidently good; it may be useful, however, to take a brief look at their origins. It will be seen that our moral standards of clinical research are of Judeo-Christian origin. This origin greatly influences our view of what is ethical and what is not. It seems unquestionable that our moral traditions have been influenced in large part by theological considerations. Perhaps one reason for the existence of today's moral uncertainties is the lessening of the theological domination of many aspects of life.

While there were early glancing references to the moral and religious problems raised by human experimentation, it is only within the last several decades that the principal Western religious groups have begun to face up to the situation. It is evident that human experimentation has raised many new and critical issues. These include the limitation on the freedom of the subject, as well as on that of the investigator (as explicitly set forth by Pius XII); on the selection of subjects; on the limitations of informed consent; and on the extent of the necessary requirements of forthright discussion and disclosure in the subject-physician-investigator triad. It also involves a balancing of risks and benefits without invoking, as the only justification, the view that ends alone justify any means. This is not to imply that concern for these problems is not shared equally by the responsible investigator and the moralist. Indeed, there is considerable evidence to show that the responsible investigator recognized them for what they were and accepted them as serious problems before the theologians did so. Evidence for this lies in the physicians' ancient ethical concepts that showed that scientific validity and moral propriety are reconcilable—indeed, have been reconciled—in modern clinical investigation [263].

For background, it seems appropriate to examine the attitudes of the principal religions toward these moral issues in terms of what their respective theologians have had to say about them [227]. This can be done here only very briefly. One can seek for the source of accepted moral responsibilities in the several views of the nature of man. It will be evident that the Roman Catholic leaders have examined these questions with great care and have arrived at firm conclusions. It is interesting to observe that their attitudes on most such questions are remarkably similar to the Jewish. Modern Protestant theological considerations are not very helpful in the present quest.

WORLD RELIGIONS

In primitive, predeistic times, those things that were held sacred were permeated with magical beliefs; thus, many ethical principles have their lowly precursors in tribal customs. One can find parallels in present-day medicine!

In the Greek and Roman views, man was dualistic: he consisted of spirit and body. He was considered unique because of his ability to reason and to formulate general concepts. Reason was identified with God, whereas the body was associated or identified with evil. The body imprisoned the soul. Individuality was not important because it was derived from the body, not the mind. Philosophers held the body in slight regard; thus there was little compassion for and a disregard of the weak, the unwell, the hopelessly ill. A man received a physician's care only if it seemed likely that his state could be improved.

In India, the Hindu's philosophy chose to deny this world and life; the goal was escape from an unreal world. The aim was to avoid harmful acts rather than actively to express compassion and love. In recent years some Hindus have turned toward Western science and the Christian ethic of love in actions as shown, for example, in Gandhi's concern for the social and economic betterment of his people.

Buddhist hospitals in India were established 400 years before the first Christian hospital was founded. Buddha believed in mercy for the suffering, self-discipline, and kindness; nevertheless, the sick man was not of particular value. Kindness was for the benefit of him who grants it, not for him who suffers; a man's primary goal was his own redemption. Mercy helps to free the individual from rebirth and continued suffering, a view very different from the Christian compassion and reverence for life.

Chinese religious ethics are based on a concept of world order; a man's obligation is to reflect this order in his life. The ethical ideal is that of conformity and propriety. China achieved great medical development about the same time as India; it declined some centuries later. The extension of Buddhism to China in the first century A.D. stimulated medical inquiry, but did not lead to the founding of hospitals. Under the influence of Confucius, subjection to authority produced a fatal inertia that turned tradition into a prison. Basic causes of the lack of progress in scientific medicine and the relief of suffering have been described by Garlick as lack of an active ethic and the denial of reality to the physical world in the case of India, worship of the past and submission to an authoritarian ethic in the case of China [227].

The Judeo-Christian view is derived from the Old Testament statements that man was created by God in His image. Both mind and body were so created, and both are good. In this concept, there is no such thing as a good mind and an evil body. The mind can express itself only through the body. The finite nature of man leads to suffering; it is not unreal and is to be relieved.[1] Life is valuable and was created for a valuable purpose. God gave man dominion over other living creatures. In the Christian view, man is unique, with free will, infinitely valuable, in contrast to the indifferent and fatalistic attitudes of Greek and Roman and Eastern religious thought. To the Greek, compassion was *kalon,* a virtue; with the coming of Christianity, however, it became *deon,* a duty. Moral laws then became divine commands, ethical duty a religious requirement.

Earlier mention was made of the possibility that the value of our ethical code is self-evident. It is not self-evident to those who believe in the Marxist ideology, in which the existence of God and the sanctity of life are denied. This ideology covers a third of the

[1] It would be interesting to study the power of placebos in the presence of these several philosophies [18].

world's population. In this view, the only rights a man has are those given him by the state; a healthy state requires healthy individuals. However wrong some of these views are, there is logic in the concept that if man exists for the state the state can dispose of him as it wishes.

ROMAN CATHOLIC VIEWS

Roman Catholic theologians have given sustained examination to moral and ethical issues of every kind. The great sweep of their cumulative thinking concerning experimentation and morals has been expressed best by Pius XII.

On September 14, 1952, Pope Pius XII reviewed the "Moral Limits of Medical Research and Treatment" and there presented the view of the Roman Church. This must represent Christendom, since the Protestant theologians have had so little to say on this subject. With one notable exception, the Roman Catholic and the Jewish views are quite similar. Thus, the Roman view concerning science and morals, with the exception to be noted, can stand for the theologians' view of human experimentation. The Pope made it evident that he was concerned, not with the theoretical or practical limits of medical possibilities, but rather with the limits of moral rights and duties. Thus, his presentation is "moral" rather than technical. In his presentation he made it very clear that he was sympathetic toward the "bold spirit of research [which] incites one to follow newly discovered roads, to extend them, to create new ones and to renew methods."

His discussion is organized about three main principles: (1) the interests of medical science; (2) the interests of the individual patient to be treated; and (3) the interests of the community, the *"bonum commune."*

THE INTERESTS OF MEDICAL SCIENCE

The value of scientific research must not be minimized and may be independent of questions of usefulness. Knowledge as such and the full understanding of any truth are not morally objectionable.

In agreement with this principle, research and the acquisition of new, wider, and deeper knowledge and understanding are in themselves in accord with the moral order. This does not mean, however, that all methods, or even a single method, derived from scientific and technical research offer every moral guarantee. Moreover, it does not mean that every method becomes allowable merely because it increases and deepens our knowledge. Sometimes it is not possible to use a method without injuring the rights of others or without violating some moral rule of absolute value. Even though one envisages and pursues such increase of knowledge for the general benefit of mankind, the method is not admissible morally. It is not admissible because science is not the highest value to which all other orders of value are to be subordinated. Therefore science itself, as well as its acquisitions, must be inserted into the order of values. There are well-defined limits beyond which even medical science cannot venture without violating higher moral rules. For example, the confidential relations between doctor and patient, the right of the patient to the life of his body and the soul with its psychic and moral integrity—these are some of the values that stand above science.

Although one recognizes in the interests of science the true value that the moral law allows man to preserve, increase, and widen scientific knowledge, nevertheless one cannot grant that a doctor's intervention is to be determined by scientific interest without limitations.

THE INTERESTS OF THE PATIENT AS JUSTIFICATION

Basic considerations can be stated in the following form. The medical treatment of the patient requires taking a certain step; some believe that this in itself proves that research is morally legal. An alternative view is that some new method hitherto neglected or perhaps little used will give possible, probable, or even certain results and is therefore worthy of consideration.

Pius XII asks whether anyone can fail to see that truth and falsehood are intermingled in these statements. It is true that in a very large number of cases the interests of the patient do provide moral justification for the doctor's conduct. Here, again, the question concerns the absolute value of this principle, but does this make evident the fact that what the doctor wants to do conforms to the moral law? As a private person, the doctor can take no measure or try any course of action without the consent of the patient. The doctor's only rights or power over the patient are those which the latter gives him, explicitly or implicitly and tacitly. The patient cannot, however, confer rights he does not possess. The decisive point here is the moral permissibility of the patient's right to dispose of himself. Here is the moral limit to the doctor's action taken with the consent of the patient.

The patient is not absolute master of himself, of his body, or of his soul. Therefore, he cannot freely dispose of himself as he pleases. The reason for which he acts is of itself neither determining nor sufficient. The patient has the right, limited by natural finality, to use the faculties and powers of his human nature. He is a user and not a proprietor; he does not have unlimited power to destroy or mutilate his body or its functions. Nevertheless, in line with the principle of totality, the patient can, by virtue of his right to use the services of his organism as a whole, allow individual parts to be destroyed or mutilated to the extent required for the good of his being as a whole. He may do this to ensure his being's continued existence or to undo serious and lasting damage that cannot otherwise be avoided or repaired. In the view of the Church, the patient has no right to involve his physical or psychic integrity in medical experiments or research when these entail serious destruction, mutilation, wounds, or perils.

In exercising his right to dispose of himself, his faculties, and his organs, the individual must observe the hierarchy of the orders of values or, within a single order of values, the hierarchy of particular rights insofar as the rules of morality demand. For example, a man cannot perform on himself, or allow doctors to perform, acts of a physical or somatic nature that conceivably could relieve heavy physical or psychic burdens or infirmities, but that at the same time include permanent loss or even considerable and durable reduction of his freedom, that is, of his human personality in its typical and characteristic function. An act of this kind degrades a man to the level of a being who reacts only to acquired reflexes, a living automaton. The moral law does not condone such a reversal of values. In this case, it sets up its limits to the "medical interests of the patient." We can ask where the doctor finds a moral limit in research into and use of new methods and procedures in the "interests of the patient"? His limit is the same as that for the patient. It is fixed by the judgment of sound reason, set by the demands of the natural moral law. The limit is the same for the doctor as for the patient because, as already stated, the doctor as a private individual disposes only of the rights given to him by the patient, bearing in mind that the patient can give only that which he himself possesses.

These remarks can be extended to the legal representatives of the person who is incapable of caring for himself and his affairs. For example, this applies to children below the age of reason, to the feebleminded, and to the insane. These legal representatives can be authorized to act by private decision or by public authority, but they have no rights over the body and life of those they represent other than those people would themselves have if they were capable. The same limits obtain as those described above.

THE INTERESTS OF THE COMMUNITY AS JUSTIFICATION

The moral justification of the doctor's right to try new approaches, new methods, and new procedures invokes a third interest: the interest of the community, of human society, the common good. There is no doubt that such a common good does indeed exist; neither can we question the fact that it calls for and justifies research. The two interests already spoken of—that of science and that of the patient—are very closely allied to the general interest.

For the third time one returns to the question: Is there any moral limit to the medical interests of the community in content or in extension? Are there full powers over the living man in every serious medical case? Can public authority, responsible as it is for the common good, endow the doctor with the power to experiment on the individual in the interests of science and the community in order to discover and try out new methods and procedures when these experiments transgress the right of the individual to dispose of himself? A further question: In the interests of the community, can public authority really limit or suppress the right of the individual over his body and his life and his psychic integrity? In all of this, it is assumed that the scientific questions asked are not trivial, but rather are honest efforts to promote the theory and practice of medicine, not a maneuver serving as a scientific pretext to mask other ends in order to achieve them with impunity.

Concerning these questions, many people have been and are still of the opinion that the answer must be in the affirmative. In order to support their contention, they emphasize their view that the individual is subordinated to the community and that the individual's good must give way to the common good and be sacrificed to it. They hold that the sacrifice of an individual for research and investigation profits the individual in the long run.

The Nuremberg trials exposed a terrifying number of documents testifying to the sacrifice of the individual in the "medical interests of the community." In the record of these trials one can find testimony and reports showing how, with the consent and sometimes even under the formal order of public authority, certain research centers systematically ordered individuals from the concentration camps to be delivered for medical experiments. It is not possible to read these reports without feeling profound compassion for the victims, many of whom went to their deaths.

Is the interest of the individual subordinate to the community's medical interests? Or is there here a transgression, conceivably in good faith, against the most elementary demands of the natural law?

It would be necessary to close one's eyes to reality to believe that one could presently find anyone in the medical world to defend the ideas that gave rise to the facts just stated. To convince oneself of this, it is necessary only to follow for a short time the reports of such medical efforts and experiments. One can only ask himself, who has or who could have authorized any doctor to try such experiments? In the experiments referred to, there is not a word concerning their moral legality. In the cases described at Nuremberg, this is based on error, insofar as the moral justification of the experiments depends on the mandate of public authority, that is to say, on the subordination of the individual to the community, of the individual's welfare to the common welfare. It must be agreed that man's personal being is not finally ordered to be of usefulness to society; on the contrary, the community exists for man.

The Church's view is that God has intended community life to be the means of regulating the exchange of mutual needs and aids that man, in the full development of his personality, requires according to his individual and social abilities. The community, considered as a whole, is not a physical unity subsisting in itself; rather, it is the individual members who are the integral parts of it. The physical organism of living beings, of plants, animals, or man considered as a whole has a unity subsisting in itself. Each of the members of the body—for example, the hand, the foot, the heart, or the eye—is an integral part, destined by all its being to be inserted in the entire organism. It has no finality outside the organism, for it is wholly absorbed by the totality of the organism to which it is attached.

The story is entirely different in the moral community and in every organism of a purely moral character. Here the whole has no unity subsisting in itself, but it does have a simple unity of finality and action. Individuals are merely collaborators and instruments for the realization of the community's common ends.

What about the physical organism concerned? The user of this organism, which possesses the subsisting unity, can dispose directly and immediately of the individual parts, members, and organs within this range of their natural finality. He also can intervene as frequently and to the extent that the good of the whole demands to paralyze, destroy, mutilate, and separate the members. When the whole, on the other hand, has only a unity of finality and action, the public authority doubtless holds direct authority and the right to make demands upon the activities of the parts. However, in no case can it dispose of its physical being, for every direct attempt upon its essence constitutes an abuse of the power of authority.

Medical experiments immediately and directly affect the physical being, either of the whole or of the several organs of the human organism, but the public authority has no power in this sphere. Therefore it cannot pass on to research workers and doctors a non-existent authority. The doctor must receive authorization from the state when he acts upon the organism of the individual "in the interests of the community." He is then acting, not as a private individual, but as a functionary of the public power. The public power, however, cannot pass on a right that it does not possess, except in the cases already mentioned where it acts as a deputy or as the legal representative of a minor for as long as he cannot make his own decision or where it acts on behalf of a person of feeble mind or a lunatic.

With regard to the execution of a condemned man, the state does not deny the individual's right to life. In this case, the public power deprives the condemned man of the enjoyment of life in expiation of a crime by reason of which he has already deprived himself of his right to life.

To return to the principle of totality, this asserts that the part exists for the whole and that the good of the part therefore remains subordinate to the good of the whole. One must respect the principle of totality in itself; to apply it correctly, however, certain premises must be understood. The basic premise is that of clarifying the question of fact. Are the objects to which the principle is applied related to the whole or to its parts? A second premise deals with the clarification of the nature or the extension and the limitation of this relationship. Is the level one of essence or merely one of action, or both? Does it apply to the part only in certain aspects or in all of its relationships? Where it applies, does it absorb the part completely or still leave it a limited finality, that is, a limited independence? The answers to these questions can never be inferred from the principle of totality itself; they must be drawn from other facts and other knowledge. This is affirmed by the very principle of totality, where the relationship of a whole to its part holds; in the exact measure it holds good, the part is subordinated to the whole, and the whole in its own interest can dispose of the part. Too often people ignore these considerations when they invoke the principle of totality. This is true, not only in the field of theoretical study and the field of application of law, sociology, physics, biology, and medicine, but also in the fields of logic, psychology, and metaphysics.

It is obvious that the application of new methods to living man must be preceded by research on cadavers or experimentation on animals. Sometimes, of course, this procedure is impossible, insufficient, or not feasible from a practical point of view. In such a case, medical research must work on its immediate object, the living man, in the interests of science, in the interests of the patient, and in the interests of the community. Nevertheless, the limitations established by moral principles must be borne in mind. One cannot ask that any danger or risk be excused before giving moral authorization to the use of new methods; that would exceed human possibilities and would paralyze serious scientific research, and not infrequently be to the detriment of the patient. In such cases, the weighing of the danger must be left to the judgment of the tried and competent physician. As the foregoing explanation has shown, however, there is a degree of danger not condoned by morality. In questionable cases when means already known have failed, it sometimes happens that a new method as yet insufficiently tried offers, with dangerous elements, appreciable chances of success. If the patient gives his consent, the use of such a procedure is lawful, but this way of acting cannot be upheld as a line of conduct in ordinary cases.

Some may object that the ideas set forth here present a serious obstacle to scientific research and work. In this respect, the field of medicine cannot differ from other fields of mass research. The great moral demands force the impetuous flow of human thought and will into certain channels. They increase the flow in efficiency and usefulness. They dam it so that it does not overflow and cause ravages that can never be compensated for by the good it seeks. Moral demands are a brake; they contribute to the best that man has produced for science, the individual, and the community. So ends the exposition of the Roman Catholic view as expressed by Pius XII.

Some amplifying points of view have been expressed by Father Lynch [287]. Medical experimentation, of course, envisages two main purposes: (1) diagnostic and therapeutic benefit for the individual patient and (2) benefit to science in general. Thus, two distinct moral problems exist. The first is more easily solved than the second, although the first can present difficulties as, for example, when there is a "standard" treatment situation. There is the further desire to go beyond or to improve upon this, certainly necessary if progress is to be made. This is attended by a considerable number of moral pitfalls. In connection with this problem one can say that if a proved remedy would entail exceptional expense, pain, uncertainty, or other inconvenience, a patient may be justified in choosing instead a procedure whose effectiveness is not yet completely established, but that has circumvented the considerable disadvantage one might suppose to be inherent in the proved procedure. The patient, in other words, may legitimately run the risk, even though it be considerable, of a less certain remedy if there is sufficient serious reason for him to do so.

The second purpose is more complex. Two fundamental philosophical truths—not exclusively Roman Catholic, although they have repeatedly been stated authoritatively by the Roman Church—are, first, denial of that extremist attitude that can be identified as totalitarian wherein the individual would be subjected to the community or state by subordinating all individual rights to the prior claim of what has been called the common good. This is totalitarianism. The second principle denies what might be called extreme individualism. It imposes certain fundamental limitations on one's right to dispose of one's bodily members or one's own life. There is dignity in one's human nature, and man thus enjoys a large measure of independence from his equals, from his fellow men. Nevertheless, he must admit his essential dependence on his Creator. Thus, as already emphasized, man is not complete and absolute master of his life and being. He is not a proprietor of himself, but is instead "a steward entrusted with the care of 'property' which belongs solely to God." There is clearly the natural law against suicide. This is not to deny that there are circumstances under which a man is justified in risking his life by actions that are necessary for the achievement of some great good. If in this situation death occurs, it is an unintended by-product of an act legitimately performed for another purpose and is not morally evil. Even if one were to deal with the laudable purpose of the advancement of medical science, no one would be justified in making his own death the intended means to that end.

Both Pius XI and Pius XII affirmed the principle that man is responsible to God, not only for life itself, but also for his physical integrity. Only within certain limits may he legitimately mutilate his body or suppress its natural functions. Implicit in these statements is the concession of a limited right of self-disposition. Just how far a man may go in this direction is still a matter for speculation among theologians. In the principle of totality as expressed in the foregoing by Pius XII, one can find justification for legitimate destructive surgery when this is necessary for preservation of the whole; one can find equal condemnation of unnecessary surgery.

Let us return to our main theme. In investigative procedures designed exclusively for the benefit of mankind, the more pertinent question concerns the ordination, if any, of our bodies and members to the good of our fellow man. One should observe here that the term used is "ordination" and not "subordination," for to admit subordination would logically lead to corollaries of an inadmissible totalitarian character. At the same time, it would seem to be theologically evident beyond doubt that the principle of charity —that is, love of one's fellow man—does legitimize a certain degree of bodily self-sacrifice for altruistic motives. In the Roman Catholic view it is quite permissible, for sufficient reason, to carry out blood transfusions, skin grafts, and organ transplants. Indeed, such donors have been singled out for explicit commendation in Papal documents. In fact, many moralists of high standing have vigorously defended some forms of organ transplantation from a living donor, with no qualifications beyond those that good medical practice would indicate. Finally, while one may never intend his own death as a means of saving another's life, it is unquestionably permissible deliberately to perform an heroic act with two immediate consequences: the saving of another's life and the unintended, but in the circumstances inevitable, loss of one's own. In none of these instances does any bodily benefit accrue to the donor subject—quite the opposite, especially where the sacrifice of an organ and risk to life are concerned.

Clearly, Pius XII's "immanent teleology" of our corporal being does allow a certain ordination for the benefit of others. In experimental medicine it is also plain that as the clear need for investigative procedures becomes evident and urgent, one is morally justified in submitting to considerably more than a little risk to bodily integrity or even to life. The problem is where to draw the line. The moralist, like a good physician, must weigh all aspects of individual situations to decide whether there is sufficient reason to justify the risk in the contemplated procedure.

To aid in a decision as to the morality of experimentation not planned to benefit the subject, Lynch has stated three generic norms [287]. (1) When bodily damage and risk are insignificant, there is no reason to object to the proposed procedure. (2) There is no right to consent to an experimental procedure that entails certain death. Although Lynch suggests that a criminal condemned to death might legitimately choose this form of execution, there are grave reasons for denying this possibility, as we have indicated on page 76. (3) In the great intermediate area where the danger to health or life may range from moderate to very serious, the maximum limit of permissible risk is not yet sharply defined.

There is a remarkable similarity in the Roman Catholic and Jewish attitudes toward the moral and ethical problems encountered in human experimentation, although there exists a startling exception, a restriction by the Jewish theologians, to be discussed later. The similarity is doubtless derived from a common Judeo-Christian heritage. Characteristically, as mentioned, the Roman Catholics have delved deeply into these matters and have clearly stated their position. There is, of course, less uniformity of view amongst the Jewish theologians, since these derive from a considerable number of sects.

JEWISH VIEWS [2]

The total Jewish position is based upon the assumption that all of the divine commandments, as presented in Leviticus 18:5, were intended that man might live by them. The saving of a life, the *pikuah nefesh,* holds priority over all other divine commandments. It abrogates all other commandments except murder, such sexual sin as incest and adultery, and idolatry [373]. The authority, Rabbi Ishmael (Folkman), disagreed with his colleagues and held that even the law against idolatry might be suspended by the need to save a life, if it was done privately; however, if an act of public idolatry were required, a Jew should choose martyrdom. So long as the three prohibitions are observed, the view of Judaism is that any medical practice designed to save a life is in accordance with Jewish law.

Priority in medical experimentation given to *saving* life and not to the advancement of science would come under the general view just described. Rabbinic authorities do not object to medical or surgical procedures that would not harm the patient or that would be expected to leave him no worse off than he would have been if they had not been used. Obviously, patient care enjoys a higher priority than pure science in the Jewish ethical system. This is consistent with the Hippocratic Oath and other dicta, "Above all, no harm!" The concept of a "controlled experiment" is utterly foreign to the rabbinic authorities. Folkman and Guttmann have given particular consideration to these matters and have pointed out that the ancients did not, any more than we ourselves do, know exactly what the results of any medical or surgical procedure might be; all of their efforts in this field were experimental.

[2] I must acknowledge at once my great indebtedness to Professor Irving M. Levey, to Jerome D. Folkman, Ph.D., D.D., Rabbi, and through him, to Professor Alexander Guttmann. Especially I am indebted to the report of the Committee on *Judaism and Medicine* of the Central Conference of American Rabbis, which presents the current position of Reform Judaism, as I understand it.

Taking into account this framework, one can state that the ethical limit of experimental medicine would be the point at which harm to the patient might exceed the consequences of no treatment at all. This presupposes that the goal is diagnosis or therapy and leaves untouched the difficult question of experimentation, not for the specific benefit of the subject involved but for patients in general, that is, for science and society. It is evident that patient care has priority over scientific research; this is a basic ethical principle of modern Jewish life.

Folkman and Guttmann have grappled with the problems that stem from the use of a placebo on a control group in a medical investigation. No prior authoritative Jewish statement on this subject exists. They have formulated the following point of view. An experimental drug may be used in man if the probabilities are that he will be helped rather than harmed and if the possibility of harm is less than the results to be expected if no treatment is given. The problem is more difficult when a placebo is to be employed. In their view, the use of a placebo entails *g'nevat dat,* usually translated as deception, which literally means "theft of knowledge"—a violation of the Eighth Commandment, "Thou shalt not steal." One wonders if these theologians may be unaware that a placebo is not "nothing," but rather, a very powerful therapeutic tool, perhaps half or more as effective in controlling severe pain as a large dose of morphine [18]. Surely, there is no requirement, as mentioned earlier, to use always the most powerful therapeutic agent, with its customarily greater entailment of harmful side effects. It would be interesting and perhaps informative to debate the matter. It has been suggested that if the subjects were told that half would receive an experimental drug and half a placebo, this would not constitute *g'nevat dat,* deception. It might, however, skew the results and give a false or imperfect answer; it might lead to self-deception, a less than admirable state.

Earlier reference was made to a startling restriction of medical experimentation or practice. Jewish authorities agree that tissues or organs may be removed from a dead person and transplanted to a survivor, but "This does not apply to the donation of an organ to a living person by another living person no matter how close the relationship" [351], for this would constitute an act of mutilation of the living donor, strongly forbidden in Jewish law [351]. Thus, the highly successful transplantation of a kidney between identical twins is forbidden.[3] To a layman, this violates the Jewish injunction that saving a life, the *pikuah nefesh,* holds priority over all other divine commandments. It also can be construed as violation of the principle of totality: a gangrenous leg may be amputated to save a life. In the identical twin transplant situation, it has been well established by many physicians and also by the decision of the Supreme Judicial Court of Massachusetts that the well twin, if denied the right to save the life of his brother by the donation of a kidney, could suffer irreparable psychological damage. The well twin would lose a kidney, but would at the same time receive spiritual gain, and his mental health would be preserved—the principle of totality.

Very like the Roman Catholic view, the Central Conference of American Rabbis cannot condone the hastening of death, but at the same time they do not see any virtue "in prolonging life when it has become nothing more than a biological process." In such cases, "death may be allowed to come." The moral right of a suffering patient to die peacefully and with dignity is recognized when there is no hope of a restoration of his spiritual and intellectual life. Euthanasia, however, is contrary to the spirit and teaching of Judaism.

A NOTE ON SCIENCE AND ETHICS

Only one aspect of science and ethics will be considered here; for a larger view, see Glass [179]. Perhaps a sounder title for this section would be "Science versus Ethics." There is the point of view that science can only measure without dealing with values; on the other hand, there are those who believe that science is concerned

[3] Some rabbis deny this; yet the Report [351] of the Central Conference of American Rabbis was utterly clear on this point as recently as 1965, under the chairmanship of Rabbi Jerome D. Folkman.

not only with measurements, but also with value judgments. It is rather clear, as one examines the arguments, that the dispute between the two camps is not likely soon to be settled, for the adherents of one view invoke teleology, while the others believe that an understanding of "Darwinism" will reveal the proper answer. Prejudice and one's orientation—discipline and background—appear to weigh heavily in a given individual's assessment. There may be some usefulness in taking a brief look at the propositions advanced, for the subject is certainly pertinent to the theme of this book. Some relevant concepts can be set down, but it would be presumptuous for this writer to attempt a truly philosophic examination of the matter, which must be left to the philosophers.

SOME GENERAL PROPOSITIONS

1. In determining what constitutes our ethical concerns, the role of religion is declining and the influence of science is increasing.

2. Scientists must participate in defining and determining the ethical base of the work done.

3. There is a great deal of evidence to show that medical science has influenced medical ethics. A recent Ciba symposium offered many illustrations of this [430]. A specific example is the propriety of using a well twin as a kidney donor. It was agreed that the operation on the donor was not therapy, that it was not making a sick person well but a well man sick, but that it was nevertheless morally acceptable [317]. As another example is that study of the use of prisoners will finally determine the proper ethical degrees of freedom for future experimentation in that area. In still another example, however ill-advised it may have been in concept and in practice to utilize animal tissues in transplantation into man, the ethical motivation—the wish to spare human donors—is understandable.

4. There is an inseparable link between science and values. Ethics must be taken into account in determining the limitations of our scientific activities, and science must be considered in determining our ethical freedoms.

5. It has been said that science has no ethical basis, that it is no more than a cold, impersonal way of arriving at the objective truth about natural phenomena. One can challenge this view on the basis that by examining critically the nature, origins, and methods of science one may "logically arrive at a conclusion that science is ineluctably involved in questions of values, is inescapably committed to standards of right and wrong, and unavoidably moves in the large toward social aims" [179]. Glass has skillfully argued that there *is* a scientific basis for making ethical decisions: one has only to follow the Darwinian principle of survival through natural selection from the subcellular level all the way up through organs and individuals and into the community. Science "is also man's means of adjustment to nature, man's instrument for the creation of an ideal environment. Since it is pre-eminently an achievement of social man, its primary function is not simply that of appeasing the individual scientist's curiosity about his environment—on the contrary it is that of adjusting man to man, and of adjusting social groups in their entirety to nature, to both the restrictions and the resources of the human environment."

Glass contends that science itself is ". . . an evolutionary product and a human organ produced by natural selection . . ." He does not hold the view that either the processes or concepts of science are strictly objective. "They are as objective as man knows how to make them, that is true; but man is a creature of evolution, and science is only his way of looking at nature. As long as science is a *human* activity, carried on by individual men and by groups of men, it must at bottom remain inescapably subjective."

"Science is ultimately as subjective as all other human knowledge, since it resides in the mind and the senses of the unique individual person." Glass holds that sentences constructed with "is" usually have a verifiable meaning; those constructed with "ought" never have. One may observe that failure to act is in itself a choice. The writer's prejudice is clearly indicated in the foregoing propositions.

Bentley [34] believes that to consider science in the determination of ethical considerations is a "will-o'-the-wisp," for, he argues, you cannot derive an "ought" from an "is." He believes that science, in establishing facts, does not thereby give knowledge of what should or should not be done. To make this transition one needs teleology: ". . . if you are convinced," he says, "that the developing universe disclosed by science has an ascertainable purpose, then you begin to get a standard by which to judge good and bad. But the actual decision involves something science cannot supply, concerned as it is with the measurable and not with values."

Platt argues with Glass that science is at once concerned with values in the Darwinian approach [347]. He points out that the ethics of human sexual behavior are founded on the fact that human infants mature slowly and that this is, indeed, the basis of our monogamous society. Bentley rebuts this by accepting it as the factual basis, but he insists that the valuation of monogamy involves something more. In Platt's view, valuation is shown in our survival, while Bentley insists that generally speaking our survival is good, but that value judgment is not derived alone from the facts before one. It seems unlikely that the two viewpoints will soon be reconciled.

SOME LIMITING PROPOSITIONS

To turn to an easier problem, the following views may be set down.

1. New procedures are necessarily experimental. The investigator's judgment is an act of faith; he relies on his conscience. When a modicum of success is achieved and others wish to follow the new scientific lead, the supporting agency is confronted with an ethical problem. It is clear that it must make value judgments, *for* one experimental team and *against* another in the pioneer days. Limitations are thus imposed [212].

2. Professional organizations have an obligation to express their views on these matters and to insist forthrightly that complex pioneer work should be carried out only at designated centers; as Himsworth says [212], "a 'free-for-all' is professionally unethical

and should not be allowed." In this connection, see the statement of the Board of Medicine of the National Academy of Sciences concerning heart transplants, 1968, page 306.

3. The profession is responsible for the acts of its members. Kilbrandon holds that this requirement is no more unreasonable than the establishment of educational standards for its members [250].

"STATISTICAL" MORALITY

Socrates: Genuine knowledge pertains only to universals.
Bacon: Philosophy discards individuals.

At the Dartmouth conference on "The Great Issues of Conscience in Modern Medicine" of 1960, Warren Weaver described statistical morality [422] as derived from "the prejudice against even permitting any one known specific individual to sacrifice his life for the common good," and yet "we have to, in a great many circumstances, submit a lot of individuals to a partial risk" with the result that even though "the risk is only one in a million, when a million are involved, one man will be dead with our acquiescence. . . . It is a comfort to our conscience that we don't know *where* it occurred or *when* it occurred. But that individual is just as dead as though we knew all about it." In such deep waters we strive for balance, but sometimes emerge with little more than questions and tangled arguments.

For example, in discussing new and uncertain risk against probable benefit, Adrian spoke of the increase in Britain of mass radiography of the chest [2]. Four and a half million examinations were made in 1957. It has been calculated that while the effects of the radiation on bone marrow might possibly have caused as many as 20 cases of leukemia in that year, nevertheless the examinations revealed 18,000 cases of pulmonary tuberculosis needing supervision, as well as thousands of other abnormalities. Although the 20 deaths from leukemia were only a remote possibility, Lord Adrian asks: if they were a certainty, would they have been too high a price to pay for the early detection of tuberculosis in 18,000 people?

One can see some fascinating similarities and equally fascinating differences when comparisons are made between the attitudes and goals of those whose concern is accident law, on the one hand, and those involved in human experimentation, on the other hand. Calabresi has made penetrating studies in this area [57]. For example, the issue in medical experimentation is the risking of lives to save other lives, but almost always in accident law the issue is loss of life because prevention costs too much, is too much trouble, or interferes with the pleasure of many; here again, considerations of statistical morality are evident. Calabresi points out that grade crossings cost a certain number of lives each year. These deaths could easily be prevented, but the cost of eliminating all such crossings is simply "too much." He continues: automobiles cost 50,000 lives each year and most of these could doubtless be saved if slower and less transportation were accepted, but that the cost in terms of pleasure and profit would be "too high." Automobiles are driven on relatively cheap, but also relatively dangerous, tires. Other risky economies are condoned until the missionary zeal of a Nader calls attention to the fact that the automobile is unsafe at any speed. In other words, "our commitment to human life is not, in fact, as great as we say it is; our commitment to life-destroying material progress and comfort is greater."

When the consideration is a faceless number in jeopardy, even if that number is known to be large, the matter is often treated with indifference; as Calabresi remarks, "Somehow a man is less a man to us when he is simply a number." If the situation involves a specific man trapped in a coal mine, however, no cost or effort is spared to rescue him, for "We know the man trapped in a coal mine, just as we often know the patient subjected to experimentation; the statistical accident victim we do not know—so we can ignore him." Thoughtful people must have known for a long time that health and life are sometimes lost in medical experimentation, but very little was said publicly about the matter. It was only when live cancer cells were injected into 22 *specific*, sick and elderly patients without their knowledge and when I [28] at about the same time, quite by coincidence, presented a 10-year study of ethics in medical experimentation, giving *specific* examples, that a considerable public furor occurred.[4] No such furor arose during the preceding decade when I not infrequently spoke and wrote in general terms on the same subject. The somewhat extreme reaction of praise by some and condemnation by others occurred only when I dealt with specific examples.

To return to Calabresi's analysis of the situation, there appears to be "a deep conflict between our fundamental need constantly to reaffirm our belief in the sanctity of life, and our practical placing of some values (including future lives) above an individual life." How can we resolve this conflict? Several factors must be incorporated into any satisfactory resolution; these can be suggested tentatively. Perhaps man is not very much interested in mankind in general; he cannot relate to many people, but *can* identify himself with a single individual. Another, quite different, ingredient in any understanding of the problem surely is the fact that accidents are the result of chance, carelessness, or such factors beyond control as the unseen crack in the axle, whereas human experimentation involves risk deliberately taken.

When many accidents occur as a consequence of some particular situation, restrictive, hopefully corrective, law is applied, sometimes with half-way measures such as warning devices at grade crossings, in place of corrective elimination. Restrictive law has not

[4] Two or three other rather more obvious factors were doubtless in part responsible for this disturbance. When the results of the 10-year study were first presented at the Brook Lodge Conference on Problems in Clinical Research of March 22, 1965 [51], a press conference was immediately called by two medical colleagues to refute my study. The two colleagues were allowed to make prepared statements; I was not. The conference was abruptly terminated after the two colleagues had made their statements. The press enjoys a disagreement among doctors; they made the most of it. Furthermore, my publication was regarded by a good many colleagues as a breach of medical custom. Still another factor, perhaps the most important, is the comment by many that they felt threatened by this report, that they feared curtailment of their present or future research activities. Some certainly disliked having attention called to their patently unethical activities in the past. This last "reason" contains its own commentary on the situation.

yet been applied to human experimentation in any very comprehensive way. One of the very few certainties in this complex field is that such restrictions will be imposed if certain abuses such as the case material mentioned in Chap. 4 are not soon corrected. It is probably always a mistake to invoke legal action in any rapidly changing situation such as presently exists in human experimentation. Hopefully, scientists and physicians will be able to correct practices that need correction before coercive and restrictive legislation is imposed.

SITUATION ETHICS

Our purpose, as I hope I have already made clear, is to examine, as well as one can do so briefly, a world in which there are basically only two inhabitants: the investigator and his human subject. In this world there are a number of imponderables, not the least of which is situation ethics, so eloquently described by Joseph Fletcher [161]. If I may be permitted an oversimplification, it is a world in which circumstances alter cases, a pragmatic world in which matters are judged by results. I realize I can easily fall into disfavor with the philosophers. Bertrand Russell has already likened the situation to a bath that heats up so imperceptibly that one knows not when to scream. We should look at one example from the world of experimentation, for we dare not overlook the relevance of the situation to the ethics thereof.

When the wonders of penicillin were new, but recognized, and the supply heartbreakingly meager, a small shipment finally arrived in North Africa during World War II. The hospital beds were overflowing with wounded men. Many had been wounded in battles; many had also been wounded in brothels. Which group would get the penicillin? By all that is just, it would go to the heroes who had risked their lives, who were still in jeopardy, and some of whom were dying. They did not receive it, nor should they have; it was given to those infected in brothels. Before indignation takes over, let us examine the situation. First, there were desperate shortages of manpower at the front. Second, those with broken bodies and broken bones would not be swiftly restored to the battle line even with penicillin, whereas those with venereal disease, on being treated with penicillin, would in a matter of days free the beds they were occupying and return to the front. Third, no one will catch osteomyelitis from his neighbor; the man with venereal disease remains, until he is cured, a reservoir of infection and a constant threat. In terms of customary morality, a great injustice was done; in view of the circumstances, I believe that the course chosen was the proper one.

ENDS AND MEANS

Lasting progress in understanding the problems inherent in human experimentation can come only if one searches out the areas where men of good will differ, where sound principles seem to be in conflict. I have tried from time to time to identify these, for example, the conflict between the rights of the individual and the rights of society. We have now a far more subtle confrontation: ends and means.

A prevalent school of moralists declares that the end does not and will never justify the means. Moore [309] disagrees categorically: "What I wish first to point out is that 'right' does and can mean nothing but 'cause of a good result,' and is thus identified with 'useful': whence it follows that the end always will justify the means, and that no action which is not justified by its results can be right." This is obviously pragmatism. It is also comforting to know that Lao Tsu said long ago that true philosophy is like a pickle on the knee. I think I know what he meant: that it is difficult to keep a balance, that systems are prone to tumble. When the experts so easily harass each other, I am not on safe ground. Since Fletcher has thoroughly convinced me, who earlier thought to the contrary, that *only* the end justifies the means [161], I should like to explain how my conversion came about, for the debate is most relevant to certain basic problems in human experimentation.

If the end does not justify the means, what does? Fletcher answers, "Nothing." Human experimentation without a definite purpose is meaningless; worse, it is unethical. Unless there is an end to serve, action is haphazard: ". . . means without ends are empty and ends without means are blind . . . it is the coexistence of its means and ends that puts it in the realm of ethics." This is no place for a universal: not any end will justify any means. Our concern is greater for the end than for the means; at the same time, however, the means must be "appropriate" to the end. The means used "ought to fit the end, ought to be fitting"; they are not neutral. In the situationist's circumstances-alter-cases view, ". . . *ends* like means, are relative . . . all ends and means are related to each other in a contributory hierarchy . . . *Not only means but ends too are relative,* only extrinsically justifiable. They are good only if they happen to contribute to some other good than themselves."

The usual procedure of self-justification is to say that the progress of science "requires" the experimentation done on the uninformed, unconsenting patient. Some medical editors hold that objection to publication of certain unethical studies "would block progress." These typical remarks have been voiced many times, so often, in fact, that one wonders where the medical schools have failed. Rarely, such remarks are made by men who apparently could not care less about ethical failure. Far more often they are made by young and old who have, owing to failure to consider them, failed to see clearly the issues involved. It is often said that one lives in a materialistic age and in a materialistic world. Considerable numbers of individuals are in the unhappy and untenable position of accepting the results of unethical experimentation while disapproving the means.

If any further example were needed, atomic fission dramatically emphasized the inseparability of science and ethics. We can hardly separate the moral equivalents bound up in means and ends in this area. However, we can, for example, take a pragmatic stand and say with Russell that means are determined by science, whereas ends are set by desire. We can say with Kant that people must always be treated as ends, never as means alone. In Bronowski's view [50], this is "the scientist's ethic, and the poet's, and every creator's: that the end for which we work exists and is judged only by the means which we use to reach it."

Bronowski recalls [50] that at the end of his short life the mathematician and philosopher Clifford had this to say nearly a hundred years ago:

> If I steal money from any person, there may be no harm done by the mere transfer of possession; he may not feel the loss, or it may even prevent him from using the money badly. But I cannot help doing this great wrong towards Man, that I make myself dishonest. What hurts society is not that it should lose its property, but that it should become a den of thieves; for then it must cease to be society. This is why we ought not to do evil that good may come; for at any rate this great evil has come, that we have done evil and are made wicked thereby.

"Dass wir uns ans Schwere halten müssen ist eine Gewissheit die uns nicht verlassen wird."

"That we must seek to do the difficult is a certainty that shall never leave us."

RAINER MARIA RILKE, *Letters to a Young Poet*

Appendix A

Codes

470–360 B.C. *Hippocratic Oath.* (p. 217)

1803 *Percival's Code.* (p. 218)

1833 *William Beaumont's Code.* (p. 219)

1846–1967 American Medical Association Codes (1846, 1847, 1946, 1949, 1958, 1966, and 1967). (p. 221)

1856 *Claude Bernard's Personal Code.* (p. 226)

1946–1949 The *Nuremberg Code.* (p. 227)

1948 *Declaration of Geneva.* The second general assembly of the World Medical Association, Geneva. (p. 235)

1949 *International Code of Medical Ethics.* The general assembly of the World Medical Association, London. (p. 236)

1950 *Wiggers's Code.* (p. 238)

1952 *Resolutions on Disapproval of Participation in Scientific Experiments by Inmates of Penal Institutions.* Adopted by the House of Delegates, American Medical Association. (p. 225)

1954 *Principles for Those in Research and Experimentation.* The general assembly of the World Medical Association. (p. 240)

1955 *Report on Human Experimentation.* Public Health Council of the Netherlands. (p. 241)

1955 *Ethical and Religious Directives for Catholic Hospitals.* Selections related to experimentation on human subjects. The Catholic Hospital Association of the United States and Canada. (p. 245)

1957 *Statement of Principles Involved in the Use of Investigational Drugs in Hospitals.* Approved by Board of Trustees, American Hospital Association. (p. 246)

1958 Article Seven. *Draft Covenant on Civil and Political Rights.* The Third Committee of the General Assembly of the United Nations. Reaffirmed by the General Assembly, 1966. (p. 247)

1962 *Use of Volunteers as Subjects of Research.* Army regulation no. 70–25. Department of the Army, United States of America. (p. 252)

CODES

> These principles are not laws to govern but are principles to guide to correct conduct.
>
> THOMAS PERCIVAL, 1803

> Principles, yes, but not rules . . . principles or maxims or general rules are *illuminators*. But they are not *directors*.
>
> JOSEPH FLETCHER, 1966

No attempt has been made to include the scores of codes that exist; rather, our purpose has been to give examples over the years, in the hope that chronological tracing—except for grouping of the American Medical Association and the Public Health Service's several statements—would show an interesting growth of responsibility on the part of those engaged in experimentation in man. This is clearly so. A further aim has been to give in detail examples of how various groups have faced the great problems common in this field.

In society great effort is made to set down accurately the commitments of one to another. In the business world this is possible and necessary; the instrument is called a contract. In medical practice great difficulties stand in the way of such regulation. In human experimentation the "contractural" problems become enormous. Nevertheless, many attempts have been made to spell out in the form of codes the limitations imposed. Perusal of a considerable number of such codes can be useful in indicating troublesome areas that others have encountered. On the other hand, rigid codes can never anticipate all of the possible contingencies in any given situation and, if trouble arises, an endless vista of possible legal actions opens up. Notwithstanding this, lawyers have been, for whatever reasons—leaving aside cynicism—much more interested in applying codes to given medical situations than scientists, who are better aware of the possible pitfalls in codes than lawyers. In general, lawyers seem to believe that the philosophy of the business contract can be carried over to the scientific. In any case, it would be wrong to assume that documents and codes can ever assume a responsibility that can be borne only by the able and wise and compassionate investigator. Rules will not curb the unscrupulous.

As already mentioned, it is not possible that very many "rules" can be laid down to govern experimentation in man. In most cases these are, if they are rigid, more likely to do harm than good. There is the leeway required for the exercise of sound judgment, without which a code becomes unworkable; there can also be too much leeway, which invites evasion. Cahn puts it [56] clearly: "General propositions do not decide concrete cases . . . universals are futile in human affairs unless someone has sense and judgment to apply them productively, and . . . nothing is altogether 'pure' in this world except perhaps a pure fool."

Such abuses as have occurred are usually, in one's experience, owing to ignorance and inexperience, not to an ambitious and vicious disregard of the patient's rights. The most effective protection for all concerned must be based upon recognition and understanding of the various aspects of the problem. Here are presented the principal examples of "Rules for Investigation in Man" and "Codes for Investigators" that have been offered in the past. Eventually, we must narrow and hopefully close the broad gap, between the law of the land and its interpretation on the one hand and on the other hand scientifically and ethically and morally sanctioned experimentation in man. This legal development can be helpful and directed toward progress, or it can be harmfully restrictive. Which it is to be will be determined by the breadth of understanding we are willing to expend in the complex area of rules and laws.

The basic purpose of most codes is to facilitate a clear understanding between the investigator and the subject of the purposes, the benefits, and the risks involved in a proposed experiment.

HIPPOCRATIC OATH* 470–360, B.C.

I swear by Apollo the physician, and Aesculapius, and Hygeia, and Panacea and all the gods and goddesses, that, according to my ability and judgment, I will keep this Oath and this stipulation—to reckon him who taught me this art equally dear to me as my parents, to share my substance with him, and relieve his necessities if required; to look upon his offspring in the same footing as my own brothers, and to teach them this art, if they shall wish to learn it, without fee or stipulation, and that by precept, lecture, and every other mode of instruction, I will impart a knowledge of the art to my own sons, and those of my teachers, and to disciples bound by stipulation and oath according to the law of medicine, but to none others. *I will follow that system of regimen which, according to my ability and judgment, I consider for the benefit of my patients, and abstain from whatever is deleterious and mischievous.* I will give no deadly medicine to anyone if asked, nor suggest any such counsel; and in like manner I will not give to a woman a pessary to produce abortion. With purity and holiness I will pass my life and practice my art. I will not cut persons labouring under the stone, but will leave this to be done by men who are practitioners of this work. Into whatever houses I enter, I will go into them for the benefit of the sick, and will abstain from every voluntary act of mischief and corruption; and, further, from the seduction of females or males, of freemen and slaves. Whatever, in connection with my professional practice, or not in connection with it, I see or hear, in the life of men, which ought not to be spoken of abroad, I will not divulge, as reckoning that all such should be kept secret. While I continue to keep this Oath unviolated, may it be granted to me to enjoy life and the practice of the art, respected by all men, in all times! But should I trespass and violate this Oath, may the reverse be my lot!

Comment. Since only physicians can accept the responsibility for most human experimentation, beyond the simplest procedures, the Oath of Hippocrates has been a basic guide: the physician agrees to work to the best of his ability for the good of his patients and to "abstain from whatever is deleterious and mischievous." "Life is short and the art long, the occasion instant, experiment perilous, decision difficult." (Hippocrates, *Aphorisms*)

* "The . . . physician's oath, the earliest and most impressive document in medical ethics, is not usually regarded as a genuine Hippocratic writing, but is thought to be an ancient temple oath of the Asclepiads" [175].

PERCIVAL'S CODE, 1803

Whenever cases occur, attended with circumstances not heretofore observed, or in which the ordinary modes of practice have been attempted without success, it is for the public good, and in especial degree advantageous to the poor (who, being the most numerous class of society, are the greatest beneficiaries of the healing art) that *new remedies* and *new methods* of *chirurgical treatment* should be devised. But in the accomplishment of the salutary purpose, the gentlemen of the faculty should be scrupulously and conscientiously governed by sound reason, just analogy, or well authenticated facts. And no such trials should be instituted, without a previous consultation of the physicians or surgeons, according to the nature of the case.

Comment. Thus it was evident 166 years ago that the growth of medicine required "new remedies" and "new methods" and that departure from established custom must take place only when "scrupulously and conscientiously governed by sound reason, just analogy, or well authenticated facts," and that the innovator must, prior to the study, consult with his peers. Echoes of all of these points are present in the most up-to-date codes.

WILLIAM BEAUMONT'S CODE, 1833

In a very real sense, Beaumont's studies (1822–1833) of Alexis St. Martin led to a clear delineation in his work of a fundamental code [425]. This is the oldest American code; personal though it was, it set a high standard for subsequent statements.

1. There must be recognition of an area where experimentation in man is needed (study of the functions of the stomach, for example).

2. Some experimental studies in man are justifiable when the information cannot otherwise be obtained.

3. The investigator must be conscientious and responsible. ("I have availed myself of the opportunity afforded . . . from motives my conscience approves.")

4. A well-considered, methodical approach is required so that as much information as possible will be obtained whenever a human subject is used. No random studies are to be made.

5. The voluntary consent of the subject is necessary. William Beaumont and Alexis St. Martin even made a legal contract: *

6. The experiment is to be discontinued when it causes distress to the subject. ("Its extraction [gastric juice] is generally attended by that peculiar sensation at the pit of the stomach, termed sinking, with some degree of faintness, which renders it necessary to stop the operation.")

7. The project must be abandoned when the subject becomes dissatisfied.

* Alexis St. Martin made two agreements with William Beaumont [15, 327]. In the first he bound himself for a term of one year to "serve, abide and continue with the said William Beaumont, wherever he shall go or travel or reside in any part of the world his covenant servant and diligently and faithfully . . . submit to assist and promote by all means in his power such philosophical or medical experiments as the said William shall direct or cause to be made on or in the stomach of him, the said Alexis, either through and by means of the aperture or opening thereto in the side of him, the said Alexis, or otherwise, and will obey, suffer and comply with all reasonable and proper orders of or experiments of the said William in relation thereto and in relation to the exhibiting and showing of his said stomach and the powers and properties thereto and of the appurtenances and the powers, properties and situation and state of the contents thereof."

Comment. Wiggers [425] makes this observation: "The ethical principles . . . of William Beaumont gradually grew into an unwritten code consonant with the moral dictates and laws of all civilized countries."

AMERICAN MEDICAL ASSOCIATION CODES, 1846, 1847, 1946, 1949, 1958, 1966, 1967

At the National Medical Conventions held at New York in May 1846, a committee was authorized to prepare a report on medical ethics. This was presented a year later by John Bell, M.D., at Philadelphia in May 1847. This report, resting "on the basis of religion and morality," was concerned principally with the relationships of physicians to each other and to their patients and to the society in which they lived. Only glancing references were made to the obligation "to prevent disease and to prolong life . . . to add to the civilization of an entire people." It was also stated that "The right of free inquiry, common to all, does not imply the utterance of crude hypotheses, the use of figurative language . . . the involution of old truths, for temporary effect and popularity" [32]. "If able teachers and writers, and profound inquirers, be still called for to expound medical science, and to extend its domain of practical application and usefulness, they cannot be procured by intuitive effort on their own part . . . They must be the product of a regular and comprehensive system."

THE AMERICAN MEDICAL ASSOCIATION, 1946

In order to conform to the ethics of the American Medical Association, three requirements must be satisfied: (1) the voluntary consent of the person on whom the experiment is to be performed; (2) the danger of each experiment must be previously investigated by animal experimentation, and (3) the experiment must be performed under proper medical protection and management.

Comment. The difficulties of obtaining valid consent have been described elsewhere (page 18). Item (2) could hardly be adhered to in psychological studies, for example, or in a study of disease not present or producible in an animal.

THE AMERICAN MEDICAL ASSOCIATION, 1949

In 1949, the American Medical Association presented the graduates in medicine of that year a booklet, *Principles of Medical Eth-*

ics. Nothing is said in it about research or experimentation in man. This stands in contrast to the brief statement on ethics made a hundred years earlier. One can speculate whether the present omission is oversight or reluctance to acknowledge the existence of a difficult field. Whatever the situation in 1949, the detailed statement of 1966 (to follow) faces up to some of the problems of experimentation.

THE AMERICAN MEDICAL ASSOCIATION, 1966

At the 1966 Annual Convention of its House of Delegates, the American Medical Association endorsed the ethical principles set forth in the 1964 *Declaration of Helsinki* of the World Medical Association concerning human experimentation. These principles conform to and express fundamental concepts already embodied in the *Principles of Medical Ethics* of the American Medical Association.

The following guidelines, enlarging on these fundamental concepts, are intended to aid physicians in fulfilling their ethical responsibilities when they engage in the clinical investigation of new drugs and procedures.

1. A physician may participate in clinical investigation only to the extent that his activities are a part of a systematic program competently designed, under accepted standards of scientific research, to produce data which is scientifically valid and significant.
2. In conducting clinical investigation, the investigator should demonstrate the same concern and caution for the welfare, safety and comfort of the person involved as is required of a physician who is furnishing medical care to a patient independent of any clinical investigation.
3. In clinical investigation *primarily for treatment*
   A. The physician must recognize that the physician-patient relationship exists and that he is expected to exercise his professional judgment and skill in the best interest of the patient.
   B. Voluntary consent must be obtained from the patient, or from his legally authorized representative if the patient lacks the capacity to consent, following: (a) disclosure that the physician intends to use an investigational drug or experimental procedure, (b) a reasonable explanation of the nature of the drug or procedure to be used, risks to be expected, and possible therapeutic benefits, (c) an offer to answer any inquiries concerning

the drug or procedure, and (d) a disclosure of alternative drugs or procedures that may be available.

i. In exceptional circumstances and to the extent that disclosure of information concerning the nature of the drug or experimental procedure or risks would be expected to materially affect the health of the patient and would be detrimental to his best interests, such information may be withheld from the patient. In such circumstances such information shall be disclosed to a responsible relative or friend of the patient where possible.

ii. Ordinarily, consent should be in writing, except where the physician deems it necessary to rely upon consent in other than written form because of the physical or emotional state of the patient.

iii. Where emergency treatment is necessary and the patient is incapable of giving consent and no one is available who has authority to act on his behalf, consent is assumed.

4. In clinical investigation *primarily for the accumulation of scientific knowledge*

A. Adequate safeguards must be provided for the welfare, safety and comfort of the subject.

B. Consent, in writing, should be obtained from the subject, or from his legally authorized representative if the subject lacks the capacity to consent, following: (a) a disclosure of the fact than an investigational drug or procedure is to be used, (b) a reasonable explanation of the nature of the procedure to be used and risks to be expected, and (c) an offer to answer any inquiries concerning the drug or procedure.

C. Minors or mentally incompetent persons may be used as subjects only if:

i. The nature of the investigation is such that mentally competent adults would not be suitable subjects.

ii. Consent, in writing, is given by a legally authorized representative of the subject under circumstances in which an informed and prudent adult would reasonably be expected to volunteer himself or his child as a subject.

D. No person may be used as a subject against his will.

Comment. Item 1. A physician ". . . may participate in clinical investigation only to the extent that his activities . . . produce data which is [are] scientifically valid and significant." Much research, even when soundly motivated and in competent hands, fails to be of significance; thus, a strict reading of Item 1 would designate that work and that investigator as unethical in the given instance. This, of course, is absurd. Item 3, B is weakened by the casual assumption that risks are known and can be communicated. Item 3, B, i is not in accord with the rulings of the Food and Drug Administration, although in the writer's view Item 3, B, i is the sounder. Concerning Items 3, B, ii and 4, B: It is not the view, at this time, of the Massachusetts General Hospital Subcommittee on Human Studies (Ethics) that it is generally advisable, necessary, or wise to obtain consent *in writing* for experimental studies. Item 4, C: It is by no means certain that United States law, if tested, will allow experimentation in children when it is not for their direct benefit. English law does not permit such experimentation. (See page 63 for a discussion of this point.)

This code of the American Medical Association, like nearly all, if not all, other codes slides right over the most difficult questions: Examples: (1) What to do about consent to a new procedure where the hazards are not known? (2) The difficulties in assuring that morality will be preserved are great when a "standard" treatment, i.e., an accepted treatment, is available while a new and untried one promises to be better. To forbid trial of the new would mean that no progress is possible. To go beyond the accepted treatment, if the new is found to have serious hazards, could result in harm to the patient, not only by denying him the standard treatment but also by exposing him to the hazards of the new treatment (see page 90).

"The Blue Sheet" *Drug Research Reports* (1967) says that "the AMA's patient-consent guidelines are tougher on researchers in some ways than the views of the Food and Drug Administration." This report then comments, astonishingly, as though this were news, that the American Medical Association would "make use of subjects against their will explicitly unethical." The writer had supposed, since the Nazi outrages, that such use was universally considered to be unethical.

RESOLUTIONS ON DISAPPROVAL OF PARTICIPATION IN SCIENTIFIC EXPERIMENTS BY INMATES OF PENAL INSTITUTIONS

Adopted by the House of Delegates of the American Medical Association, 1952. [This resolution of disapproval is presented out of chronological sequence, since it is not, strictly speaking, a code, but rather an addendum to the code.]

Whereas, during recent years, numerous medical and scientific experiments and research projects have been conducted partly or wholly in federal and state penal institutions; and

Whereas, volunteers among the inmates of such institutions have been permitted to participate in scientific experimental work and to submit to the administration of untested and potentially dangerous drugs; and

Whereas, some of the inmates who have so participated have not only received citations, but have in some instances been granted parole much sooner than would otherwise have occurred, including several individuals convicted of murder and sentenced to life imprisonment; and

Whereas, the Illinois State Medical Society's delegation to the American Medical Association's clinical session whole-heartedly supports research and progress in the fight against disease but does believe that persons convicted of vicious crimes should not qualify for pardon or early parole in this manner; now therefore be it

Resolved, that the House of Delegates of the American Medical Association express its disapproval of the participation in scientific experiments of persons convicted of murder, rape, arson, kidnapping, treason, or other heinous crimes, and also urges that individuals who have lost their citizenship by due process of law be considered ineligible for meritorious or commendatory citation; and be it further

Resolved, that copies of this resolution be transmitted to the Surgeons General of all federal services, the governors of all states, all officials of state and federal penal institutions and parole boards.

CLAUDE BERNARD'S PERSONAL CODE, 1856

Christian morals forbid only one thing, doing ill to one's neighbors. So, among experiments that may be tried on man, those that can only do harm are forbidden, those that are harmless are permissible, and those that may do good are obligatory.

Comment. These are splendid sentiments, but it is difficult to understand why they are so often quoted. How does one make such distinctions? The harm inherent in an experiment is often not evident at the beginning of its conduct, but is exposed only as the work proceeds. One can not agree that all "harmless experiments are permissible" unless they are properly organized and give promise of value they are unethical. Finally, proof of good may come only after much trial and error. If the investigator has made an honest mistake in judgment and the experiment does not turn out well, careful and responsible though he may have been, is he to be condemned?

THE NUREMBERG CODE, 1946–1949

At the Nuremberg hearings certain kinds of information were gathered concerning the activities of the German experimentalists. This was weighed, discussed, and argued by counsel, resulting in the formulation of a standard under which the prisoners were tried; seven were condemned to death and nine were sentenced to prison. The so-called Nuremberg Code emerged from these events. While the Nuremberg Code is not itself a precedent in the usual legal sense, the conclusions arrived at there are now beginning to assume the aura of established convention. This trend was strengthened when the Charter of the United Nations validated the procedures adopted at the war crimes trials.

The goal of this code was to set down ". . . certain basic principles [that] must be observed in order to satisfy moral, ethical and legal concepts." These principles have already achieved wide acceptance as guides to action. Moreover, in the increasing reference to Nuremberg's Ten Points, one can foresee their adoption by common consent as a form of Western credo for the investigator. This tendency has been somewhat slowed by the emergence of the Declaration of Helsinki, discussed elsewhere. There are reasons for reexamining the propositions advanced in the code. On first reading, they sound simple and to the point, but on reflection one encounters certain difficulties.

1. The voluntary consent of the human subject is absolutely essential. This means that the person involved should have legal capacity to give consent; should be so situated as to be able to exercise free power of choice, without the intervention of any element of force, fraud, deceit, duress, overreaching, or other ulterior form of constraint or coercion; and should have sufficient knowledge and comprehension of the elements of the subject matter involved as to enable him to make an understanding and enlightened decision. This latter element requires that before the acceptance of an affirmative decision by the experimental subject there should be made known to him the nature, duration, and purpose of the experiment; the method and means by which it is to be conducted; all inconveniences and hazards reasonably to be expected; and the effects upon his health or person which may possibly come from his participation in the experiments.

The duty and responsibility for ascertaining the quality of the consent rests upon each individual who initiates, directs or engages in the experiment. It is a personal duty and responsibility which may not be delegated to another with impunity.

2. The experiment should be such as to yield fruitful results for the good of society, unprocurable by other methods or means of study, and not random and unnecessary in nature.

3. The experiment should be so designed and based on the results of animal experimentation and a knowledge of the natural history of the disease or other problem under study that the anticipated results [will] justify the performance of the experiment.

4. The experiment should be so conducted as to avoid all unnecessary physical and mental suffering and injury.

5. No experiment should be conducted where there is an *a priori* reason to believe that death or disabling injury will occur; except, perhaps, in those experiments where the experimental physicians also serve as subjects.

6. The degree of risk to be taken should never exceed that determined by the humanitarian importance of the problem to be solved by the experiment.

7. Proper preparations should be made and adequate facilities provided to protect the experimental subject against even remote possibilities of injury, disability, or death.

8. The experiment should be conducted only by scientifically qualified persons. The highest degree of skill and care should be required through all stages of the experiment of those who conduct or engage in the experiment.

9. During the course of the experiment the human subject should be at liberty to bring the experiment to an end if he has reached the physical or mental state where continuation of the experiment seems to him to be impossible.

10. During the course of the experiment the scientist in charge must be prepared to terminate the experiment at any stage, if he has probable cause to believe, in the exercise of the good faith, superior skill and careful judgment required of him that a continuation of the experiment is likely to result in injury, disability, or death to the experimental subject.

Of the ten principles which have been enumerated our judicial concern, of course, is with those requirements which are purely legal in nature—or which at least are so clearly related to matters legal that they assist us in determining criminal culpability and punishment. To go beyond that point would lead us into a field that would be beyond our sphere of competence. However, the point need not be labored. We find from the evidence that in the medical experiments which have been proved, these ten principles were much more frequently honored in their breach than in their observance. Many of the concentration camp inmates who were the victims of these atrocities were citizens of countries other than the German Reich. They were non-German nationals, including Jews and "asocial persons," both prisoners of war and civilians, who had been imprisoned and forced to submit to these tortures and barbarities without so much as a semblance of trial. In every single instance appearing in the record, subjects were used who did not consent to the experiments; indeed, as to some of the experiments, it is not even contended by the defendants that the subjects occupied the status of volunteers. In no case was the experimental subject at liberty of his own free choice to withdraw from any experiment. In many cases experiments were performed by unqualified persons; were conducted at random for no adequate scientific reason, and under revolting physical conditions. All of the experiments were conducted with unnecessary suffering and injury and but very little, if any, precautions, were taken to protect or safeguard the human subjects from the possibilities of injury, disability, or death. In every one of the experiments the subjects experienced extreme pain or torture, and in most of them they suffered permanent injury, mutilation, or death, either as a direct result of the experiments or because of lack of adequate follow-up care.

Obviously all of these experiments involving brutalities, tortures, disabling injury, and death were performed in complete disregard of international conventions, the laws and customs of war, the general principles of criminal law as derived from the criminal laws of all civilized nations, and Control Council Law No. 10. Manifestly human experiments under such conditions are contrary to "the principles of the law of nations as they result from the usages established among civilized peoples, from the laws of humanity, and from the dictates of public conscience."

Comment. Curran regards this as a legal code [123] It is subject to serious criticism, as are most other codes, because of its bland assumption that consent is there for the asking. Unfortunately, this is not the case. This complex and important matter requires detailed and thoughtful examination, which it will receive elsewhere in the section headed "Consent" (page 18.)

The defense of the defendants at Nuremberg, a number of whom were doctors of medicine, was presented under two heads. It was claimed (1) that the law applied was expressed after the fact of the alleged crime and (2) that the defendants' acts were done under the order of higher authority.

This code attempts to set forth general principles covering human experimentation, which, it is often said, are "universally accepted by civilized men." One wonders why the defense did not make more of the fact that compliance with Rule 1—The voluntary consent of the human subject is absolutely essential—is, in the majority of complex cases, quite unrealizable in any complete sense. A realistic view recognizes that informed consent cannot be achieved unless the subject knows what he is consenting to, something that it is often not possible to know. Thus, one can ask how there can be universal acceptance of something unachievable? The probable answer is that neither defense nor prosecution at the time fully recognized the often insurmountable obstacles to getting completely informed consent.

The second category of defense, that experimentation was carried out on the order of higher authority, was refuted by the declaration, albeit *post hoc,* that "The duty and responsibility for ascertaining the quality of consent rests upon each individual who initiates, directs or engages in the experiment. It is a personal duty and responsibility which may not be delegated to another with impunity."

Article 7 of the Draft Covenant on Civil and Political Rights of the United Nations evolved from the same milieu as the Nuremberg Code; the article says, "No one shall be subjected to torture or to cruel, inhuman or degrading treatment or punishment. In particular, no one shall be subjected without his free consent to medical or scientific experimentation." As Curran has pointed out [123], the Draft Covenant was the only international precept until the World Medical Association in 1964 adopted the Declaration of Helsinki, to be discussed later.

Certain criticisms can be made of the Nuremberg Code. It is said in the elaboration of Rule 1 that the subject should have ". . . sufficient knowledge and comprehension of the elements of the subject matter involved as to enable him to make an understanding and enlightened decision." Of course, this is often impossible. It says further that the experimental subject should have ". . . made known to him . . . hazards reasonably to be expected; and the effects upon his health or person which may possibly come from his participation in the experiment." Unhappily, these are often unknown; when the risk is not known to the investigator, he certainly cannot communicate it to the subject. Some hold that any consent thus obtained is not valid. The section on "Consent" (page 18) will deal with further related difficulties.

Concerning the amplification of Rule 1, reflection also reveals certain difficulties. For one thing, a rigid interpretation of this would effectively cripple, if not eliminate, most research in the field of mental disease, which is one of our two or three greatest medical problems. However, Ivy served as chief medical consultant to the War Crimes Trials and presumably had a hand in formulating the 10 points and has said [226] elsewhere, "The ethical principles involved in the use of the mentally incompetent are the same as for mentally competent persons. The only difference involves the matter of consent. Since mental cases are likened to children in an ethical and legal sense, the consent of the guardian is required." If this was the intention of the Nuremberg Tribunal, it is regrettable that the matter was not explicitly stated. Thus all research on the mentally ill or with children not for their direct benefit would be excluded. So also prohibited would be research on unconscious persons [161a].

Strict observance of Rule 1 casts considerable doubt on the propriety, not only of studying mental disease, but also on the use of placebos, often important to progress in studies where judgment is involved in decision. The essential nature of the inclusion of placebos in much of such work has been discussed elsewhere [18, 20]. Explicit observance of Rule 1 would require detailed explanation to the participating subject, with the inevitable result that he would become self-conscious and introspective. An abundance of evidence in the study of subjective responses has shown that such introspection has given misleading results [20]. The use of placebos in therapy—nearly all therapy involves some experimentation

—occasionally necessary for the guidance of the able, responsible physician as well as the treatment of the patient, could hardly be tolerated under a strict observance of the point in question.

To continue, how is the investigator to draw a practical line in the prior information to be given his patient, between "reasonably to be expected" and possible hazards, when these will often be quite unknown in first experiments?

It is easy enough to say, as Rule 1 does, that the subject ". . . should have sufficient knowledge and comprehension of the elements of the subject matter involved as to enable him to make an understanding and enlightened decision." Practically, this is often quite impossible, as we have seen, for the complexities of essential medical research have reached the point where the full implications and possible hazards cannot always be known to anyone and are often communicable only to a very few informed investigators —and sometimes not even to them, when no one really knows what the hazards may be. Certainly, the full implications of work to be done are often not really communicable to lay subjects. As mentioned in an earlier section, this throws a serious burden on the responsible investigator. Once again, Rule 1 states a requirement very often impossible of fulfillment.

In Rule 2, the phrase "for the good of society" is unsavory. To disclaim "random" experiments could be construed as antagonistic to pilot experiments or against experiments not immediately useful. Rule 2 is vague and frowns on random experiments, yet anesthesia, x-rays, radium, and penicillin, to mention a few products of random experimentation, seem to justify the disallowed approach. Bernard observes that most of the epoch-making discoveries in science have been unexpected [35]. Surely, there is something to be said for the random experiment. This writer, at last, would not know how to define experiments "unnecessary in nature." Doubtless, cardiac catheterization and frontal lobotomy would each have been placed in such a category at the beginning of its use. Perhaps lobotomy would now be so characterized by many, although it would not have been a few years ago.

Ladimer suggests that Rule 2 be revised to read, "The experiment should be such as to yield fruitful results not inconsistent with the moral and legal context of society." It is his belief that the change would remove any totalitarian overtone [263].

In Rule 3, one can ask whether, if the anticipated results fail to justify the performance of the experiment, the investigator has necessarily been guilty of wrong behavior. Who can guarantee the success of any new experiment?

Rule 5 suggests that self-experimentation by the investigator in situations fraught with serious risk may justify the hazardous undertaking. This will hardly withstand scrutiny. As I have pointed out elsewhere, serious risk can rarely be taken properly except where the subject's illness requires it and where he promises to profit from it himself. If an experiment is morally wrong, it will not be made right by the self-experimentation of the investigator. The implication in Rule 5 that it might be justified is bizarre, to say the least.

Rule 5 has been criticized by Welt [423] as follows:

> It is not clear whether this rule means that such studies may be performed only with the experimentalist as the subject; or whether the fact that the investigator is willing to serve as the subject makes it permissible to use lay subjects as well. One could argue with either interpretation. If the intent is the former, one might legitimately raise the question as to whether lay subjects who are capable of consent of a high quality should not have the same opportunities for risk should they want them. If the latter interpretation is correct the rule is unacceptable because the motivation of the investigator may be overpowering and lead him to an erroneous or, at least, quite different value judgment than that which might apply to the lay subject. In contrast one might more justifiably state that a minimal requirement of any experiment should be the willingness of the investigator to serve as a subject.

Rule 6 says clearly that ends must justify means. If this amounts to a balancing of interests where the subject himself stands to profit, it may be allowed, as just mentioned in the discussion of Rule 5. This has been considered further in the chapter on legal aspects. In any case, the final evaluation of the results of experimentation are often not immediately apparent.

As Curran has pointed out, the most serious *legal* issue in the Nuremberg Code is the problem of justification of a given experimental study [123]. There is, throughout the entire subject of human experimentation, a concern for human rights and human dignity; it is inevitable that at times this comes in conflict with concern for curing the ills of mankind. Experiment is indeed perilous and decision difficult.

Telford Taylor, who served as chief counsel for the War Crimes Trials, says [303] of the 10 points derived from the Nuremberg Trials ". . . the judgment lays down ten standards to which physicians must conform." Must? Most investigators would do so if only they knew how to comply.

These comments are by no means intended to scoff at this valiant effort to codify permissible experimentation in man. Rather, they are intended to indicate, more clearly than the 10 points do, how difficult it is to be precise in this field.

DECLARATION OF GENEVA

The Second General Assembly of the World Medical Association, Geneva, Switzerland, September, 1948

PHYSICIAN'S OATH

Now being admitted to the profession of medicine I solemnly pledge to consecrate my life to the service of humanity. I will give respect and gratitude to my deserving teachers. I will practice medicine with conscience and dignity. The health and life of my patient will be my first consideration. I will hold in confidence all that my patient confides in me. I will maintain the honor and the noble traditions of the medical profession. My colleagues will be as my brothers. I will not permit considerations of race, religion, nationality, party politics, or social standing to intervene between my duty and my patient. I will maintain the utmost respect for human life from the time of its conception. Even under threat I will not use my knowledge contrary to the laws of humanity. These promises I make freely and upon my honor.

INTERNATIONAL CODE OF MEDICAL ETHICS

The General Assembly of the World Medical Association, London, England, 1949

"As ye would that men should do to you, do ye even so to them," is a Golden Rule for all men. A Code of Ethics for physicians can only amplify or focus this and other golden rules and precepts to the special relations of practice. As a stream cannot rise above its source, so a code cannot change a low-grade man into a high-grade doctor, but it can help a good man to be a better man and a more enlightened doctor. It can quicken and inform a conscience, but not create one. Only in a few things can it decree "thou shalt" or "thou shalt not," but in many things it can urge "thou shouldst," or "thou shouldst not." While the highest service they can give to humanity is the only worthwhile aim for those of any profession, it is so in a special sense for physicians, since their services concern immediately and directly the health of the bodies and minds of men.

A doctor must always maintain the highest standards of professional conduct.

A doctor must not allow himself to be influenced merely by motives of profit.

The following practices are deemed unethical:

a) Any self-advertisement except such as is expressly authorized by the national code of medical ethics.
b) Taking part in any plan of medical care in which the doctor does not have complete professional independence.
c) To receive any money in connection with services rendered to a patient other than the acceptance of a proper professional fee, or to pay any money in the same circumstances without the knowledge of the patient.

Under no circumstances is a doctor permitted to do anything that would weaken the physical or mental resistance of a human being except from strictly therapeutic or prophylactic indications imposed in the interest of his patient.

A doctor is advised to use great caution in publishing discoveries. The same applies to methods of treatment whose value is not recognized by the profession.

When a doctor is called upon to give evidence or a certificate he should only state what he can verify.

A doctor must always bear in mind the importance of preserving life from conception until death.

A doctor owes his patient complete loyalty and all the resources of his science. Whenever an examination or treatment is beyond his capacity he should summon another doctor who has the necessary ability.

A doctor owes to his patient absolute secrecy on all which has been confided to him or which he knows because of the confidence entrusted to him.

A doctor must give the necessary treatment in emergency, unless he is assured that it can and will be given by others.

A doctor ought to behave to his colleagues as he would have them behave to him.

A doctor must not entice patients from his colleagues.

A doctor must observe the principles of "The Declaration of Geneva" approved by The World Medical Association.

WIGGERS'S CODE, 1950

Basic Ethical Principles for the Conduct of Human Experiments

1. Human experiments should not be projected until their necessity has been unquestionably established and a feasible humane procedure for their conduct has been formulated.

2. The scientific, ethical, and legal considerations pertaining to contemplated studies on human subjects should, whenever possible, be reviewed and approved by a group of colleagues who will not participate in the investigation. The nature of the experiments and reasons for their performance should be explained.

3. The voluntary consent of the human subject must be obtained.

4. The results for the good of society should be unprocurable by other means, including animal experimentation.

5. The anticipated results, as based on animal experimentation and scientific knowledge of the problems, must justify the performance of the experiment.

6. The experiment should not be random and the degree of risk should never exceed that determined by the humanitarian importance of the problem.

7. All unnecessary physical and mental suffering should be avoided.

8. The investigation should be so conducted that legal liability under malpractice or personal injury laws never comes into question.

9. No experiment should be conducted in which there is an *a priori* reason to believe that death or disabling injury will occur.

10. The subject of the experiments should be protected against even remote possibilities of injury, disability, or death.

11. Experimenters should possess the highest degree of skill and competence, gained whenever possible from previous practice on animals.

12. The human subject should be at liberty to terminate the experiment at any time.

13. The scientist in charge must be prepared to terminate the experiment at any stage if he has probable cause to believe that a continuation is likely to result in injury, disability, or death to the subject.

14. The experimenter should have sufficient experience with apparatus and technique employed to assure other investigators as well as himself that data obtained are accurate and not falsified through experimental errors.

15. Finally, in the case of experiments that seem to involve some risk, the good faith of the responsible investigator would be demonstrated by submitting himself as an experimental subject before using

the experimental technique on volunteers. [Good faith, yes; but such an act will not make an unethical procedure ethical.]

In laboratories of basic science, experimental medicine, and experimental surgery, rules are posted for the proper conduct of experiments performed on animals. The publication of similar rules according to which experiments may be conducted on human subjects might allay any suspicion in the minds of the lay public that human beings are being improperly used for experimental purposes.

PRINCIPLES FOR THOSE IN RESEARCH AND EXPERIMENTATION

The General Assembly of the World Medical Association, 1954

1. Scientific and Moral Aspects of Experimentation
   The word experimentation applies not only to experimentation itself but also to the experimenter. An individual cannot and should not attempt any kind of experimentation. Scientific qualities are indisputable and must always be respected. Likewise, there must be strict adherence to the general rules of respect of the individual.
2. Prudence and Discretion in the Publication of the First Results of Experimentation
   This principle applies primarily to the medical press and we are proud to note that in the majority of cases this rule has been adhered to by the editors of our journals. Then there is the general press which does not in every instance have the same rules of prudence and discretion as the medical press. The World Medical Association draws attention to the detrimental effects of premature or unjustified statements. In the interest of the public, each national association should consider methods of avoiding this danger.
3. Experimentation on Healthy Subjects
   Every step must be taken in order to make sure that those who submit themselves to experimentation be fully informed. The paramount factor in experimentation on human beings is the responsibility of the research worker and not the willingness of the person submitting to the experiment.
4. Experimentation on Sick Subjects
   Here it may be that in the presence of individual and desperate cases one may attempt an operation or a treatment of a rather daring nature. Such exceptions will be rare and require the approval either of the person or his next of kin. In such a situation it is the doctor's conscience which will make the decision.
5. Necessity of Informing the Person Who Submits to Experimentation of the Nature of the Experimentation, the Reasons for the Experiment, and the Risks Involved
   It should be required that each person who submits to experimentation be informed of the nature of, the reason for, and the risk of the proposed experiment. If the patient is irresponsible, consent should be obtained from the individual who is legally responsible for the individual. In both instances, consent should be obtained in writing.

REPORT ON HUMAN EXPERIMENTATION

Public Health Council of the Netherlands, 1955

. . . "Human Experimentation" is defined as any "intervention in the psychic and/or somatic integrity of man which exceeds in nature or extent those in common practice." Such an intervention may be an act either of commission or of omission.

The nature of experimentation is that one or more circumstances are deliberately altered to such an extent that the influence of the alterations can be studied by observation.

It is not the problem nor the experimental character which forms the basis of admissibility of an experiment, but rather the medical actions involved. Hence, the committee's study centered on *medical activities on man*.

Scientific knowledge can be enlarged by observation and experimentation, singly or in combination. Medical evolution has proceeded from its earlier emphasis on observation to a strong modern emphasis on experimentation. Scientific developments may make some, hitherto inadmissible, types of observation recognized under new conditions.

All physicians must, of course, be ever alert to any opportunity to improve or perfect their methods. Experimental activities may be carried out to increase medical knowledge generally, to achieve specific diagnostic or therapeutic results, or to increase the ability and experience of the investigator.

Human experimentation, *per se*, cannot be considered inadmissible. Under proper conditions, it is indispensable to medical progress. An example of this is any diagnostic or therapeutic activity designed to promote or restore the health of a specific patient. On the other hand, diagnostic activities not strictly necessary for identifying the malady may approach the inadmissible. In this connection, the committee warns against "a certain perfectionism" in which the desire for completeness in examination leads the physician into extending the diagnostic experimentation.

When a research project for purely scientific purposes or simply to provide additional experience is undertaken its acceptance is based upon the following criteria:

a. the approval of the subject;
b. risk, pain, or inconvenience and duration of experiment;
c. the standards to be followed.

APPROVAL OF THE SUBJECT

It is generally agreed that if the experiment is not solely, primarily, or to any degree a direct benefit to the subject, his approval is required. This approval should neither be conditioned by idealistic impulses (nurses and medical students); nor by special conditions (prisoners, etc.). Even under ideal conditions, the subject's consent has only relative importance.

However the committee felt that when a physician undertakes "new treatment" on his own patient, the relationship of confidence between physician and patient is in no way violated if the physician increases his knowledge or experience without first informing the patient, with the understanding that recovery is not delayed and there is no detrimental effect.

After all, hospitals exist not only to treat patients, but also to increase medical knowledge and skill. Animal experimentation always [sic] precedes that on humans. The public should understand that the interests of the patients require a certain amount of experimentation.

RISK

"Risk" is defined as "any danger that is greater than the inevitable peril." Surgical procedures inevitably involve a risk, therefore, proper investigation and use of powerful new medicaments cannot be carried out without a degree of inevitable risk to the patient.

A distinction is made between the research expert and the investigator who is also the patient's attending physician. The Committee was of the opinion that "medical activities involving risk to the experimental subject should not be carried on by the practicing physician; the practicing physician who also is the investigator is not the person qualified to objectively judge the risk involved."

When experimentation is conducted in institutions such as homes for children, convalescents or old people, etc., the responsibility must be shared by the attending physician in addition to the investigator.

The Committee recognizes the inherent right of a person to accept a voluntary risk, and the right of the investigator to make use of this attitude to achieve altruistic objectives but ethics must act as a check wherever a great risk is involved. Dangerous experiments are never justifiable if the aim is only advancement of medical knowledge; they must also entail some benefit for humanity. [One would suppose that "advancement of medical knowledge" would "entail some benefit for humanity"!]

The Committee recognized that in time of war or epidemic, dangerous experiments may be justified. However, in normal times, "human experiments involving dangerous risks of life cannot be reconciled with the nature and objective of the medical profession." Hence it recognized that the nature of the problem does not make it possible to have clearly defined standards governing experimentation; "the conscience of the investigator will have to determine the course of conduct" . . . and even the "individual conscience cannot be relied upon unconditionally". . . . For, "scientific experimentations demand from the investigator an objective attitude, a certain distance and restraint toward his object of experimentation which is actually in conflict with the relationship of physician and patient."

STANDARDS

Nevertheless, it is felt that standards should be sought that will govern individual conscience in making decisions; guarantee acceptable scientific procedures; and provide all the precautions necessary.

The Committee recommends the following guarantees and standards:

a. study of relevant publications to avoid unnecessary repetitions of experiments;
b. the physicians conducting experiments should have special knowledge of the problem and be completely responsible;
c. good organization and execution.
d. Every available aid for special or emergency treatment of the experimental subject should be available.

Prior to experimentation the following aspects should be considered

1. Can the experiment wholly or partly, be carried out on animals?
2. What is the minimum requirement to obtain the observation? Is its importance and duration ethically justifiable?
3. What is the minimum requirement in alterating [sic] the conditions of the experiment?
4. Are the requirements for the observation and the alterations of conditions the same?
5. What arrangements are planned? Is the project the fruit of mature thought and expert advice?
6. How will the results be used in obtaining a definite conclusion?

Risk, inconvenience or pain for the subject should be governed by these principles:

a. The investigator's responsibility is more important than the willingness of the subject to accept the conditions.
b. The investigator should consult other experts on the research project in order to intensify the sense of responsibility.
c. The subject must be fully informed and must consent freely.

d. If considerable risk is involved, the experiment is not in accord with the object and purpose of medicine.
e. A practicing physician should not become an investigator on his own patient, if the experiment involves danger. A body of advisers should be consulted. [But desperate situations sometimes require desperate experimental therapy.]
f. Experiments should be discontinued if the subject so desires or if unexpected danger is encountered, activities the consequences of which cannot be undone, and which therefore cannot be discontinued, are therefore disapproved.
g. Any suffering or danger not strictly inevitable must be prevented.
h. Experiments on children; in institutions for children, old people, etc.; on the insane; or on prisoners, which involve dangerous risks, inconvenience or pain are not approved. All experiments on the dying under any circumstances are disapproved.
i. The "utmost restraint" must be exercised in experiments on patients deemed to have an incurable malady, even though they volunteer as subjects. [And thereby possibly deny such patients their one chance to be saved.]
j. Unnecessary examinations should be avoided, and diagnostic activities that may be dangerous are justified only if they result in effective therapy. In routine examinations, new methods that are dangerous should be strictly limited.

To interpret and apply these principles and standards, the Committee recommended establishment of a permanent advisory committee of men experienced in human experimentation.

The Committee feels there has been some deterioration of ethical standards in experimentation which it wants to check, insofar as possible, by preventive and educational measures.

Publication of articles describing human experiments that are contrary to medical ethics is strongly criticized, and it is recommended that medical journals refuse to publish articles based on unethical experiments.

Among the general recommendations of this Committee are:

1. that the Council of The World Medical Association be informed of this report, and
2. that any further revision of "medical ethics" should take this report under consideration for the possible incorporation of some of these recommendations.

This summary of a report submitted to the Netherlands Minister of Social Affairs and Health in 1955 was prepared for the *World Medical Journal* in 1957.

ETHICAL AND RELIGIOUS DIRECTIVES FOR CATHOLIC HOSPITALS

Selections Related to Experimentation on Human Subjects

The Catholic Hospital Association of the United States and Canada, 1955

13. Risk of life and even the indirect taking of life are morally justifiable for proportionate reasons. Life is taken indirectly when death is the unavoidable accompaniment or result of a procedure which is immediately directed to the attainment of some other purpose, e.g., to the removal of a diseased organ.

40. Any procedure harmful to the patient is morally justified only insofar as it is designed to produce a proportionate good.

Ordinarily the "proportionate good" that justifies a directly mutilating procedure must be the welfare of the patient himself. However, such things as blood transfusions and skin grafts are permitted for the good of others. Whether this principle of "helping the neighbor" can justify organic transplantation is now a matter of discussion. Physicians are asked to present practical cases for solution, if such cases exist.

42. Experimentation on patients without due consent and not for the benefit of the patients themselves is morally objectionable. Even when experimentation is for the genuine good of the patient, the physician must have the consent, at least reasonably presumed, of the patient or his legitimate guardian.

48. Unnecessary procedures, whether diagnostic or therapeutic, are morally objectionable. A procedure is unnecessary when no proportionate reason requires it for the welfare of the patient; *a fortiori* unnecessary is any procedure that is contraindicated by sound medical standards. This directive applies especially, but not exclusively, to unnecessary surgery.

STATEMENT OF PRINCIPLES INVOLVED IN THE USE OF INVESTIGATIONAL DRUGS IN HOSPITALS

Approved by Board of Trustees, American Hospital Association, 1957

Hospitals are the primary centers for clinical investigations on new drugs. By definition these are drugs which have not yet been released by the Federal Food and Drug Administration for general use.

Since investigational drugs have not been certified as being for general use and have not been cleared for sale in interstate commerce by the Federal Food and Drug Administration, hospitals and their medical staffs have an obligation to their patients to see that proper procedures for their use are established.

Procedures for the control of investigational drugs should be based upon the following principles:

1. Investigational drugs should be used only under the direct supervision of the principal investigator who should be a member of the medical staff and who should assume the burden of securing the necessary consent.

2. The hospital should do all in its power to foster research consistent with adequate safeguard for the patient.

3. When nurses are called upon to administer investigational drugs, they should have available to them basic information concerning such drugs—including dosage forms, strengths available, actions and uses, side effects, and symptoms of toxicity, etc.

4. The hospital should establish, preferably through the pharmacy and therapeutics committee, a central unit where essential information on investigational drugs is maintained and whence it may be made available to authorized personnel.

5. The pharmacy department is the appropriate area for the storage of investigational drugs, as it is for all other drugs. This will also provide for the proper labeling and dispensing in accord with the investigator's written orders.

ARTICLE SEVEN. DRAFT COVENANT ON CIVIL AND POLITICAL RIGHTS

The Third Committee of the General Assembly of the United Nations, 1958 [The following material has been presented in considerable detail since it emphasizes the difficulties and the necessity of precise use of language in this area.]

3. Article 7 of the draft Covenant on Civil and Political Rights, as submitted by the Commission on Human Rights, reads as follows:

No one shall be subjected to torture or to cruel, inhuman or degrading treatment or punishment. In particular, no one shall be subjected with his free consent to medical or scientific experimentation involving risk, where such is not required by his state of physical or mental health. Reaffirmed by the General Assembly, 1966.

4. The Committee discussed this article at its 847th to 856th meetings.

AMENDMENTS SUBMITTED

5. Amendments were submitted by the Netherlands, Pakistan, the Philippines, Ecuador, Guatemala, Australia and Greece and Italy. Sub-amendments to the revised amendment of Greece and Italy were submitted by Canada and Mexico (see paragraph 14).

6. The amendment of the Netherlands called for the deletion of the words: "involving risk, where such is not required by his state of physical or mental health" from the second sentence.

7. The amendment of Pakistan consisted in replacing the full stop after the words "treatment or punishment" by a comma and in replacing the words "In particular, no one shall be" by the words "or even." At the 854th meeting, the representative of Pakistan withdrew the amendment.

8. The Philippine amendment called for the insertion of the word "unusual" between the words "inhuman" and "or degrading" in the first sentence. The representative of the Philippines withdrew this amendment at the 853rd meeting.

9. The Ecuadorian amendment consisted in the deletion of the words "involving risk" from the second sentence. The representative of Ecuador withdrew this amendment at the 853rd meeting, on the understanding that a separate vote would be taken on the words "involving risk" in the Netherlands amendment.

10. The amendments of Guatemala called for:

(1) The amendment of article 7 to read as follows:

No person shall be subjected to torture or to cruel, inhuman or degrading treatment or punishment.

(2) The insertion of an additional article reading as follows: *Article 8.* No person shall be subjected without his free and spontantous consent to medical or scientific experimentation. Medical experimentation shall not be permitted in the case of a person who is incapable of giving his free and spontaneous consent, unless the main and essential purpose of the experimentation is the restoration of the physical and mental health of the said person and in that case the consent shall be obtained from those persons who in accordance with the law of the country concerned are the legal representatives of the person who is incapacitated from giving his consent.

The subsequent articles were to be renumbered accordingly.

At the 853rd meeting, the representative of Guatemala withdrew these amendments.

11. The Australian amendment called for the replacement of the full stop after the word "punishment" by a comma and the replacement of the text thereafter by the following words: "and in particular no one shall be subjected to such treatment in the form of medical or scientific experimentation."

12. The revised amendment of Greece and Italy called for the replacement of the second sentence by the following: "No one shall, *inter alia,* be subjected without his free consent to medical or scientific experimentation."

13. Canada submitted a sub-amendment to the revised amendment of Greece and Italy replacing the words "No one shall, *inter alia,* be subjected" by the following: *"Inter alia,* no one shall be made to undergo any form of torture or cruel treatment by being subjected." The representative of Canada accepted a suggestion by the representative of Ireland to the effect that the words "inhuman or degrading" should be inserted between the words "cruel" and "treatment."

14. The representative of Mexico re-introduced the original amendment of Greece and Italy, submitting it as a sub-amendment to the revised text. The original Greek-Italian amendment consisted in the replacement of the second sentence of the article by the following text:

> No one shall be made to undergo any form of torture or cruel treatment by being subjected without his free consent to medical or scientific experimentation when such experimentation is not required by his state of physical or mental health.

At the 855th meeting, the Mexican representative withdrew this sub-amendment.

ISSUES DISCUSSED

15. The word "unusual" proposed in the Philippine amendment gave rise to some discussion. It was argued that while cruel, degrading and inhuman treatment or punishment might be "unusual," the converse was not necessarily true. The amendment was supported by some representatives who felt that it might be applicable to certain actual practices which, although not intentionally cruel, inhuman or degrading, nevertheless affected the physical or moral integrity of the human person. On the other hand, it was objected that the term "unusual" was vague. What was "unusual" in one country might not be so in other countries.

16. Most of the discussion centered on the second sentence. Some felt that the sentence was unnecessary, since what it sought to prohibit was already covered by the first sentence. Moreover, it weakened the article in that it directed attention to only one of the many forms of cruel, inhuman or degrading treatment, thereby lessening the importance of the general prohibition laid down in the first sentence. On the other hand, most representatives attached special importance to the second sentence which, they pointed out, was intended to prevent the recurrence of atrocities such as those which had been committed in Nazi concentration camps during the Second World War. In their view the second sentence, far from being superfluous, served to complement the provisions of the first.

17. Several suggestions were made with a view to meeting the objection that the second part of the article was emphasized at the expense of the first. One was to replace the words "in particular" in the second sentence by the words *"inter alia,"* as proposed by Greece and Italy. Others thought that the substance of the second sentence might be embodied in a separate paragraph or, as proposed by Guatemala, in a separate article. However, these proposals were opposed by those who regarded the first and second sentences as closely linked and wished, therefore, to preserve the unity of the article. The amendment of Pakistan sought to resolve the difficulty by combining the two clauses of the article in a single sentence, thereby making the act covered in the second clause an addition to that covered in the first. The main objection to this amendment was that it weakened the second clause. As the debate developed, it became apparent that there was wide agreement that the second sentence should be retained. Some representatives, however, felt that, as drafted, it lacked precision and

clarity. The main problem was how to find a formulation which, while outlawing criminal experimentation, would not hinder legitimate scientific or medical practices. There was general agreement that the Covenant should not attempt to lay down rules concerning medical treatment, as that was a matter which should be left to national legislation and the medical profession.

18. One approach to the problem, exemplified by the Australian amendment, was to limit explicitly the scope of the provision to scientific and medical experimentation which constituted torture or cruel, inhuman or degrading treatment. However, the Australian proposal was opposed on the grounds that, by not referring to "free consent," it failed to provide a satisfactory criterion for determining whether a given experiment was of the prohibited type or not. It was also pointed out that the proposed text sought to cover only experiments of a cruel, inhuman or degrading nature, while permitting other experiments conducted without the consent, or even the knowledge, of the subject.

19. Another approach, proposed by the Netherlands, was simply to eliminate from the text any references to legitimate medical practices. It was pointed out that the term "experimentation" did not cover medical treatment required in the interest of the patient's health. Hence, the clause "where such is not required by his state of physical or mental health" should be deleted, as it only served to confuse the meaning and intent of the provision by implying that medical or scientific practices having the welfare of the patient in view came within its scope. A similar approach was proposed by Greece and Italy in their revised amendment, except that the words "in particular" were to be replaced by *"inter alia."* However, several representatives preferred the term "in particular," since it linked the second sentence to the first more closely, making it clear that what was referred to was medical or scientific experimentation which amounted to torture or cruel, inhuman, or degrading treatment.

20. Some doubts were raised as to the desirability of retaining the words "without his free consent" if the intention of the provision was solely to prohibit criminal experimentation. It was argued that the words were not only redundant, but might open the door to abuses in that it would be possible to justify experimentation of a criminal nature on the pretext that the subject had given his "consent." Such practices should be forbidden even if undertaken with the free consent of the subject. In reply, it was argued that consent given under pressure could never be regarded as "free" consent. It was unthinkable that anyone would freely submit himself to torture or cruel, inhuman, or degrading practices. The introduction of the notion of "free consent" provided not only a safeguard, but also a criterion for determin-

ing whether an experiment was legitimate or not. Certain kinds of treatment became cruel, inhuman or degrading only because they were administered without the subject's free consent.

VOTING ON ARTICLE 7

21. The voting on article 7 and on the amendments thereto took place at the 855th meeting, as follows:
   (a) The Canadian sub-amendment, as orally amended, was rejected by 40 votes to 12, with 15 abstentions.
   (b) After a request by the representative of the Philippines for a separate vote on the words "without his free consent" had been rejected by 46 votes to 4, with 14 abstentions, the revised amendment of Greece and Italy was rejected by 37 votes to 18, with 10 abstentions.
   (c) The Australian amendment was rejected by 40 votes to 15, with 11 abstentions.
   (d) At the request of the representative of Ecuador, the Netherlands amendment was put to the vote in parts. It was decided, by 41 votes to 8, with 16 abstentions, to delete the words "involving risk" from the text of article 7. It was decided, by 25 votes to 21, with 8 abstentions, to delete also the remaining words "where such is not required by his state of physical and mental health."
   (e) Article 7, as amended, was voted on in parts, as follows:
      (i) The first sentence was adopted unanimously.
      (ii) The second sentence, as amended, was voted on by roll-call at the request of the USSR. It was adopted by 39 votes to none, with 29 abstentions . . .
      (iii) At the request of the Ukrainian Soviet Socialist Republic, article 7 as a whole, as amended, was voted on by roll-call. It was adopted by 64 votes to none, with 4 abstentions . . .

TEXT AS ADOPTED

22. Article 7, as adopted by the Committee, read as follows:
No one shall be subjected to torture or to cruel, inhuman or degrading treatment or punishment. In particular, no one shall be subjected without his free consent to medical or scientific experimentation.

USE OF VOLUNTEERS AS SUBJECTS OF RESEARCH

Army Regulation No. 70–25.

Department of the Army, United States of America, 1962

1. *Purpose.* These regulations prescribe policies and procedures governing the use of volunteers as subjects in Department of the Army research, including research in nuclear, biological, and chemical warfare, wherein human beings are deliberately exposed to unusual or potentially hazardous conditions. These regulations are applicable world-wide, wherever volunteers are used as subjects in Department of the Army research.

2. *Definition.* For the purpose of these regulations, unusual and potentially hazardous conditions are those which may be reasonably expected to involve the risk, beyond the normal call of duty, of privation, discomfort, distress, pain, damage to health, bodily harm, physical injury, or death.

3. *Exemptions.* The following categories of activities and investigative programs are exempt from the provisions of these regulations:

   a. Research and nonresearch programs, tasks, and tests which may involve inherent occupational hazards to health or exposure of personnel to potentially hazardous situations encountered as part of training or other normal duties, e.g., flight training, jump training, fire drills, gas drills, and handling of explosives.

   b. That portion of human factors research which involves normal training or other military duties as part of an experiment, wherein disclosure of experimental conditions to participating personnel would reveal the artificial nature of such conditions and defeat the purpose of the investigation.

   c. Ethical medical and clinical investigations involving the basic disease process or new treatment procedures conducted by the Army Medical Service for the benefit of patients.

4. *Basic Principles.* Certain basic principles must be observed to satisfy moral, ethical, and legal concepts. These are—

   a. Voluntary consent is absolutely essential.

      (1) The volunteer will have legal capacity to give consent, and must give consent freely without being subjected to any force or duress. He must have sufficient understanding of the implications of his participation to enable him to make an informed decision, so far as such knowledge does not compromise the experiment. He will be told as much of

the nature, duration, and purpose of the experiment, the method and means by which it is to be conducted, and the inconveniences and hazards to be expected, as will not invalidate the results. He will be fully informed of the effects upon his health or person which may possibly come from his participation in the experiment.

(2) The consent of the volunteer will be in writing. A document setting forth substantially the above requirements will be signed by the volunteer in the presence of at least one witness not involved in the research study who will attest to such signature in writing.

(3) The responsibility for ascertaining the quality of the consent rests upon each person who initiates, directs, or conducts the experiment. It is a personal responsibility which may not be delegated.

b. The number of volunteers used will be kept at a minimum consistent with "c" below.

c. The experiment must be such as to contribute significantly to approved research and have reasonable prospects of yielding militarily important results essential to an Army research program which are not obtainable by other methods or means of study.

d. The experiment will be conducted so as to avoid all unnecessary physical and mental suffering and injury.

e. No experiment will be conducted if there is any reason inherent to the nature of the experiment to believe that death or disabling injury will occur.

f. The degree of risk to be taken will never exceed that determined to be required by the urgency or importance of the Army program for which the experiment is necessary.

g. Proper preparations will be made and adequate facilities provided to protect the volunteer against all foreseeable possibilities of injury, disability, or death.

h. The experiment will be conducted only by scientifically qualified persons. The highest degree of skill and care will be required during all stages of the experiment of persons who conduct or engage in the experiment.

i. The volunteer will be informed that at any time during the course of the experiment he will have the right to revoke his consent and withdraw from the experiment, without prejudice to himself.

j. Volunteers will have no physical or mental diseases which will make the proposed experiment more hazardous for them than for normal healthy persons. This determination will be made by the project leader with, if necessary, competent medical advice.

k. The scientist in charge will be prepared to terminate the experiment at any stage if he has probable cause to believe, in the exercise of good faith, superior skill, and careful judgment required of him, that continuation is likely to result in injury, disability or death to the volunteer.

l. Prisoners of war will not be used under any circumstances.

5. *Additional safeguards.* As added protection for volunteers, the following safeguards will be provided.

a. A physician approved by The Surgeon General will be responsible for the medical care of volunteers. The physician may or may not be the project leader but will have authority to terminate the experiment at any time that he believes death, injury, or bodily harm is likely to result.

b. All apparatus and instruments necessary to deal with likely emergency situations will be available.

c. Required medical treatment and hospitalization will be provided for all casualties.

d. The physician in charge will have consultants available to him on short notice throughout the experiment who are competent to advise or assist with complications which can be anticipated.

6. *Approval to conduct experiment.* It is the responsibility of the head of each major command and other agency to submit to The Surgeon General a written proposal for studies which come within the purview of this directive. The proposal will include for each study the name of the person to be in charge, name of the proposed attending physician, and the detailed plan of the experiment. The Surgeon General will review the proposal and forward it with his comments and recommendations on medical aspects to the Chief of Research and Development for approval. When a proposal pertains to research with nuclear, biological, or chemical agents, the Chief of Research and Development will submit the proposal, together with The Surgeon General's review, to the Secretary of the Army for approval. No research with nuclear, biological, or chemical agents using volunteers will be undertaken without the consent of the Secretary of the Army.

7. *Civilian employees.* When civilian employees of the Department of the Army volunteer under this program, the following instructions will be observed:

a. Any duty as a volunteer performed during the employee's regularly scheduled tour of duty will be considered as constructive duty for which straight time rates are payable. Time spent in connection with an experiment outside the employee's regularly scheduled tour will be considered as voluntary overtime for which no payment may be made nor compensatory time granted. The employee will be so informed before acceptance of his volunteer services.

b. Claims submitted to the Bureau of Employees' Compensation, U.S. Department of Labor, because of disability or death resulting from an employee's voluntary participation in experiments, will include a citation to title 10, United States Code, section 4503 as the Department of the Army authority for the use of such volunteer services.

c. All questions concerning hours of duty, pay, leave, compensation claims, or application of other civilian personnel regulations will be presented through channels to the Deputy Chief of Staff for Personnel, ATTN: Office of Civilian Personnel.

8. *Implementing instructions.* Heads of major commands and other agencies will issue necessary implementing instructions to subordinate units. Copies of implementing instructions will be furnished to the Chief of Research and Development.

ETHICAL STANDARDS OF PSYCHOLOGISTS

[Excerpts Relevant to Research]

American Psychological Association, 1963

The psychologist believes in the dignity and worth of the individual human being. He is committed to increasing man's understanding of himself and others. While pursuing this endeavor, he protects the welfare of any person who may seek his service or of any subject, human or animal, that may be the object of his study. He does not use his professional position or relationships, nor does he knowingly permit his own services to be used by others, for purposes inconsistent with these values. While demanding for himself freedom of inquiry and communication, he accepts the responsibility this freedom confers: for competence where he claims it, for objectivity in the report of his findings, and for consideration of the best interests of his colleagues and of society.

SPECIFIC PRINCIPLES

Principle 1. Responsibility. The psychologist,* committed to increasing man's understanding of man, places high value on objectivity and integrity, and maintains the highest standards in the services he offers.

a. As a scientist, the psychologist believes that society will be best served when he investigates where his judgment indicates investigation is needed; he plans his research in such a way as to minimize the possibility that his findings will be misleading; and he publishes full reports of his work, never discarding without explanation data which may modify the interpretation of results.
b. As a teacher, the psychologist recognizes his primary obligation to help others acquire knowledge and skill, and to maintain high standards of scholarship.
c. As a practitioner, the psychologist knows that he bears a heavy social responsibility because his work may touch intimately the lives of others.

Principle 5. Public Statements. Modesty, scientific caution, and due regard for the limits of present knowledge characterize all statements of psychologists who supply information to the public, either directly or indirectly.

* A student of psychology who assumes the role of psychologist shall be considered a psychologist for the purpose of this code of ethics.

a. Psychologists who interpret the science of psychology or the services of psychologists to clients or to the general public have an obligation to report fairly and accurately. Exaggeration, sensationalism, superficiality, and other kinds of misrepresentation are avoided.

b. When information about psychological procedures and techniques is given, care is taken to indicate that they should be used only by persons adequately trained in their use.

c. A psychologist who engages in radio or television activities does not participate in commercial announcements recommending purchase or use of a product.

Principle 6. Confidentiality. Safeguarding information about an individual that has been obtained by the psychologist in the course of his teaching, practice, or investigation is a primary obligation of the psychologist. Such information is not communicated to others unless certain important conditions are met.

a. Information received in confidence is revealed only after most careful deliberation and when there is clear and imminent danger to an individual or to society, and then only to appropriate professional workers or public authorities.

b. Information obtained in clinical or consulting relationships, or evaluative data concerning children, students, employees, and others are discussed only for professional purposes and only with persons clearly concerned with the case. Written and oral reports should present only data germane to the purposes of the evaluation; every effort should be made to avoid undue invasion of privacy.

c. Clinical and other case materials are used in classroom teaching and writing only when the identity of the persons involved is adequately disguised.

d. The confidentiality of professional communications about individuals is maintained. Only when the originator and other persons involved give their express permission is a confidential professional communication shown to the individual concerned. The psychologist is responsible for informing the client of the limits of the confidentiality.

e. Only after explicit permission has been granted is the identity of research subjects published. When data have been published without permission for identification, the psychologist assumes responsibility for adequately disguising their sources.

f. The psychologist makes provision for the maintenance of confidentiality in the preservation and ultimate disposition of confidential records.

Principle 7. Client Welfare. The psychologist respects the integrity and protects the welfare of the person or group with whom he is working.

a. The psychologist in industry, education, and other situations in which conflicts of interest may arise among various parties, as between management and labor, or between the client and the employer of the psychologist, defines for himself the nature and direction of his loyalties and responsibilities and keeps all parties concerned informed of these commitments.
b. When there is a conflict among professional workers, the psychologist is concerned primarily with the welfare of any client involved and only secondarily with the interest of his own professional group.
c. The psychologist attempts to terminate a clinical or consulting relationship when it is reasonably clear to the psychologist that the client is not benefiting from it.
d. The psychologist who asks that an individual reveal personal information in the course of interviewing, testing, or evaluation, or who allows such information to be divulged to him, does so only after making certain that the responsible person is fully aware of the purposes of the interview, testing, or evaluation and of the ways in which the information may be used.
e. In cases involving referral, the responsibility of the psychologist for the welfare of the client continues until this responsibility is assumed by the professional person to whom the client is referred or until the relationship with the psychologist making the referral has been terminated by mutual agreement. In situations where referral, consultation, or other changes in the conditions of the treatment are indicated and the client refuses referral, the psychologist carefully weighs the possible harm to the client, to himself, and to his profession that might ensue from continuing the relationship.
f. The psychologist who requires the taking of psychological tests for didactic classification, or research purposes protects the examinees by insuring that the tests and test results are used in a professional manner.
g. When potentially disturbing subject matter is presented to students, it is discussed objectively, and efforts are made to handle constructively any difficulties that arise.
h. Care must be taken to insure an appropriate setting for clinical work to protect both client and psychologist from actual or imputed harm and the profession from censure.

Principle 8. Client Relationship. The psychologist informs his prospective client of the important aspects of the potential relationship that might affect the client's decision to enter the relationship.

a. Aspects of the relationship likely to affect the client's decision include the recording of an interview, the use of interview material for training purposes, and observation of an interview by other persons.
b. When the client is not competent to evaluate the situation (as in the case of a child), the person responsible for the client is informed of the circumstances which may influence the relationship.
c. The psychologist does not normally enter into a professional relationship with members of his own family, intimate friends, close associates, or others whose welfare might be jeopardized by such a dual relationship.

Principle 13. Test Security. Psychological tests and other assessment devices, the value of which depends in part on the naivete of the subject, are not reproduced or described in popular publications in ways that might invalidate the techniques. Access to such devices is limited to persons with professional interests who will safeguard their use.

a. Sample items made up to resemble those of tests being discussed may be reproduced in popular articles and elsewhere, but scorable tests and actual test items are not reproduced except in professional publications.
b. The psychologist is responsible for the control of psychological tests and other devices and procedures used for instruction when their value might be damaged by revealing to the general public their specific contents or underlying principles.

Principle 14. Test Interpretation. Test scores, like test materials, are released only to persons who are qualified to interpret and use them properly.

a. Materials for reporting test scores to parents, or which are designed for self-appraisal purposes in schools, social agencies, or industry are closely supervised by qualified psychologists or counselors with provisions for referring and counseling individuals when needed.
b. Test results or other assessment data used for evaluation or classification are communicated to employers, relatives, or other appropriate persons in such a manner as to guard against misinterpretation or misuse. In the usual case, an interpretation of the test result rather than the score is communicated.
c. When test results are communicated directly to parents and students, they are accompanied by adequate interpretive aids or advice.

Principle 15. Test Publication. Psychological tests are offered for commercial publication only to publishers who present their tests in a professional way and distribute them only to qualified users.

a. A test manual, technical handbook, or other suitable report on the test is provided which describes the method of constructing and standardizing the test, and summarizes the validation research.

b. The populations for which the test has been developed and the purposes for which it is recommended are stated in the manual. Limitations upon the test's dependability, and aspects of its validity on which research is lacking or incomplete, are clearly stated. In particular, the manual contains a warning regarding interpretations likely to be made which have not yet been substantiated by research.

c. The catalog and manual indicate the training or professional qualifications required for sound interpretation of the test.

d. The test manual and supporting documents take into account the principles enunciated in the *Technical Recommendations for Psychological Tests and Diagnostic Techniques.*

e. Test advertisements are factual and descriptive rather than emotional and persuasive.

Principle 16. Research Precautions. The psychologist assumes obligations for the welfare of his research subjects, both animal and human.

a. Only when a problem is of scientific significance and it is not practicable to investigate it in any other way is the psychologist justified in exposing research subjects, whether children or adults, to physical or emotional stress as part of an investigation. [Ends justify means?]

b. When a reasonable possibility of injurious aftereffects exists, research is conducted only when the subjects or their responsible agents are fully informed of this possibility and agree to participate nevertheless.

c. The psychologist seriously considers the possibility of harmful aftereffects and avoids them, or removes them as soon as permitted by the design of the experiment.

d. A psychologist using animals in research adheres to the provisions of the Rules Regarding Animals, drawn up by the Committee on Precautions and Standards in Animal Experimentation and adopted by the American Psychological Association.

Principle 17. Publication Credit. Credit is assigned to those who have contributed to a publication, in proportion to their contribution, and only to these.

a. Major contributions of a professional character, made by several persons to a common project, are recognized by joint authorship. The experimenter or author who has made the principal contribution to a publication is identified as the first listed.
b. Minor contributions of a professional character, extensive clerical or similar nonprofessional assistance, and other minor contributions are acknowledged in footnotes or in an introductory statement.
c. Acknowledgment through specific citations is made for unpublished as well as published material that has directly influenced the research or writing.
d. A psychologist who compiles and edits for publication the contributions of others publishes the symposium or report under the title of the committee or symposium, with his own name appearing as chairman or editor among those of the other contributors or committee members.

Principle 18. Responsibility toward Organization. A psychologist respects the rights and reputation of the institute or organization with which he is associated.

a. Materials prepared by a psychologist as a part of his regular work under specific direction of his organization are the property of that organization. Such materials are released for use or publication by a psychologist in accordance with policies of authorization, assignment of credit, and related matters which have been established by his organization.
b. Other material resulting incidentally from activity supported by any agency, and for which the psychologist rightly assumes individual responsibility, is published with disclaimer for any responsibility on the part of the supporting agency.

Principle 19. Promotional Activities. The psychologist associated with the development or promotion of psychological books, devices, or other products offered for commercial sale is responsible for ensuring that such books, devices, or products are presented in a professional and factual way.

a. Claims regarding performance, benefits, or results are supported by scientifically acceptable evidence.
b. The psychologist does not use professional journals for the commercial exploitation of psychological products, and the psychologist-editor guards against such misuse.
c. The psychologist with a financial interest in the sale or use of a psychological product is sensitive to possible conflict of interest in his promotion of such products and avoids compromise of his professional responsibilities and objectives.

RESPONSIBILITY IN INVESTIGATIONS ON HUMAN SUBJECTS

Medical Research Council, Great Britain, 1963

During the last fifty years, medical knowledge has advanced more rapidly than at any other period in history. New understandings, new treatments, new diagnostic procedures and new methods of prevention have been, and are being, introduced at an ever-increasing rate; and if the benefits that are now becoming possible are to be gained, these developments must continue.

Undoubtedly the new era in medicine upon which we have now entered is largely due to the marriage of the methods of science with the traditional methods of medicine. Until the turn of the century, the advancement of clinical knowledge was in general confined to that which could be gained by observation, and means for the analysis in depth of the phenomena of health and disease were seldom available. Now, however, procedures that can safely, and conscientiously, be applied to both sick and healthy human beings are being devised in profusion, with the result that certainty and understanding in medicine are increasing apace.

Yet these innovations have brought their own problems to the clinical investigator. In the past, the introduction of new treatments or investigations was infrequent and only rarely did they go beyond a marginal variation on established practice. Today, far-ranging new procedures are commonplace and such are their potentialities that their employment is no negligible consideration. As a result, investigators are frequently faced with ethical and sometimes even legal problems of great difficulty. It is in the hope of giving some guidance in this difficult matter that the Medical Research Council issues this statement.

A distinction may legitimately be drawn between procedures undertaken as part of patient-care which are intended to contribute to the benefit of the individual patient, by treatment, prevention or assessment, and those procedures which are undertaken either on patients or on healthy subjects solely for the purpose of contributing to medical knowledge and are not themselves designed to benefit the particular individual on whom they are performed. The former fall within the ambit of patient-care and are governed by the ordinary rules of professional conduct in medicine; the latter fall within the ambit of investigations on volunteers.

Important considerations flow from this distinction.

PROCEDURES CONTRIBUTING TO THE BENEFIT OF THE INDIVIDUAL

In the case of procedures directly connected with the management of the condition in the particular individual, the relationship is essentially that between doctor and patient. Implicit in this relationship is the willingness on the part of the subject to be guided by the judgment of his medical attendant. Provided, therefore, that the medical attendant is satisfied that there are reasonable grounds for believing that a particular new procedure will contribute to the benefit of that particular patient, either by treatment, prevention or increased understanding of his case, he may assume the patient's consent to the same extent as he would were the procedure entirely establishd practice. It is axiomatic that no two patients are alike and that the medical attendant must be at liberty to vary his procedures according to his judgment of what is in his patients' best interests. The question of novelty is only relevant to the extent that in reaching a decision to use a novel procedure the doctor, being unable to fortify his judgment by previous experience, must exercise special care. That it is both considerate and prudent to obtain the patient's agreement before using a novel procedure is no more than a requirement of good medical practice.

The second important consideration that follows from this distinction is that it is clearly within the competence of a parent or guardian of a child to give permission for procedures intended to benefit that child when he is not old or intelligent enough to be able himself to give a valid consent.

A category of investigation that has occasionally raised questions in the minds of investigators is that in which a new preventive, such as a vaccine, is tried. Necessarily, preventives are given to people who are not, at the moment, suffering from the relevant illness. But the ethical and legal considerations are the same as those that govern the introduction of a new treatment. The intention is to benefit an individual by protecting him against a future hazard; and it is a matter of professional judgment whether the procedure in question offers a better chance of doing so than previously existing measures.

In general, therefore, the propriety of procedures intended to benefit the individual—whether these are directed to treatment, to prevention or to assessment—are determined by the same considerations as govern the care of patients. At the frontiers of knowledge, however, where not only are many procedures novel but their value in the particular instance may be debatable, it is wise, if any doubt exists, to obtain the opinion of experienced colleagues on the desirability of the projected procedure.

CONTROL SUBJECTS IN INVESTIGATIONS OF TREATMENT OR PREVENTION

Over recent years, the development of treatment and prevention has been greatly advanced by the method of the controlled clinical trial. Instead of waiting, as in the past, on the slow accumulation of general experience to determine the relative advantages and disadvantages of any particular measure, it is now often possible to put the question to the test under conditions which will not only yield a speedy and more precise answer, but also limit the risk of untoward effects remaining undetected. Such trials are, however, only feasible when it is possible to compare suitable groups of patients and only permissible when there is a genuine doubt within the profession as to which of two treatments or preventive regimes is the better. In these circumstances it is justifiable to give to a proportion of the patients the novel procedure on the understanding that the remainder receive the procedure previously accepted as the best. In the case when no effective treatment has previously been devised then the situation should be fully explained to the participants and their true consent obtained.

Such controlled trials may raise ethical points which may be of some difficulty. In general, the patients participating in them should be told frankly that two different procedures are being assessed and their cooperation invited. Occasionally, however, to do so is contra-indicated. For example, to awaken patients with a possibly fatal illness to the existence of such doubts about effective treatment may not always be in their best interest; or suspicion may have arisen as to whether a particular treatment has any effect apart from suggestion and it may be necessary to introduce a placebo into part of the trial to determine this. Because of these and similar difficulties, it is the firm opinion of the Council that controlled clinical trials should always be planned and supervised by a group of investigators and never by an individual alone. It goes without question that any doctor taking part in such a collective controlled trial is under an obligation to withdraw a patient from the trial, and to institute any treatment he considers necessary, should this, in his personal opinion, be in the better interests of his patient.

PROCEDURES NOT OF DIRECT BENEFIT TO THE INDIVIDUAL

The preceding considerations cover the majority of clinical investigations. There remains, however, a large and important field of investigations on human subjects which aims to provide normal values and their variation so that abnormal values can be recognized. This involves both ill persons and "healthy" persons, whether the latter are entirely healthy or patients suffering from a condition that has no relevance to the investigation. In regard to persons with a particular illness, such as metabolic defect, it may be necessary to know the range of abnormality compatible with the activities of normal life or the reaction of such persons to some change in circumstances such as an alteration in diet. Similarly it may be necessary to have a clear understanding of the range of a normal function and its reaction to changes in circumstances in entirely healthy persons. The common feature of this type of investigation is that it is of no direct benefit to the particular individual and that, in consequence, if he is to submit to it he must volunteer in the full sense of the word.

It should be clearly understood that the possibility or probability that a particular investigation will be of benefit to humanity or to posterity would afford no defence in the event of legal proceedings. The individual has rights that the law protects and nobody can infringe those rights for the public good. In investigations of this type it is, therefore, always necessary to ensure that the true consent of the subject is explicitly obtained.

By true consent is meant consent freely given with proper understanding of the nature and consequences of what is proposed. Assumed consent or consent obtained by undue influence is valueless and, in this latter respect, particular care is necessary when the volunteer stands in special relationship to the investigator as in the case of a patient to his doctor, or a student to his teacher.

The need for obtaining evidence of consent in this type of investigation has been generally recognized, but there are some misunderstandings as to what constitutes such evidence. In general, the investigator should obtain the consent himself in the presence of another person. Written consent unaccompanied by other evidence that an explanation has been given, understood and accepted is of little value.

The situation in respect of minors and mentally subnormal or mentally disordered persons is of particular difficulty. In the strict view of the law parents and guardians of minors cannot give consent on their behalf to any procedures which are of no particular benefit to them and which may carry some risk of harm. Whilst English law does not fix any arbitrary age in this context, it may safely be assumed that the Courts will not regard a child of 12 years or under (or fourteen years or under for boys in Scotland) as having the capacity to consent to any procedure which may involve him in an injury. Above this age the reality of any purported consent which may have been obtained is a question of fact and as with an adult the evidence would, if necessary, have to show that irrespective of age the person concerned fully understood the implications to himself of the procedures to which he was consenting.

In the case of those who are mentally subnormal or mentally disordered the reality of the consent given will fall to be judged by similar criteria to those which apply to the making of a will, contracting a marriage or otherwise taking decisions which have legal force as well as moral and social implications. When true consent in this sense cannot be obtained, procedures which are of no direct benefit and which might carry a risk of harm to the subject should not be undertaken.

Even when true consent has been given by a minor or a mentally subnormal or mentally disordered person, considerations of ethics and prudence still require that, if possible, the assent of parents or guardians or relatives, as the case may be, should be obtained.

Investigations that are of no direct benefit to the individual require, therefore, that his true consent to them shall be explicitly obtained. After adequate explanation, the consent of an adult of sound mind and understanding can be relied upon to be true consent. In the case of children and young persons the question whether purported consent was true consent would in each case depend upon facts such as the age, intelligence, situation and character of the subject and the nature of the investigation. When the subject is below the age of 12 years, information requiring the performance of any procedure involving his body would need to be obtained incidentally to and without altering the nature of a procedure intended for his individual benefit.

PROFESSIONAL DISCIPLINE

All who have been concerned with medical research are aware of the impossibility of formulating any detailed code of rules which will ensure that irreproachability of practice which alone will suffice where investigations on human beings are concerned. The law lays down a minimum code in matters of professional negligence and the doctrine of assault. But this is not enough. Owing to the special relationship of trust that exists between a patient and his doctor, most patients will consent to any proposal that is made. Further, the considerations involved in a novel procedure are nearly always so technical as to prevent their being adequately understood by one who is not himself an expert. It must, therefore, be frankly recognized that, for practical purposes, an inescapable moral responsibility rests with the doctor concerned for determining what investigations are, or are not, proposed to a particular patient or volunteer. Nevertheless, moral codes are formulated by man and if, in the ever-changing circumstances of medical advance, their relevance is to be maintained, it is to the profession itself that we must look, and in particular to the heads of departments, the specialized Societies and the editors of medical and scientific journals.

In the opinion of the Council, the head of a department where investigations on human subjects take place has an inescapable responsibility for ensuring that practice by those under his direction is irreproachable.

In the same way the Council feel that, as a matter of policy, bodies like themselves that support medical research should do everything in their power to ensure that the practice of all workers whom they support shall be unexceptionable and known to be so.

So specialized has medical knowledge now become that the profession in general can rarely deal adequately with individual problems. In regard to any particular type of investigation, only a small group of experienced men who have specialized in this branch of knowledge are likely to be competent to pass an opinion on the justification for undertaking any particular procedure. But in every branch of medicine specialized scientific societies exist. It is upon these that the profession in general must mainly rely for the creation and maintenance of that body of precedents which shall guide individual investigators in case of doubt, and for the critical discussion of the communications presented to them on which the formation of the necessary climate of opinion depends.

Finally, it is the Council's opinion that any account of investigations on human subjects should make clear that the appropriate requirements have been fulfilled and, further, that no paper should be accepted for publication if there are any doubts that such is the case.

The progress of medical knowledge has depended, and will continue to depend, in no small measure upon the confidence which the public has in those who carry out investigations on human subjects, be these healthy or sick. Only insofar as it is known that such investigations are submitted to the highest ethical scrutiny and self-discipline will this confidence be maintained. Mistaken, or misunderstood, investigations could do incalculable harm to medical progress. It is our collective duty as a profession to see that this does not happen and so to continue to deserve the confidence that we now enjoy.

EXPERIMENTAL RESEARCH ON HUMAN BEINGS

Approved by the Representative Body of the British Medical Association, 1963

1. New drugs or other therapy should not be prescribed unless prior investigation as to the possible effects upon the human body has been fully adequate.

2. Before a new drug is used in treatment, the clinician should ensure that the distributors of the drug are reputable and the claims made for the products include reference to independent evidence of its effects.

3. No new technique or investigation shall be undertaken on a patient unless it is strictly necessary for the treatment of the patient, or, alternatively, that following a full explanation the doctor has obtained the patient's free and valid consent to his actions, preferably in writing.

4. A doctor wholly engaged in clinical research must be at special pains to remember the responsibility to the individual patient when his experimental work is conducted through the medium of a consultant who has clinical responsibility for the patient.

5. The patient must never take second place to a research project nor should he be given any such impression. Before embarking upon any research the doctor should ask himself these questions:

   a. Does the patient know what it is I propose to do?
   b. Have I explained fully and honestly to him the risks I am asking him to run?
   c. Am I satisfied that his consent has been freely given and is legally valid?
   d. Is this procedure one which I would not hesitate to advise, or in which I would readily acquiesce, if it were to be undertaken upon my own wife or children?

BRADFORD HILL AND A CODE FOR THE CLINICAL TRIAL, 1963

Bradford Hill [209] has proposed the following approach to the clinical trial.

"1. *Is the Proposed Treatment Safe or, in other words, is it Unlikely to do Harm to the Patient?*" Hardly any treatment is free of some undesirable side effects. If absolute safety is demanded, no important progress can be made. The risk of giving the treatment must be balanced against the risk of withholding it. (The use of chloramphenicol could be imperative in typhoid fever, but unwise in uncomplicated whooping cough.) When possibility of injury is not known, use of the treatment could be properly explored in a serious disease situation, but not in a mild self-limiting ailment. One of the great values of the controlled clinical trial is, of course, that it exposes danger areas more rapidly than do the old trial-and-error methods. It cannot be expected that either method will efficiently reveal the disaster that occurs only once in many hundreds of cases.

"2. *Can a New Treatment Ethically Be Withheld from Any Patients in the Doctor's Care?*" In a controlled comparison of a wholly new treatment and a standard treatment, we do not know the relative values. We do know something about the value of the older treatment. One of the most difficult problems is when to withhold the established in favor of the unproved.

There is no efficient treatment for fatal cancer; therefore, any new treatment that offers any hope at all is permissible, even mandatory, unless the side effects are of such truly serious nature, usually in terms of comfort, that the new treatment is dismissed. In mild self-limiting diseases, on the other hand, there is no license to take on risky treatments. The common problems lie between these two extremes. They can be dealt with only by weighing the circumstances of a specific case.

"3. *What Patients may be Brought into a Controlled Trial and Allocated Randomly to Different Treatments?*" Random distribution of subjects can be used only if it is possible ethically to give every patient in the experimental group every treatment. This presupposes that the investigator has no knowledge of different hazards among the trials. If the doctor thinks one treatment rather than another should be administered to a given patient, that patient should not be admitted to the study. Such exclusions from a trial may limit the generality of the answer obtained, but is often necessary for ethical reasons; ". . . the ethical obligation always and entirely outweighs the experimental" [209]. Statistically, the use of random sampling numbers is better than the common alternate patient system.

Bradford Hill [209] believes ". . . that ethically the doctor is in very much the same situation if, more traditionally, he measures the relative effects of treatments by 'ringing the changes' *within* rather than *between* patients. It was, wrote Lord MacMillan, a wise statesman who said of the law that 'where it is not necessary to change it is necessary not to change."

Certain patients are best avoided in clinical trials: pregnant women, patients with complicating conditions and diseases, the very old and frail, the very young. The elimination of such individuals from a trial may limit the breadth of possible conclusions, but it is often necessary on ethical grounds. It must always be possible to drop a patient from a study when his physician deems this necessary; ". . . the ethical obligation always and entirely outweighs the experimental."

"4. *Is it Necessary to Obtain the Patient's Consent to His Inclusion in a Controlled Trial?* I have already made clear that in my opinion this question should really be worded, *When* is it necessary to ask the patient's consent to his inclusion in a controlled trial?" If pain or discomfort or danger, not part of the patient's disease, is to be produced by experimentation, it is desirable to obtain consent with understanding. Bradford Hill believes that, if there is no reason to fear a dangerous or painful effect in the situation where one does not know the relative value of two treatments, it is not necessary to expose one's ignorance and confuse the subjects.

"5. *Is it Ethical to Use a Placebo, or Dummy Treatment?" If* there is a standard treatment, this can be pitted against the new treatment, often making a placebo unnecessary. Treatment of the common cold in young adults compared an antihistamine with a placebo, since the criteria for judgments were derived from subjective sensation. The placebo was required. The patients knew that not all would receive the same treatment. Harm can be done to medicine by the overuse or unnecessary use of placebos if the public believes that patients are often used as guinea pigs.

"6. *Is it Proper for the Doctor Not to Know the Treatment Being Administered to his Patient?*" The physician must know and approve the agents employed in a given study. He need not know which patient received which agent at a given time. There is nothing unethical in having the results appraised by a colleague who is in ignorance of the identity of the tested agents. Unknowns must be revealed whenever the physician in charge believes it to be necessary. It is probable that the double-blind technique should not be used in prolonged studies where fine adjustments of dosage are required for the patient's welfare.

HARVARD UNIVERSITY HEALTH SERVICES CODE, 1963*

Rules Governing the Participation of Healthy Human Beings as Subjects in Research

The following rules and procedures, formulated by the University Health Services, were adopted by the President and Fellows on April 1, 1963. They will apply hereafter to all parts of the University except the Medical School.

These rules are not intended to cover research on sick patients.

STATEMENT OF POLICY

1. In considering the participation of human beings as research subjects, the guiding principle is that no one, whether students or other persons, should be exposed to unreasonable risk to health or well-being.

2. All persons involved in initiating, approving, or conducting research involving human subjects shall be aware of a joint responsibility for the welfare of the individuals who serve as subjects.

3. It shall be the responsibility of the individual investigator to decide when he does not have adequate knowledge of the possible consequences of his research, or of research done under his direction. When he is in doubt, he must obtain the advice of others who do have the requisite or relevant knowledge.

4. Any hazards to health of each research procedure must be first investigated through animal research, whenever such be possible and relevant.

5. Whenever medication or physical intervention is used, or whenever the subject's environment is altered beyond the limits of normality, the research must be performed under medical protection and supervision.

6. The purpose of the research, the procedures to be followed, and the possible risks involved must be carefully and fully explained to the subject; the investigator must be satisfied that the explanation has been understood by the subject; and the consent of the subject must be obtained in writing without duress or deception.

Where unreasonable risks to the subject are *not* involved, and a full account of purpose and procedure in advance might bias the results, as in some psychological and social research, such an account may be post-

* The then Dean, George Packer Berry, and I opposed the adoption of this code on the grounds that it was unwisely rigid in some areas, not clear enough in others, and that certain important problems were not faced at all. We were overruled by the Corporation.

poned to a later appropriate time or may be omitted—as for example in public opinion research, or observation of children in educational or play situations, provided there is no ethical problem.

7. A research project shall not be represented to potential research subjects as being sponsored by Harvard University or by a given department of the University except by explicit arrangements with appropriate administrative authorities. It is appropriate for the researcher to make known his position at Harvard. It is the subject's right to know, if he so desires, the source of support for the research in which he is being asked to participate.

8. The individual's personal privacy and the confidentiality of information received from him must be protected.

9. An individual's time should not be invaded to the extent that it creates conflicts with his other obligations; whenever possible the research project should contribute to the subject's knowledge of himself and/or his knowledge of the topic under investigation.

10. Remuneration may be offered to an individual for the time involved in a study provided the investigator is satisfied that under the circumstances the remuneration is not so large as to constitute an improper inducement.

11. Any individual may request termination of his participation in an experiment at any time, and this request will be honored promptly and without prejudice.

PROCEDURE

The Dean of each Faculty shall be responsible to the Corporation that research involving healthy human subjects by members of his faculty is conducted with care and propriety. The procedures used in the Faculty of Medicine are described in a statement, dated January 1, 1958. All other Faculties will observe the following procedures. The Deans may delegate this responsibility to department chairmen who may in turn delegate it to other responsible members of their Department.

1. All officers of the University shall evaluate research using human subjects, to be conducted or directed by them, in terms of ethical and legal standards as well as according to scientific criteria, keeping in mind that the acceptance of individual responsibility for one's actions constitutes the foundation of the trust which the individual enjoys as a member of the University.

2. All research must comply with all requirements in the statement of policy listed above.

3. The following list is illustrative of the types of research procedures that are likely to involve consequences beyond the ability of

many investigators to evaluate adequately, and will, therefore, make it necessary that the investigator in any such research refer his proposal to other responsible persons for further consideration. In such cases the University Health Services through Environmental Health and Safety are prepared to provide advice and to evaluate and approve procedures. The list is not intended to be inclusive.

a. Injection, ingestion or inhalation of any potentially toxic material, including all drugs, or any usually ingested or inhaled material in excess of or in less than normal amounts.
b. Physical stimuli, in abnormal amounts, such as:

Noise	Ionizing radiation
Vibration	Non-ionizing radiation
Electric shock	Ultra violet
Heat and/or humidity	Visible light
Cold and/or wind	Infra-red radiations
Magnetic fields	Microwaves
Gravitational fields	Ambient pressure

c. Sensory deprivation.
d. Sleep deprivation.
e. Special diets that vary appreciably from generally accepted standards.
f. Psychological experiments using hypnosis, deception, or mental stresses.

4. A department whose members may need advice may appoint a committee to assist the investigator in obtaining the advice he requires. When such a committee exists, it will ordinarily be the first group to which the investigator turns, and shall have power to require that the investigator obtain approval from the University Health Services, through Environmental Health and Safety, before going ahead to recruit subjects for his research.

5. In cases where the departmental committee learns informally of a proposed research project that it believes should be referred to it, it will be appropriate for the committee to request that the proposal be submitted to it for evaluation.

6. It shall be the prerogative of both the departmental committee and the University Health Services to require for projects referred to them that parental consent be obtained before individuals under the age of 21 may participate in a research project.

7. For those cases in which it has been determined that approval by Environmental Health and Safety is required, the proposed research will be presented in proper form to that body. Approval of the use of

human beings as research subjects in such cases will be valid only for a specific project and for a maximum of one year. If further time or change in protocol is necessary, application for re-approval will be necessary. It is recommended, in order to prevent delay of the investigation, that sufficient time be allowed before the start of the project for review by Environmental Health and Safety and other responsible parties.

8. In all cases where it has been determined that a proposal is one requiring approval of the division of Environmental Health and Safety or other administrative body, no action to recruit individuals will be taken until written approval from this body has been received. The principal investigator, the departmental committee, and the Student Employment Office will receive notification of the action taken on a proposal.

9. The investigator will report immediately to the University Health Services any significant observations of change in the behavior or health of a subject during or following an experiment, and the investigator will terminate that experiment.

10. Whether a specific project has been cleared or not, the investigator should feel free to seek advice from the University Health Services at any time during the study.

11. These regulations shall be circulated to the members of the departments concerned at the beginning of each academic year.

Comment: This might be called an administration code; it appears to be designed to keep the administration out of trouble. Certainly it passes lightly over some difficult problems; for example, see item 6 below, concerning consent.

Comment.

POLICY SECTION

1. This implies that reasonable risk is acceptable; it is regrettable that this is not spelled out. This vague statement is not helpful.

6. The trouble here lies in the view that risks are known, very often not the case, and that knowledge of them can be transmitted if one will only take the trouble to do so. While consent obtained in writing may have some psychological value, it has no legal worth. It is also my interpretation of the law that, where no discernible risk is involved and where discussion of the matter might

bias the results, as in some psychological studies, then consent need not be obtained. It must be pointed out, however, that this is *not* the view of the Food and Drug Administration. Once again, there is no hint of the appalling difficulties that, in many cases, lie in the way of obtaining truly informed consent.

7. When research is carried out on Harvard property by Harvard staff, with Harvard money or money disbursed by Harvard, it would not be surprising if the subject jumped to the conclusion that the study was sponsored by Harvard.

PROCEDURE SECTION

3a. What is meant by a "normal amount" of a toxic substance for "injection, ingestion or inhalation"? This is obscure.

DECLARATION OF HELSINKI, 1964, Revised [Originally 1962]

It is the mission of the doctor to safeguard the health of the people. His knowledge and conscience are dedicated to the fulfilment of this mission.

The Declaration of Geneva of the World Medical Association (1964) binds the doctor with the words, "The health of my patient will be my first consideration"; and the International Code of Medical Ethics which declares that "Any act or advice which could weaken physical or mental resistance of a human being may be used only in his interest."

Because it is essential that the results of laboratory experiments be applied to human beings to further scientific knowledge and to help suffering humanity, the World Medical Association has prepared the following recommendations as a guide to each doctor in clinical research. It must be stressed that the standards as drafted are only a guide to physicians all over the world. Doctors are not relieved from criminal, civil, and ethical responsibilities under the laws of their own countries.

In the field of clinical research a fundamental distinction must be recognized between clinical research in which the aim is essentially therapeutic for a patient, and clinical research the essential object of which is purely scientific and without therapeutic value to the person subjected to the research.

I. Basic Principles

1. Clinical research must conform to the moral and scientific principles that justify medical research, and should be based on laboratory and animal experiments or other scientifically established facts. [The use of animals is not always feasible or possible.

2. Clinical research should be conducted only by scientifically qualified persons and under the supervision of a qualified medical man.

3. Clinical research cannot legitimately be carried out unless the importance of the objective is in proportion to the inherent risk to the subject.

4. Every clinical research project should be preceded by careful assessment of inherent risks in comparison to foreseeable benefits to the subject or to others.

5. Special caution should be exercised by the doctor in performing clinical research in which the personality of the subject is liable to be altered by drugs or experimental procedure.

II. Clinical Research Combined with Professional Care

1. In the treatment of the sick person the doctor must be free to use a new therapeutic measure, if in his judgment it offers hope of saving life, re-establishing health, or alleviating suffering.

If at all possible, consistent with patient psychology, the doctor should obtain the patient's freely given consent after the patient has been given a full explanation. In case of legal incapacity consent should also be procured from the legal guardian; in case of physical incapacity the permission of the legal guardian replaces that of the patient.

2. The doctor can combine clinical research with professional care, the objective being the acquisition of new medical knowledge, only to the extent that clinical research is justified by its therapeutic value for the patient.

III. Non-therapeutic Clinical Research

1. In the purely scientific application of clinical research carried out on a human being it is the duty of the doctor to remain the protector of the life and health of that person on whom clinical research is being carried out.

2. The nature, the purpose, and the risk of clinical research must be explained to the subject by the doctor.

3a. Clinical research on a human being cannot be undertaken without his free consent, after he has been fully informed; if he is legally incompetent the consent of the legal guardian should be procured.

3b. The subject of clinical research should be in such a mental, physical, and legal state as to be able to exercise fully his power of choice.

3c. Consent should as a rule be obtained in writing. However, the responsibility for clinical research always remains with the research worker; it never falls on the subject, even after consent is obtained.

4a. The investigator must respect the right of each individual to safeguard his personal integrity, especially if the subject is in a dependent relationship to the investigator.

4b. At any time during the course of clinical research the subject or his guardian should be free to withdraw permission for research to be continued. The investigator or the investigating team should discontinue the research if in his or their judgment it may, if continued, be harmful to the individual.

Comment. Here, as in most other codes, the impossibility of knowing what the hazards will be in a new project—plus the frequent difficulties, even impossibility, of communicating the problems involved—are ignored. There is no facing up to the frequently overwhelming difficulties in obtaining truly valid consent.

In actual fact in our society many kinds of human experimentation are often conducted by laymen; the introduction of a new type of plane constitutes a human, sometimes even a fatal experiment. Much psychological experimentation is carried out by psychologists; physicians often would not be competent to engage in it. A physician should, of course, supervise such aspects of psychological studies as the use of drugs.

The phrase in the first basic principle, ". . . research should be based on laboratory and animal experiments . . . ," cannot always be followed, certainly not generally in the study of mental disease and its treatment; neither can it be followed in study of disease not present and not producible in animals. Mead [296] makes an interesting comment in this area; there is in certain kinds of animal work the problem of ". . . how to control the tendency of the human observer to anthropomorphize, and so distort his observations."

The Nuremberg Code presents a rigid set of legalistic demands. In attempting to provide for all contingencies, it leaves the investigator badly exposed in two ways: (1) it is folly to suppose that every situation can be anticipated and provided for; (2) it asks for the impossible in several instances. These have been mentioned in the foregoing comment on the code. The Declaration of Helsinki, on the other hand, presents a series of guides. It is an ethical as opposed to a legalistic document, and is thus a more broadly useful instrument than the one formulated at Nuremberg. The Declaration of Helsinki separates professional care for the direct benefit of the subject from nontherapeutic research, which the Nuremberg Code does not. Until recently, the Western world was threatened with the imposition of the Nuremberg Code as a Western credo. With the wide adoption* of the Declaration of Helsinki, this danger is apparently now past.

* Among the organizations adopting it are the American Society for Clinical Investigation, the American College of Physicians, the American College of Surgeons, and the American Medical Association.

BRADFORD HILL'S CRITIQUE OF THE WORLD MEDICAL ASSOCIATION'S CODE (1962) AND IN PART OF THE DECLARATION OF HELSINKI (1964)

Bradford Hill [209] criticizes the Code of the Ethical Committee of the World Medical Association (1962) and takes sharp issue with the requirement that the experiment should be carried out "under the supervision of a qualified medical man." This requirement is also stated in the Declaration of Helsinki. While this is necessary in some types of experimentation, it is not invariably so, for example, in many experiments in industrial psychology. The physician may not even be qualified to carry on this kind of work. It is immaterial that the code did not intend to cover this psychological field. If the code does not make clear its intentions and limitations, what is its value?

A further general principle states "That the nature, the reason, and the risks of the experiment are fully explained to the subject of it, who should have complete freedom to decide whether or not to take part in the experiment." The Declaration of Helsinki says in almost identical language, "The nature, the purpose and the risk of clinical research must be explained to the subject by the doctor." Bradford Hill continues, "Personally, and speaking as a patient, I have no doubt whatever that there are circumstances in which the patient's consent to taking part in a controlled trial should be sought. I have equally no doubt that there are circumstances in which it need not—and even should not—be sought. My quarrel is again with a code that takes no heed—and in dealing with generalities can take no heed—of the enormously varying circumstances of clinical medicine. Surely it is often quite impossible to tell ill-educated and sick persons the pros and cons of a new and unknown treatment versus the orthodox and known? And, in fact, of course one does not know the pros and cons. The situation implicit in the controlled trial is that one has two (or more) possible treatments and that one is wholly, or to a very large extent, ignorant of their relative values (and dangers). Can you describe that situation to a patient so that he does not lose confidence in you—the essence of the doctor-patient relationship—and in such a way that he fully understands and can therefore give an *understanding* consent to his inclusion in a trial? In my opinion nothing less is of value. Just to ask the patient does he mind if you try some new tablets on him does nothing, I suggest, to meet the problem. That is merely paying lip-service to it. If the patient cannot really grasp the whole situation, or without upsetting his faith in your judgment cannot be made to grasp it, then in my opinion the ethical decision still lies with the doctor, whether or no it is proper to exhibit, or withhold, a treatment. He cannot divest himself of it simply by means of an illusory or uncomprehending consent." The Federal Food and Drug Administration notwithstanding!

"In looking back, and forward, it is proper to remember McCance's comment [293] that the physician 'forgets, indeed he may not even know, that what he would have regarded as an "unjustifiable experiment" five years ago may have become one of his standard diagnostic or therapeutic procedures.' "

It must be granted that some treatments are useful, some useless, some hazardous. The problem is how to make a discrimination. Very often the controlled clinical trial provides the best answer, but then we are immediately confronted with the question: under what circumstances can the responsible investigator make the decision to administer or to withhold the use of the agent in question? Generalizations are of little help. As Bradford Hill points out, an examination of the specific circumstances of each proposed trial is necessary. In consultation with one's peers, one can make some broad generalizations for guidance. Bradford Hill does not believe, nor does the writer, that one can go much beyond this in establishing rules of action that are applicable in all circumstances.

Further questions can be raised concerning the section of the World Medical Association's Code that states unequivocally "that children in institutions and not under the care of relatives should not be the subject of human experiments." This statement, unlike the preceding one, does not appear in the Declaration of Helsinki. Bradford Hill asks, "Does pasteurized milk contribute less than raw milk to the promotion of health and growth? Does sugar in the diet influence the incidence of caries? Is gamma globulin more, or less, effective than convalescent serum in the prevention of measles? Was it unethical to find out in the very circumstances in which it was possible (as well as important for the subjects) to do so? The guide says Yes."

"It also asserts that 'persons retained in mental hospitals or hospitals for mental defectives should not be used for human experiment' [this statement does not appear in the Declaration of Helsinki] and this would seem to me automatically to condemn as unethical clinical trials in psychiatry. Again, that may not be the intention; but it certainly has that result."

While such an "authoritative" code is intended only for guidance, a doctor will defy it at some risk when it has been so well publicized and so widely adopted.

HARVARD MEDICAL SCHOOL CODE, 1965

Rules Governing the Participation of Medical Students as Experimental Subjects

The participation of medical students as experimental subjects in research studies has raised practical and philosophical problems difficult to resolve. Misunderstandings have arisen, owing in part to inadequate communication and in part to the complex nature of the issues involved.

In discussing this situation, the principles that should govern the employment of human beings as research subjects, the motivations of medical students in volunteering, the educational implications, the matter of financial remuneration, the protection of health, the conflict with scheduled studies, the moral and legal responsibilities of the investigator and of the Medical School, and the advisability of the centralization of all pertinent records, have all been considered by the Administrative Board and the Faculty of Medicine.

After extensive study of these points, the University Health Services and the Dean's Office formulated the following policies and procedures, which have been unanimously approved by the Administrative Board and supported by the Faculty of Medicine.

STATEMENT OF POLICY

1. The guiding principle in considering the participation of medical students as subjects in experiments is the belief that no student should be exposed to risk as far as his health and well-being are concerned.
2. A student's time should not be invaded to the extent of creating conflicts with his scheduled work.
3. Inasmuch as motivation should stem from an opportunity to learn and to contribute, rather than from a financial inducement *per se*, payment should not ordinarily be made to the student for participating as a subject in an experiment. This does not preclude remuneration for collaborating in a research project nor for participation in programs in which a student may be employed during vacation periods, or under special circumstances at other times during the academic year, or as a Student Research Fellow.
4. The contact between investigator and student is recognized as an excellent opportunity for the investigator to demonstrate to the student both his personal responsibility for the student's health and safety and an active interest in furthering the student's education.

PROCEDURE

In order to simplify and to standardize the participation of medical students as experimental subjects, the following administrative procedure has been established for the mutual benefit of the student, the investigator, and the Medical School.

1. *Each project must be approved by the head of the department,* of which the investigator is a member. This provision specifically shall include approval of the desirability of the proposed study, the details of the experimental protocol, and the use of medical students as subjects. It shall imply, in addition, the assumption of responsibility for any medical expenses that the student may incur as a consequence of participation.
2. Subsequent to such approval, *a detailed protocol must be submitted to the Director of the Medical Area Health Service and to the Dean's Office.* In experiments involving the use of radioactive materials, a copy of the protocol shall be submitted also to the Secretary of the Committee on Medical Research in Biophysics.
3. Following review and commentary by these parties, *the protocol must be presented to the Administrative Board for discussion and for approval or disapproval of student participation.*
4. If approved, *the investigator must explain the details of the project to the medical student in advance, and must refer him to the Health Service for medical clearance before beginning the experiment.* The result of the Health Service's examination shall be sent in writing to the investigator.
5. *The Health Service must maintain records* of the research project in which medical students participate. These records shall include dosages of drugs or radioisotopes used on each individual and the total body irradiation received. In addition, *the investigator must report to the Health Service concerning any significant medical observations* that are made during the course of a given experiment.

Robert H. Ebert, M.D.
Dean

July 1, 1965

GROUP CONSIDERATION AND INFORMED CONSENT IN CLINICAL RESEARCH AT THE NATIONAL INSTITUTES OF HEALTH, 1966

The policy of the National Institutes of Health for the conduct of clinical research and medical care places primary responsibility on the principal investigators designated by each Institute. In accordance with the administrative guidelines established by the Director of the National Institutes of Health, research and medical care are conducted in conformity with legal, ethical, and professional standards. Only properly qualified physicians or dentists may assume responsibility for diagnosis, treatment, and clinical investigation. Under authority delegated by the Institute Director, the Clinical Director of each Institute is responsible for supervision of patient care and normal volunteer research activities on the inpatient and outpatient services of the Institute in the Clinical Center.

The National Institutes of Health recognizes that the main principles guiding clinical research are: (1) group consideration, including peer judgment; (2) informed consent of the patient or normal volunteer; and (3) the right of the patient or normal volunteer to withdraw from participation in a clinical research project at any time.

The form of obtaining and recording of both group consideration and informed consent may vary among the several Institutes and in dealing with patients as opposed to normal volunteers, but the substance of informed consent and group consideration is not to be altered materially by any such differences in procedures.

This document is a statement of principles that the National Institutes of Health believes must govern clinical research and a definition of the mechanisms that shall be provided to assist the principal investigators in putting these principles into practice.

I. CATEGORIES OF CLINICAL CENTER ADMISSIONS

Individuals admitted to the NIH Clinical Center can be categorized into two classes:

1. Normal Volunteers: Healthy persons who have volunteered to serve as normal controls for clinical investigation at the Clinical Center of the National Institutes of Health.
2. Patients: These are individuals who have been referred by their physician or dentist because they have a disease that may require further investigation, diagnosis, or treatment, or relatives of such patients on occasions when it is appropriate to investigate the fa-

milial aspects of a specific disease. Patients may also serve in a volunteer capacity when they participate in studies that are not of direct benefit to them.

II. MEDICAL CARE AND CLINICAL RESEARCH

In the care of patients every medical procedure is modified or adapted to accommodate the individual patient. It is recognized that every medical procedure carries some element of risk. In the formulation of clinical research projects, the determination as to which clinical procedures are considered as not being "established" or as involving unusual hazard should be on an individual basis, in the light of experience developed in institutions recognized by the profession for their excellence in conducting medical care and research.

III. GROUP CONSIDERATION AND REVIEW

The mechanisms for obtaining group consideration and review shall be used on a committee system functioning both at the intra-Institute and inter-Institute level.

A. Committees

1. *Medical Board Committee*
   The Medical Board shall establish a Clinical Research Committee to review proposals concerning clinical research involving normal volunteers and patients referred to it by the Director of the National Institutes of Health, the Director of the Clinical Center, or the Clinical Director of an Institute.
2. *Institute Committee*
   Each Institute shall establish a committee which will serve to review and make recommendations concerning certain clinical research projects carried out by its clinical investigators. Its function will be advisory to the Clinical Director of the Institute.

These committees will review both the scientific merit and propriety of the research proposed. They may enlist assistance on an ad hoc basis within and without the National Institutes of Health.

B. Review Mechanisms

1. *Review of Clinical Research Procedures in Normal Volunteers*
   Research projects involving the participation of normal volunteers must be submitted to the Medical Board through its Clinical Research Committee. The review procedures for normal volunteers shall be as follows:
   a. The research protocol shall be prepared by the principal in-

vestigator and shall contain sufficient information for proper review (see APPENDIX, Section VI). This protocol shall have the written approval of the Branch Chief and the Clinical Director of the Institute before it is forwarded to the Medical Board. The Medical Board in turn will make appropriate recommendations to the Director of the National Institutes of Health, through the Director of the Clinical Center and the Director of Laboratories and Clinics, NIH.

2. *Review of Clinical Research Procedures in Patients*

The National Institutes of Health recognizes two categories of research in patients.

a. Clinical studies that are diagnostic or therapeutic in intent and in which there is potential benefit to the patient concerned.

For these studies the group consideration that is provided at ward rounds by these studies the group consideration that is provided at ward rounds by the interaction of Clinical Associates, Attending Physicians, and the Service Head or Branch Chief is generally sufficient. However, when such studies represent a significant deviation from accepted practice or are associated with unusual hazard, the Branch Chief will review the proposed studies with the Clinical Director. The Clinical Director may either approve, disapprove, or refer this project to the Institute Clinical Research Committee.

b. Investigative non-diagnostic, non-therapeutic clinical research not motivated wholly toward the patient, where, in effect, the patient serves essentially as a volunteer.

All projects involving the utilization of patients for such studies shall be preceded by group consideration and have the approval of the Service Head or Branch Chief and the Clinical Director. The Clinical Director shall have the option of referring this project to the Institute Clinical Research Committee. This Committee can then either recommend approval, disapproval, or further review by the Medical Board. The Clinical Director shall retain the right to terminate any project at any time in the interest of the welfare of the patient.

The form in which protocols are presented to the Institute Clinical Research Committees may vary within the Institutes but an appropriate record must be kept of the actions of the Committee in its consideration of each project.

IV. PRINCIPLES GOVERNING PHYSICIAN-PATIENT RELATIONSHIP

1. *Information for the Patient*
   Each patient and each normal volunteer shall be given an oral explanation in terms suited to his comprehension of his role in the Clinical Center, the nature of the proposed studies and, particularly, any hazards. This information should be given to the patient on a continuing basis. A summary of this information and a record of its communication to the patient shall be played in the patient's medical record over the signature of the principal investigator.
   For normal volunteers a specific consent form [NIH-658-1 (formerly PHS-4573-1)] containing this information must be signed by the normal volunteer and the principal investigator.
2. *Patient Understanding and Agreement and Consent*
   The Director of the National Institutes of Health has approved a list of procedures which require specific written consent (see APPENDIX, Section I). For those procedures and studies not covered, voluntary agreement by the patient to participate, or when appropriate by next of kin, based upon informed consent, shall be obtained and recorded by the principal investigator.
3. *Responsibility*
   The principal investigator shall be responsible for providing information to the patient, to the referring physician and next of kin, and for obtaining consent when it is required.

Comment. See also specific details that elaborate on the foregoing, especially concerning consent, volunteers, and interpretation of the Food and Drug Administration's rulings from 1954 to 1967. These will be found in a Memorandum from the Director, National Institutes of Health, dated July 1, 1966, with additions made in January, 1967.

BEECHER'S CODE, 1966

*Some Guiding Principles for Clinical Investigation**

EXPERIMENTATION FOR THE BENEFIT OF OTHERS, NOT FOR THE PATIENT INVOLVED

Rigid codes which attempt to give detailed instructions to govern research are to be avoided. It is not possible to outline all contingencies; the consequent shortcomings when revealed during work invite legal action.

Insofar as it is possible, it is essential to get the informed consent of the patient involved prior to study. It must be recognized that in any complete sense this often is not possible. Nevertheless, informed consent is a goal toward which we strive. When the principle is effectively followed, the subject at least knows he is involved in an experiment and can withdraw if he chooses to do so. An even greater safeguard for the patient than consent is the presence of an informed, able, conscientious, compassionate, responsible investigator, for it is recognized that patients can, when imperfectly informed, be induced to agree, unwisely, to many things. It may be trite to say it, but firm application of the golden rule would go very far to eliminate difficulties here.

When a procedure is not for the diagnosis or treatment of his own condition, this must be made clear to the patient.

A considerable amount of specious rationalization can be avoided if it is recognized that patients will, if agreeably approached, consent to experimentation involving inconvenience and some discomfort, if these do not last long. On the other hand, "normal," i.e., ordinary, patients will not willingly risk their health or their life for "science"; only the extremely rare individual, as one perhaps seeking martyrdom will do this.

The patient can overrule the physician as to what factors are or are not relevant to his consent. There is no right to withhold from a prospective volunteer any fact which may influence his decision.

The investigator has no right to choose martyrs for science. (Kety, 1957, 1958.)

Experimentation on children and wards is often permissible and desirable; however, children and ignorant persons, or those who are mentally unsound, confused, unconscious, or anesthetized, present particularly difficult problems which require thorough discussion, explanation, and attempts to obtain as perfect understanding and con-

* The code of the Massachusetts General Hospital's Committee on Research and the Individual was only a slightly modified version of this, made in 1967.

sent as possible prior to the experimentation, through the subject, when this is possible, and the parents or guardians.

A considerable safeguard is to be found in the practice of having at least two physicians involved in experimental situations: first, there is the physician concerned with the care of the patient, his first interest is the patient's welfare; and, second, the physician-scientist whose interest is the sound conduct of the investigation. Perhaps too often a single individual attempts to encompass both roles. Some believe that the physician, as experimenter (in a procedure not for the patient's direct benefit), does not have a doctor-patient relationship which in a diagnostic or therapeutic situation would give him the right to withhold information if he judged it in the best interest of the patient. The subject is complicated.

When difficult ethical problems arise, they are best presented to a group of the investigator's peers for discussion and counsel.

The gain anticipated from an experiment must be commensurate with the risk involved. Sometimes large risks are to be taken for large gains, but such risks should be taken in almost all cases only when the patient promises to profit directly from the risk involved in needed therapy.

A poorly designed human study, one which does not yield scientifically interpretable data, is unethical.

Useful work on civil prisoners has been conducted in an ethical fashion in the past and will be in the future. It is to be emphasized, however, that in any work on a captive group, whether it be civil prisoners (military prisoners are *never* acceptable subjects for experimentation), medical students, one's own laboratory personnel, ward patients, or other captive groups may be useful, but at the same time, because of the possibilities for subtle coercion, the use of such subject material can be dealt with only with scrupulous care to preserve the subject's rights. Research is not to be carried to the point where it violates the fundamental rights of the individual.

As a general principle, it is better to avoid using as subjects persons about to die or those who are in danger of sudden death, because the death might cast a cloud on a careful investigator and on a meritorious project when, in fact, the death had nothing to do with the experimentation.

A study is ethical or not at its inception; it does not become ethical because it succeeds in producing valuable data.

When it is discovered that data have been unethically obtained, they are not to be published under ordinary circumstances. While the specific loss to medicine might be great, it is never as great in any reasonably conceivable circumstances as the moral loss sustained by medicine when unethically obtained data are published. Suppression of unethically obtained data will do much to curb the enthusiasm to carry on the unacceptable practices of the careless or the occasional unscrupulous investigator. A parallel case can be seen in the Mapp Decision of the United States Supreme Court, where it was recently ruled that evidence unconstitutionally obtained is never admissible in a court, however valuable the data might be in the pursuit of justice.

In the publication of experimental results, it must be made unmistakably clear that the proprieties have been observed in the study.

EXPERIMENTAL THERAPY FOR THE DIRECT BENEFIT OF THE PATIENT

Several of the remarks in the foregoing section are clearly applicable here; they will not be repeated.

To treat the ill is to experiment; experimentation is a common necessity in fitting the remedy to the disease. The patient gives his permission in the act of going to the physician for relief. The usual doctor-patient relationship prevails.

The coupling of the scientific method to traditional medical observation has enormously increased the understanding and successful treatment of disease. This is often accomplished through the controlled clinical trial, best supervised by a group rather than the investigator alone.

The controlled clinical trial in therapy is usually permissible under ordinary circumstances only when there is uncertainty as to which of two procedures is the better. (An exception to this might be permissible in certain simple situations where, for example, no discernible risk is present and a pain-relieving agent is pitted against a placebo.) It is permissible to give half of a group the new treatment and half the previously accepted treatment. This should ordinarily be explained to the subjects and consent obtained.

When a new and promising procedure is to be used, it is considerate and usually wise to explain this to the patient and to get his concurrence if the value of the procedure is debatable. It is prudent to get the agreement of one's peers to the proposed plan of action.

The parent or guardian can of course give consent to treatment of a child when this is for the child's benefit. (They have no such right according to English law if the procedure is not for the child's direct benefit. The issue is less clear in American law; the only precedents are the decisions of the Massachusetts Supreme Judicial Court that children at the age of understanding may donate organs for transplantation [thus avoiding guilt feelings in the donor if he had refused], and the *Bonner v. Moran* case [1941] involving a 15-year-old boy who donated skin to his cousin who had suffered severe burns. This was done at the behest of an aunt without the knowledge of the mother, who was ill and knew nothing of the plans. The court's implication was that, if the mother had consented, this would have been satisfactory.)

Preventive therapy administered to the well is covered by the same ethical and legal considerations as the treatment of disease.

NORMAL AND PATIENT VOLUNTEERS

It is held by some that there is no difference between this group and those discussed above. There is, however, the practical point that members of this group are aware that they are the subjects of experimentation, and participate or not according to their own wishes, unfortunately not always the case with patients.

An individual cannot soundly volunteer for an experiment unless he first understands what he is volunteering for.

Patients are abnormal by virtue of disease or injury. It is often important to learn the limits of normal states through study of normal individuals, who, of course, will not benefit directly from the procedures carried out.

REQUIREMENTS FOR REVIEW TO INSURE THE RIGHTS AND WELFARE OF INDIVIDUALS

Public Health Service Policy and Procedure No. 129, Revised July 1, 1966

I. BACKGROUND

Culminating several years of study by various Public Health Service staff and advisory groups, the National Advisory Health Council passed the following resolution on December 3, 1965:

"Be it resolved that the National Advisory Health Council believes that Public Health Service support of clinical research and investigation involving human beings should be provided only if the judgment of the investigator is subject to prior review by his institutional associates to assure an independent determination of the protection of the rights and welfare of the individual or individuals involved, of the appropriateness of the methods used to secure informed consent, and of the risks and potential medical benefits of the investigation."

II. POLICY

The Surgeon General accepted the resolution of the National Advisory Health Council and promulgated the following policy statement on February 8, 1966:

"No new, renewal, or continuation research or research training grant in support of clinical research and investigation involving human beings shall be awarded by the Public Health Service unless the grantee has indicated in the application the manner in which the grantee institution will provide prior review of the judgment of the principal investigator or program director by a committee of his institutional associates. This review should assure an independent determination: (1) of the rights and welfare of the individual or individuals involved, (2) of the appropriateness of the methods used to secure informed consent, and (3) of the risks and potential medical benefits of the investigation. A description of the committee of the associates who will provide the review shall be included in the application."

III. REVISED POLICY

By decision of the Surgeon General, the application of this policy has been extended to all grants and awards of the Public Health Service in the support of the research, training, or demonstration projects, including the projects supported through general research support and those of fellows and trainees. The policy is not applicable to grants in support of construction, alterations, renovations, or research resources—it is obviously applicable to the PHS projects using these facilities and resources.

This policy will be included in all pertinent grant program policy and instruction statements, and will be among the conditions of award agreed upon by grantee institutions and the Public Health Service. The policy applies to all investigations involving human subjects, including clinical research.

A. Assignment of Responsibility

Safeguarding the rights and welfare of human subjects involved in research supported by PHS grants is the responsibility of the institution to which the grant is awarded. The institution must assure the Public Health Service that in the case of investigations and activities supported directly by the PHS, it will provide group review and decision, maintain surveillance, and provide advice for investigators on safeguarding the rights and welfare of human subjects. The institution also has the responsibility to provide whatever professional attention or facilities may be required for the safety and well-being of human subjects. The institution shall be responsible for developing the administrative mechanism for review, surveillance, and advice; however, the PHS requires that, prior to inception of each course of investigation, objective decisions be made on the three points cited in the Surgeon General's policy statement (above) by an appropriate committee of associates of the investigator having no vested interest in the specific project involved. The grantee institution may utilize staff, consultants, or both to carry out the review. Any group responsible for review should possess not only specific scientific competence to comprehend the scientific content of the investigations reviewed, but also other competencies pertinent to the judgments that need to be made.

The grantee is required to make and keep written records of the group reviews and decisions on the use of human subjects and to obtain and keep documentary evidence of informed consent relating to investigations carried out with the assistance of PHS financial support.

B. Timing of Review

While this policy requires that review be conducted prior to the use of human beings as subjects, there are advantages to both the PHS and the grantee in having the review conducted *prior to* application for PHS support. The PHS encourages the institution to do so, if the review can be accomplished without causing unreasonable delay in the application process and if the application is of the type that normally contains a reviewable scientific protocol.

IV. PROCEDURAL REVISIONS—ASSURANCES OF APPLICANTS AND GRANTEES

Upon issuance of this policy statement, the PHS will require necessary assurances from the grantee institutions which sponsor investigations involving human subjects, including clinical research. These assurances will cover both the general principles of safeguarding human rights and welfare in the conduct of research and the specific points of the Surgeon General's policy. The assurance should provide explicit information on the policy and procedure it employs for review and decision on the propriety of plans of research involving human subjects. The descriptions will include the competencies represented in the committees of associates utilized for review, the sources of consultants (if used), the administrative mechanisms by which surveillance is provided for projects involving human subjects—particularly to deal with changes in protocol or emergent problems of investigations, the means of guidance and advice provided for investigators, and the manner in which the institution will assure itself that the advice of the committee of associates will be followed. Copies of documents of institutional policies on these issues should be attached to the memorandum of assurance.

Assurances can be provided which apply only to individual major components of universities or other large institutions in those instances where assurances covering the total institution are impracticable or inadvisable.

Each assurance and its attachments shall be transmitted to the Public Health Service, in care of the Chief, Division of Research Grants. When the Public Health Service has reviewed and accepted the assurance, the Chief, Division of Research Grants, shall so notify both the responsible official of the grantee institution involved and all Public Health Service extramural research program offices.

Each grantee shall report currently any changes in its policies, its procedures, or the competencies represented on its committee of associates.

For each application that includes or is likely to include investigation involving human subjects, including clinical research, the applicant institution should make reference to the certification as follows:

"The investigations encompassed by this application have been or will be approved by the committee of associates of the investigator(s) in accordance with this institution's assurance on clinical research dates ——————."

Until an institution-wide assurance has been accepted by the PHS, the institution can fulfill requirements of this policy for individual studies by submitting an assurance with each application for PHS financial support, stating that prior to inception of investigations, the requirements of section III A of this Policy and Procedure Order will be followed. The statement must also describe the composition of the group which will conduct the review.

This interim procedure will be acceptable until November 1, 1966. After that date no new, supplemental, renewal, or continuation application for a Public Health Service grant or award to support investigations involving human subjects will be accepted for review unless the PHS has approved an institution-wide assurance.

Nothing in the institution-wide assurance or in the interim policy procedure used in some cases until November 1, 1966, should inhibit PHS staff, advisory groups, or consultants (1) from identifying concern for the welfare of human subjects, and communicating this concern to the grantee institution, or (2) from recommending disapproval of the application if the gravity of the hazards and risks so indicate.

In the case of awards to U.S. citizens receiving fellowships for training abroad, special conditions or circumstances relating to the place at which the training is being provided may upon occasion justify modification of these requirements. Requests from the sponsor for approval of such modifications must be reviewed by the Office of Internation Research, NIH, and approved by the PHS bureau chief concerned.

REQUIREMENTS FOR REVIEW TO INSURE THE RIGHTS AND WELFARE OF INDIVIDUALS: CLARIFICATION

Public Health Service, December 12, 1966

This report is to clarify issues raised by PHS grantees and staff regarding the meaning of the requirements of PPO #129, Revised, July 1, 1966, subject: "Investigations Involving Human Subjects, Including Clinical Research: Requirements for Review to Insure the Rights and Welfare of Individuals."

This policy refers to all investigations that involve human subjects, including investigations in the behavioral and social sciences. The grantee institution is responsible for assuring that the investigations are in accord with the laws of the community in which the investigations are conducted and for giving due consideration to pertinent ethical issues. Appropriate groups of associates within the institution, and outside consultants if needed, are to be utilized to provide the necessary review. Institutions may designate separate groups in order to assure competence and independence of review for particular areas.

The principles of this policy apply most directly and comprehensively in those instances of social, behavioral, and medical science investigations where a procedure may induce in the subject an altered state or condition potentially harmful to his personal welfare. Surgical procedures, the administration of drugs, the requirement of strenuous physical exertion, and participation in psychologically or socially harmful activities are examples of experimental arrangements which require thorough scrutiny by institutional review groups. Such procedures require continuing overview and full documentation for the record.

Aside from the above types of procedures, there is a large range of social and behavioral research in which no personal risk to the subject is involved. In these circumstances, regardless of whether the investigation is classified as behavioral, social, medical, or other, the issues of concern are the fully voluntary nature of the participation of the subject, the maintenance of confidentiality of information obtained from the subject, and the protection of the subject from misuse of the findings. For example, a major class of procedures in the social and behavioral sciences does no more than observe or elicit information about the subject's status, by means of administration of tests, inventories, questionnaires, or surveys of personality or background. In such instances, the ethical considerations of voluntary participation, confidentiality, and propriety in use of the findings are the most generally relevant ones. However, such procedures may in many instances not require the fully informed consent of the subject or even his knowledgeable participation. In such instances full and specific documentation is necessary for the record.

Many investigations in the social and behavioral sciences involve procedures designed to alter the status of the individual as, for example, studies of human learning, social perception, or group effectiveness. In such research the effects, if any, on the subject may be transitory or even more or less permanent, but they must be judged clearly not to be harmful or not to involve the risk of harm.

Whatever the nature of the investigation, the concern for the protection of the subject and for the assurance of voluntary participation becomes most critical when the subject is not of age or competence to make an adequate judgment in his own behalf.

These are only some examples of issues which may arise. The fundamental point is that every project must be considered on an individual basis to clarify which, if any, such issues are present and to insure that these are adequately resolved by the specific design of its procedures. For this reason, it is essential that the grantee institution be responsible for the clarification and resolution of all ethical and other pertinent issues. The appropriate mechanism for this purpose is the utilization of groups of associates, established at the institution to provide competent, independent review. Based on its knowledgeable scrutiny of the specifics of the investigation involved, such a review group can decide which issues are germane and ascertain the adequacy of provisions for protecting the rights and welfare of human subjects in research, the appropriateness of the methods used to secure informed consent, and the risks and potential benefits of the investigation.

CONSENT FOR USE OF INVESTIGATIONAL NEW DRUGS ON HUMANS: STATEMENT OF POLICY

Food and Drug Administration Federal Regulation 11415, August 30, 1966

(a) Section 505 (i) of the act provides that regulations on use of investigational new drugs on human beings shall impose the condition that investigators "obtain the consent of such human beings or their representatives, except where they deem it not feasible or, in their professional judgment, contrary to the best interest of such human beings."

(b) This means that the consent of such human beings (or the consent of their representatives) to whom investigational drugs are administered primarily for the accumulation of scientific knowledge, for such purposes as studying drug behavior, body processes, or the course of a disease, must be obtained in all cases and, in all but exceptional cases, the consent of patients under treatment with investigational drugs must be obtained.

(c) "Under treatment" applies when the administration of the investigational drug for either diagnostic or therapeutic purposes constitutes responsible medical judgment, taking into account the availability of other remedies or drugs and the individual circumstances pertaining to the person to whom the investigational drug is to be administered.

(d) "Exceptional cases," as used in paragraph (b) of this section, which exceptions are to be strictly applied, are cases where it is not feasible to obtain the patient's consent or the consent of his representative, or where, as a matter of professional judgment exercised in the best interest of a particular patient under the investigator's care, it would be contrary to that patient's welfare to obtain his consent.

(e) "Patient" means a person under treatment.

(f) "Not feasible" is limited to cases where the investigator is not capable of obtaining consent because of inability to communicate with the patient or his representative; for example, where the patient is in a coma or is otherwise incapable of giving informed consent, his representative cannot be reached, and it is imperative to administer the drug without delay.

(g) "Contrary to the best interests of such human beings" applies when the communication of information to obtain consent would seriously affect the patient's disease status and the physician has exercised a professional judgment that under the particular circumstances of this patient's case, the patient's best interests would suffer if consent were sought.

(h) "Consent" or "informed consent" means that the person involved has legal capacity to give consent, is so situated as to be able to exercise free power of choice, and is provided with a fair explanation of all material information concerning the administration of the investigational drug, or his possible use as a control, as to enable him to make an understanding decision as to his willingness to receive said investigational drug. This latter element requires that before the acceptance of an affirmative decision by such person the investigator should make known to him the nature, duration, and purpose of the administration of said investigational drug; the method and means by which it is to be administered; all inconveniences and hazards reasonably to be expected, including the fact, where applicable, that the person may be used as a control; the existence of alternative forms of therapy, if any; and the effects upon his health or person that may possibly come from the administration of the investigational drug. Said patient's consent shall be obtained in writing by the investigator.

WOLFENSBERGER'S CODE, 1967

(Abstracted from Wolfensberger [428])

Guidelines for ethical conduct of research should be based on clearly identifiable and internally consistent principles. It is important that issues be stated with maximum clarity, so that problems for which no specific solutions have been previously formulated can be handled in the light of the broader principles . . .

1. The more deleterious an experimental effect may be to a subject, the more precautions the researcher should take.

2. Risk-sharing between experimenter and subject in no way releases the experimenter from any obligation toward his subject.

3. The more serious or extensive the right that the researcher wants a subject to surrender, the more consideration and effort should be devoted to the problem of consent or release.

4. No consent for level-1* research should be required at this time to use a procedure which, although it may be experimental and nonvalidated in nature, is used primarily for treating a person therapeutically, *if* (i) the procedure is considered justifiable and appropriate by qualified peers, and (ii) a consent (to treatment) appropriate to the occasion and to the risk inherent in the procedure has been obtained.

5. No consent appears necessary if the right needed by the experimenter is already possessed by him or by the legal body that he represents; then consent by that legal body, rather than by the subject, must be obtained. For example, a member of the armed forces loses certain rights of autonomy, which in turn might be delegated by the proper authorities to an experimenter without the subject's consent or knowledge.† However, it would appear to be desirable to obtain the personal consent of each subject if this is at all feasible; furthermore, if there is uncertainty as to whether the legal body in question possesses the rights required by the experimenter, then, in proportion to the extent of the rights involved, the experimenter should exert efforts to obtain opinions on this question from a group of impartial referees who could be considered qualified to judge.

* Level-1 research involves experimental activities and procedures, but are not consciously recognized or formally labeled as research, as, for example, in diagnosis or treatment.

† While the trial of new weapons or new planes certainly involves human risk, our society accepts this. I do not for a moment believe that a similar acceptance even in wartime would be countenanced by society if the project were labeled or were by implication an experiment. Consider, for example, the uproar that ensued when a member of the Congress charged that American soldiers were being used as guinea pigs in certain liver function studies during World War II.

6. I propose that except under extraordinary circumstances no consent is required where (level-1) research is conducted on record-file data if (i) such data are grouped, or their anonymity is otherwise assured, so that no subject is identified and no definite statement can be made about any specific subject; and (ii) the manipulation of the research data does not lead to consequences detrimental to a subject.

7. Where level-2* research is involved (that is, risks are extrinsic), and where only modest and reasonable amounts of rights (i) and (ii) (privacy and personal resources) are concerned, consent may be obtained by means of a routine release form. Thus agencies such as institutions, public clinics, and university hospitals might explain to their clients, during the intake process, the research orientation of the agency and the type of research that might be typically involved, and ask for the clients' cooperation and signature. Much would depend on the manner in which this approach was handled. My personal experience is that it may be best to inform the subject or his agents as early as possible, both orally and in writing, of four things: (i) there is little likelihood that the research will benefit the subject; (ii) the subject's participation may benefit many others like him in the future, and research is the only way to improve certain services, conditions, and treatments; (iii) the research will entail no undue (that is, considered unreasonable by most people) discomfort, consumption of time, or loss of privacy; and there is no direct risk; and (iv) participation is voluntary.

Such a routine release may not be legal in all states, but it can be very important in certain agencies, such as institutions for the retarded. If a broad release were not obtained, even the most harmless and minor participation in research would require a specific release. In some research-oriented institutions, a resident may be called upon several times a year to serve as a subject, and obtaining a specific release each time would be prohibitively cumbersome. Moreover, after placing residents many parents are no longer accessible, do not visit or answer mail, and may live many hundreds of miles distant. In short, unless either the superintendent were the guardian—and the trend is away from this practice—or a general release were obtained upon admission, little or no research on mental retardation could be conducted in such institutions. The implications of such a situation would be vast and horrendous. . . .

8. When level-2 research calls for right (iv), a borderline case exists. Then a decision to obtain a specific release may be based on the degree

* Level-2 research consists of clearly identified and conceptualized research; it involves manipulation of subjects.

of discomfort or pain involved and on purely psychosocial considerations such as a subject's familiarity with the procedures and the public emotion that research could generate.

9. A specific and relatively detailed release for research either on level 3 or entailing right (iii) appears to be mandatory.

10. The more reason there is to question a subject's ability to give a free, informed consent, the more care should be taken to assure that consent is free and informed, or that the responsible agent's release is appropriate; here the advice of the Medical Research Council appears sound: one should obtain consent not only in written form but also in the presence of witnesses who can provide consensual agreement regarding the subject's understanding and freedom of choice.

It is not sufficient for the researcher to exercise restraint in eliciting consent; he must also ascertain to a reasonable degree that a subject, even a volunteer, does not *perceive* himself coerced when he is not. For instance, no matter what a prisoner is told, he is likely to believe that by not volunteering to serve in a cancer-cell-injection experiment he may delay his parole; thus he may be under a subtle form of coercion. College students are particularly apt to believe that refusal to volunteer as subjects in an instructor's experiment will jeopardize their progress—and they are often right. The researcher should go out of his way to create an atmosphere and structure that permit a truly free choice.

Finally, not ethics but wisdom dictates that, when emotionally charged situations and issues are involved (such as research with "live cancer," and handicapped children), the researcher should consider raising his safeguards to a level above that required by ethical considerations alone . . .

A CODE FOR SELF-EXPERIMENTATION, 1968

National Institutes of Health

The National Institutes of Health have led for years in the development of guides to protect all participants in human experimentation. Some of the hazards of self-experimentation have already been described. While self-experimentation could have been considered as dealt with by implication in earlier statements from the National Institutes of Health, the area has now been explicitly covered by a memorandum from the Director of the Clinical Center under date of January 9, 1968. The purpose of this memorandum is to provide the same safeguards for the investigator-subject as for the normal volunteer. This grew out of a statement of the Medical Board which was approved by the Director of the National Institutes of Health, December 18, 1967, in which approval was given for the creation of a framework within which the investigator could be one of the subjects in his own studies. The stipulations are as follows:

There are certain procedures which an investigator can properly carry out on a subject which he cannot carry out on himself; e.g., certain types of catheterization. It should also be noted that an investigator who utilizes himself repeatedly may, by the sum of the investigations, do harm to himself that a single study would not do. Experience has shown that investigators tend to be less rigorous in providing themselves with the precautionary techniques they utilize with their subjects.

The requirements for approval of self-experimentation are:

(1) There is to be no self-experimentation without group consideration.

The project must be reviewed and approved by the

(a) Institute Clinical Director
(b) Clinical Research Committee of the Medical Board
(c) Medical Board
(d) Director, NIH.

Each research protocol proposal that will utilize any of the investigators listed on the project as a subject must contain a specific statement to that effect.*

* NIH policy also requires that any research protocol utilizing an employee,

(2) Investigators who serve as volunteers for experiments must meet the same standards of eligibility as other normal volunteers: a complete history, physical examination, and routine laboratory workup must be done by a Clinical Center patient-care physician before an investigator utilizes himself. This preliminary evaluation, along with an account of the research study, must be entered in a standard NIH medical record.†

(3) Exceptions to the above requirements should be made for simple procedures: e.g., collection of urine, small samples of blood, or other minor tests which are permissible in the case of normal volunteers, without the requirement for an approved research project protocol.

---

whether the employee is an investigator or not, must have the specific approval of the Medical Board and the Director, NIH.

† Inasmuch as NIH regulations require the registration of all normal controls as Clinical Center patients, the clinical investigator serving as a normal control should also be registered as a patient.

CARDIAC TRANSPLANTATION IN MAN

A Statement by the Board on Medicine,
National Academy of Sciences, 1968
(Prepared under the Chairmanship of Walsh McDermott)

Progress in medicine depends largely on the cautious extension to man of a body of carefully integrated knowledge derived from programs of basic and developmental research in the laboratory. Extension to man is itself an investigative process that must meet the same meticulous scientific standards that obtain in the laboratory, and the extension can appropriately be started only when the total body of knowledge has reached a certain point. It is clear that this point has been reached in the case of cardiac transplantation.

Careful, detailed laboratory investigations in a number of centers have demonstrated the feasibility of a surgical technique for cardiac transplanation. With the skillful use of immunosuppressive agents, investigators have succeeded in maintaining the life of laboratory animals subjected to cardiac transplants for periods up to a year or more. Moreover, considerable relevant knowledge has been acquired from carefully controlled clinical investigations involving the transplantation of a kidney in a human being.

But, in contrast to the transplant of a paired organ of man such as the kidney, cardiac transplantation raises new, complex issues that must be faced promptly. In the case of a kidney transplant, the donation of the organ is not crucial to the donor; in the event of failure, the recipient may be kept alive for extended periods until another attempt is made. In the case of cardiac transplantation, the life of the donor cannot be maintained. Further, the recipient's life cannot be salvaged if the transplanted heart does not function. Highly important is the fact that the length of time that the recipient can survive is as yet conjectural, even if the immediate result is favorable as indicated by prompt resumption of function by the transplanted heart. Thus the procedure cannot as yet be regarded as an accepted form of therapy, even an heroic one. It must be clearly viewed for what it is, a scientific exploration of the unknown, only the very first step of which is the actual surgical feat of transplanting the organ. In this connection, it is clear that there are considerably more institutions whose staffs include men with the surgical expertise appropriate for the first step of the investigation—the actual transplantation—than have available the full capability to conduct the total study in terms of all relevant scientific observations.

Because of these special circumstances it is the considered view of the

Board of Medicine of the National Academy of Sciences that for the present, cardiac transplantation should only be carried out in those institutions in which all of the following criteria can be met:

1. The surgical team should have had extensive laboratory experience in cardiac transplantation, and should have demonstrated not only technical competence but a thorough understanding of the biological processes that threaten functional survival of the transplant, i.e., rejection and its control. Investigators skilled in immunology, including tissue typing and the management of immunosuppressive procedures, should be readily available as collaborators in the transplantation effort.

2. As in any other scientific investigation, the overall plan of study should be carefully recorded in advance and arrangements made to continue the systematic observations throughout the whole lifetime of the recipient. The conduct of such studies should be within an organized framework of information exchange and analyses. This would permit prompt access by other investigators to the full positive and negative results. Thus the continued care of each recipient would be assured the continuing benefit of the most up-to-date information. Such an organized communication network would also permit the findings to be integrated with the work of others and assist in the planning of further investigative efforts. In this way, it would be possible to ensure that progress will be deliberate, and that the experience from each individual case will make its full contribution to the planning of the next.

3. As the procedure is a scientific investigation and not as yet an accepted form of therapy, the primary justification for this activity in respect to both the donor and recipient is that from the study will come new knowledge of benefit to others in our society. The ethical issues involved in the selection of donor and recipient are a part of the whole complex question of the ethics of human experimentation. This extremely sensitive and complicated subject is now under intensive study by a number of well-qualified groups in this country and abroad. Pending the further development of ethical guidelines, it behooves each institution in which a cardiac transplantation is to be conducted to assure itself that it has protected the interests of all parties involved to the fullest possible extent.

Rigid safeguards should be developed with respect to the selection of prospective donors and the selection of prospective recipients. An independent group of expert, mature physicians—none of whom is directly engaged in the transplantation effort—should examine the prospective donor. They should agree and record their unanimous opinion as to the donor's acceptability on the basis of the evidence of crucial and irreversible bodily damage and imminent death. Similarly the prospective recipient should be examined by an independent group of competent physicians and clinical scientists including a cardiologist and an expert in immunology. In this instance the consulting group should also record their opinion as to the acceptability of the recipient for transplantation on the basis of all the evidence including the presence of far-advanced, irreversible cardiac damage and the likelihood of benefit from the procedure.

* * *

Enumeration of the above criteria is based on the conviction that in order to obtain the scientific information necessary for the next phase in this form of organ transplantation, only a relatively small number of careful investigations involving cardiac transplantation need be done at this time. Therefore, the Board strongly urges that institutions, even though well-equipped from the standpoint of surgical expertise and facilities but without specific capabilities to conduct the whole range of scientific observations involved in the total study, resist the temptation to approve the performance of the surgical procedure until there has been an opportunity for the total situation to be clarified by intensive and closely integrated study.

ETHICAL GUIDELINES FOR ORGAN TRANSPLANTATION AMERICAN MEDICAL ASSOCIATION, 1968

The Judicial Council of the AMA offers the following statement for guidance of physicians as they seek to maintain the highest level of ethical conduct in their practice.

1. In all professional relationships between a physician and his patient, the physician's primary concern must be the health of his patient. He owes the patient his primary allegiance. This concern and allegiance must be preserved in all medical procedures, including those which involve the transplantation of an organ from one person to another where both donor and recipient are patients. Care must, therefore, be taken to protect the rights of both the donor and the recipient, and no physician may assume a responsibility in organ transplantation unless the rights of both donor and recipient are equally protected.

2. A prospective organ transplant offers no justification for relaxation of the usual standards of medical care. The physician should provide his patient, who may be a prospective organ donor, with that care usually given others being treated for a similar injury or disease.

3. When a vital, single organ is to be transplanted, the death of the donor shall have been determined by at least one physician other than the recipient's physician. Death shall be determined by the clinical judgment of the physician. In making this determination, the ethical physician will use all available, currently accepted scientific tests.

4. Full discussion of the proposed procedure with the donor and the recipient or their responsible relatives or representatives is mandatory. The physician should be objective in discussing the procedure, in disclosing known risks and possible hazards, and in advising him of the alternative procedures available. The physician should not encourage expectations beyond those which the circumstances justify. The physician's interest in advancing scientific knowledge must always be secondary to his primary concern for the patient.

5. Transplant procedures of body organs should be undertaken (a) only by physicians who possess special medical knowledge and technical competence developed through special training, study, and laboratory experience and practice, and (b) in medical institutions with facilities adequate to protect the health and well-being of the parties to the procedure.

6. Transplantation of body organs should be undertaken only after careful evaluation of the availability and effectiveness of other possible therapy.

7. Medicine recognizes that organ transplants are newsworthy and that the public is entitled to be correctly informed about them. Normally, a scientific report of the procedures should first be made to the medical profession for review and evaluation. When dramatic aspects of medical advances prevent adherence to accepted procedures, objective, factual, and discreet public reports to the communications media may be made by a properly authorized physician, but should be followed as soon as possible by full scientific reports to the profession.

In organ transplantation procedures, the right of privacy of the parties to the procedures must be respected. Without their authorization to disclose their identity the physician is limited to an impersonal discussion of the procedure.

Reporting of medical and surgical procedures should always be objective and factual. Such reporting will also preserve and enhance the stature of the medical profession and its service to mankind.

Appendix B

Report of

THE AD HOC COMMITTEE TO EXAMINE THE DEFINITION OF BRAIN DEATH

now presented as

A DEFINITION OF IRREVERSIBLE COMA

respectfully submitted to
Robert H. Ebert, Dean

BY

HENRY K. BEECHER, M.D., *Chairman*

RAYMOND D. ADAMS, M.D.
A. CLIFFORD BARGER, M.D.
WILLIAM J. CURRAN, L.L.M., S.M. HYG.
DEREK DENNY-BROWN, M.D.
DANA L. FARNSWORTH, M.D.
JORDI FOLCH-PI, M.D.
EVERETT I. MENDELSOHN, PH.D.
JOHN P. MERRILL, M.D.
JOSEPH MURRAY, M.D.
RALPH POTTER, TH.D.
ROBERT SCHWAB, M.D.
WILLIAM SWEET, M.D.

July 3, 1968

HARVARD MEDICAL SCHOOL

A DEFINITION OF IRREVERSIBLE COMA

BACKGROUND

Our primary purpose is to define irreversible coma as a new criterion for death. There are two reasons why there is need for a definition: (1) Improvements in resuscitative and supportive measures have led to increased efforts to save those who are desperately injured. Sometimes these efforts have only partial success so that the result is an individual whose heart continues to beat but whose brain is irreversibly damaged. The burden is great on patients who suffer permanent loss of intellect, on their families, on the hospitals, and on those in need of hospital beds already occupied by these comatose patients. (2) Obsolete criteria for the definition of death can lead to controversy in obtaining organs for transplantation.

Irreversible coma has many causes, but *we are concerned here only with those comatose individuals who have no discernible central nervous system activity*. If the characteristics can be defined in satisfactory terms, translatable into action—and we believe this is possible—then several problems will either disappear or will become more readily soluble.

More than medical problems are present. There are moral, ethical, religious, and legal issues. Adequate definition here will prepare the way for better insight into all of these matters as well as for better law than is currently applicable.

CHARACTERISTICS OF IRREVERSIBLE COMA

An organ, brain or other, that no longer functions and has no possibility of functioning again is for all practical purposes dead. Our first problem is to determine the characteristics of a *permanently* nonfunctioning brain.

A patient in this state appears to be in a deep coma. The condition can be satisfactorily diagnosed by points 1, 2, and 3 to follow. The electroencephalogram (point 4) provides confirmatory data, and when available it should be utilized. In situations where for one reason or another electroencephalographic monitoring is not available, the absence of cerebral function has to be determined by purely clinical signs, to be described, or by absence of circulation as judged by standstill of blood in the retinal vessels, or by absence of cardiac activity.

1. *Unreceptivity and unresponsitivity.* There is a total unawareness to externally applied stimuli and inner need and complete unresponsiveness—our definition of irreversible coma. Even the most

intensely painful stimuli evoke no vocal or other response, not even a groan, withdrawal of a limb, or quickening of respiration.

2. *No movements or breathing.* Observation covering a period of at least one hour by physicians is adequate to satisfy the criteria of no spontaneous muscular movements or spontaneous respiration or response to stimuli such as pain, touch, sound, or light. After the patient is on a mechanical respirator, the total absence of spontaneous breathing may be established by turning off the respirator for 3 minutes and observing whether there is any effort on the part of the subject to breathe spontaneously. (The respirator may be turned off for this time, provided that at the start of the trial period the patient's carbon dioxide tension is within the normal range, and provided also that the patient had been breathing room air for at least 10 minutes prior to the trial.)

3. *No reflexes.* Irreversible coma with abolition of central nervous system activity is evidenced in part by the absence of elicitable reflexes. The pupil will be fixed and dilated and will not respond to a direct source of bright light. Since the establishment of a fixed, dilated pupil is clear-cut in clinical practice, there should be no uncertainty as to its presence. Ocular movement (to head turning and to irrigation of the ears with ice water) and blinking are absent. There is no evidence of postural activity (decerebrate or other). Swallowing, yawning, vocalization are in abeyance. Corneal and pharyngeal reflexes are absent.

As a rule the stretch or tendon reflexes cannot be elicited; i.e., tapping the tendons of the biceps, triceps and pronator muscles, quadriceps and gastrocnemius muscles with the reflex hammer elicits no contraction of the respective muscles. Plantar or noxious stimulation gives no response.

4. *Flat electroencephalogram.* Of great confirmatory value is the flat or isoelectric EEG. We must assume that the electrodes have been properly applied, that the apparatus is functioning normally, and that the personnel in charge is competent. We consider it prudent to have one channel of the apparatus used for an electrocardiogram. This channel will monitor the ECG so that if it appears in the electroencephalographic leads because of high resistance, it can be readily identified. It also establishes the presence of the active heart in the absence of the EEG. We recommend that another channel be used for a noncephalic lead. This will pick up space-borne or vibration-borne artifacts and identify them. The simplest form of such a monitoring noncephalic electrode has two leads over the dorsum of the hand, preferably the right hand, so the ECG will be minimal or absent. Since one of the requirements of this state is that there be no muscle activity, these two

dorsal hand electrodes will not be bothered by muscle artifact. The apparatus should be run at standard gains 10 μV mm, 50 μV 5mm. Also it should be isoelectric at double this standard gain which is 5 μv mm or 25 μV mm. At least 10 full minutes of recording are desirable, but twice that would be better.

It is also suggested that the gains at some point be opened to their full amplitude for a brief period (5 to 100 seconds) to see what is going on. Usually in an intensive care unit artifacts will dominate the picture, but these are readily identifiable. There shall be no electroencephalographic response to noise or to pinch.

All the above tests shall be repeated at least 24 hours later with no change.

The validity of such data as indications of irreversible cerebral damage depends on the exclusion of two conditions: hypothermia (temperature below 90° F [32.2° C]) or central nervous system depressants, such as barbiturates.

OTHER PROCEDURES

The patient's condition can be determined only by a physician. When the patient is hopelessly damaged as defined above the family, all colleagues who have participated in major decisions concerning the patient, and all nurses involved should be so informed. Death is to be declared and *then* the respirator turned off. The decision to do this and the responsibility for it are to be taken by the physician-in-charge, in consultation with one or more physicians who have been directly involved in the case. It is unsound and undesirable to force the family to make the decision.

LEGAL COMMENTARY

The legal system of the United States is greatly in need of the kind of analysis and recommendations for medical procedures in cases of irreversible brain damage as described. At present, the law of the United States, in all 50 states and in the federal courts, treats the question of human death as a question of fact to be decided in every case. When any doubt exists, the courts seek medical expert testimony concerning the time of death of the particular individual involved. However, the law makes the assumption that the medical criteria for determining death are settled and not in doubt among physicians. Furthermore, the law assumes that the traditional method among physicians for determination of death is to ascertain the absence of all vital signs. To this extent, *Black's Law Dictionary* (fourth edition, 1951) defines death as

The cessation of life; the ceasing to exist; *defined by physicians* as a total stoppage of the circulation of the blood, and a cessation of the animal and vital functions consequent thereupon, such as respiration, pulsation, etc. [*italics added*].

In the few modern court decisions involving a definition of death, the courts have used the concept of the total cessation of all vital signs. Two cases are worthy of examination. Both involved the issue of which one of two persons died first.

In *Thomas v. Anderson* (96 Cal App 2d 371, 211 P 2d 478), a California District Court of Appeal in 1950 said, "In the instant case the question as to which of the two men died first was a question of fact for the determination of the trial court . . ."

The appellate court cited and quoted in full the definition of death from *Black's Law Dictionary* and concluded, ". . . death occurs precisely when life ceases and does not occur until the heart stops beating and respiration ends. Death is not a continuous event and is an event that takes place at a precise time."

The other case is *Smith v. Smith* (229 Ark, 579, 317 SW 2d 275), decided in 1958 by the Supreme Court of Arkansas. In this case the two people were husband and wife involved in an auto accident. The husband was found dead at the scene of the accident. The wife was taken to the hospital unconscious. It is alleged that she "remained in coma due to brain injury" and died at the hospital seventeen days later. The petitioner in court tried to argue that the two people died simultaneously. The judge writing the opinion said the petition contained a "quite unusual and unique allegation." It was quoted as follows:

That the said Hugh Smith and his wife, Lucy Coleman Smith, were in an automobile accident on the 19th day of April, 1957, said accident being instantly fatal to each of them at the same time, although the doctors maintained a vain hope of survival and made every effort to revive and resuscitate said Lucy Coleman Smith until May 6th, 1957, when it was finally determined by the attending physicians that their hope of resuscitation and possible restoration of human life to the said Lucy Coleman Smith was entirely vain, and

That as a matter of modern medical science, your petitioner alleges and states, and will offer the Court competent proof that the said Hugh Smith, deceased, and said Lury Coleman Smith, deceased, lost their power to will at the same instant, and that their demise as earthly human beings occurred at the same time in said automobile accident, neither of them ever regaining any consciousness whatsoever.

The court dismissed the petition as a *matter of law*. The court quoted *Black's* definition of death and concluded, "Admittedly, this condition did not exist, and as a matter of fact, it would be too much of a strain of credulity for us to believe any evidence offered to the effect that Mrs. Smith was dead, scientifically or otherwise, unless the conditions set out in the definition existed."

Later in the opinion the court said, "Likewise, we take judicial notice that one breathing, though unconscious, is not dead."

"Judicial notice" of this definition of death means that the court did not consider that definition open to serious controversy; it considered the question as settled in responsible scientific and medical circles. The judge thus makes proof of uncontroverted facts unnecessary so as to prevent prolonging the trial with unnecessary proof and also to prevent fraud being committed upon the court by quasi "scientists" being called into court to controvert settled scientific principles at a price. Here, the Arkansas Supreme Court considered the definition of death to be a settled, scientific, biological fact. It refused to consider the plaintiff's offer of evidence that "modern medical science" might say otherwise. In simplified form, the above is the state of the law in the United States concerning the definition of death.

In this report, however, we suggest that responsible medical opinion is ready to adopt new criteria for pronouncing death to have occurred in an individual sustaining irreversible coma as a result of permanent brain damage. If this position is adopted by the medical community, it can form the basis for change in the current legal concept of death. No statutory change in the law should be necessary since the law treats this question essentially as one of fact to be determined by physicians. The only circumstance in which it would be necessary that legislation be offered in the various states to define "death" by law would be in the event that great controversy were engendered surrounding the subject and physicians were unable to agree on the new medical criteria.

It is recommended as a part of these procedures that the judgment of the existence of these criteria is solely a medical issue. It is suggested that the physician in charge of the patient consult with one or more other physicians directly involved in the case before the patient is declared dead on the basis of these criteria. In this way, the responsibility is shared over a wider range of medical opinion, thus providing an important degree of protection against later questions which might be raised about the particular case. It is further suggested that the decision to declare the person dead, and then to turn off the respirator, be made by physicians not involved in any later effort to transplant organs or tissue from the deceased individual. This is advisable in order to avoid any appearance of self-interest by the physicians involved.

It should be emphasized that we recommend the patient be declared dead before any effort is made to take him off a respirator, if he is then on a respirator. This declaration should not be delayed until he has been taken off the respirator and all artificially stimulated signs have ceased. The reason for this recommendation is that in our judgment it will provide a greater degree of legal protection to those involved. Otherwise, the physicians would be turning off the respirator on a person who is, under the present strict, technical application of law, still alive.

DISCUSSION

Irreversible coma can have various causes: cardiac arrest; asphyxia with respiratory arrest; massive brain damage; intracranial lesions, neoplastic or vascular. It can be produced by other encephalopathic states such as the metabolic derangements associated, for example, with uremia. Respiratory failure and impaired circulation underlie all these conditions. They result in hypoxia and ischemia of the brain.

From ancient times down to the recent past it was clear that when the respiration and heart stopped, the brain would die in a few minutes; so the obvious criterion of no heartbeat as synonymous with death was sufficiently accurate. In those times the heart was considered the central organ of the body; it is not surprising that its failure marked the onset of death. This is no longer valid when modern resuscitative and supportive measures are used. These improved activities can now restore "life" as judged by the ancient standards of persistent respiration and continuing heartbeat. This can be the case even when there is not the remotest possibility of an individual recovering consciousness following massive brain damage. In other situations "life" can be maintained only by means of artificial respiration and electrical stimulation of the heartbeat, or in temporarily by-passing the heart, or, in conjunction with these things, reducing with cold the body's oxygen requirement.

In an address on "The Prolongation of Life," (1957), Pope Pius XII raised many questions; some conclusions stand out: (1) In a deeply unconscious individual vital functions may be maintained over a prolonged period only by extraordinary means. Verification of the moment of death can be determined, if at all, only by a physician. Some have suggested that the moment of death is the moment when irreparable and overwhelming brain damage occurs. Pius XII acknowledged that it is not "within the competence of the Church" to determine this. (2) It is incumbent on the physician to take all reasonable, ordinary means of restoring the spontaneous vital functions and consciousness, and to employ such extraordinary means as are available to him to this end. It is not obligatory, however, to continue to use extraordinary means indefinitely in hopeless cases. "But normally one is held to use only ordinary means—according to circumstances of persons, places, times, and cultures—that is to say, means that do not involve any grave burden for oneself or another." It is the view of the Church that there comes a time when resuscitative efforts should stop and death be unopposed.

SUMMARY

The neurological impairment to which the term "brain death syndrome" and "irreversible coma" have become attached indicates diffuse disease. Function is abolished at cerebral, brainstem and often spinal levels. This should be evident in all cases from clinical examination alone. Cerebral, cortical, and thalamic involvement are indicated by a complete absence of receptivity of all forms of sensory stimulation and a lack of response to stimuli and to inner need. The term "coma" is used to designate this state of unreceptivity and unresponsitivity. But there is always coincident paralysis of brainstem and basal ganglionic mechanisms as manifested by an abolition of all postural reflexes, including induced decerebrate postures; a complete paralysis of respiration; widely dilated, fixed pupils; paralysis of ocular movements, swallowing, phonation, face and tongue muscles. Involvement of spinal cord, which is less constant, is reflected usually in loss of tendon reflex and all flexor withdrawal or nocifensive reflexes. Of the brainstem–spinal mechanisms which are conserved for a time, the vasomotor reflexes are the most persistent, and they are responsible in part for the paradoxical state of retained cardiovascular function, which is to some extent independent of nervous control, in the face of widespread disorder of cerebrum, brainstem and spinal cord.

Neurological assessment gains in reliability if the aforementioned neurological signs persist over a period of time, with the additional safeguards that there is no accompanying hypothermia or evidence of drug intoxication. If either of the latter two conditions exist, interpretation of the neurological state should await the return of body temperature to normal level and elimination of the intoxicating agent. Under any other circumstances, repeated examinations over a period of 24 hours or longer should be required in order to obtain evidence of the irreversibility of the condition.

References

1. Adelstein, L. J. The implied contract. *Bull. Los Angeles City Med. Ass.* 88:26, 1958.
2. Adrian, E. D. Priorities in medical responsibility (Jephcott Lecture). *Proc. Roy. Soc. Med.* 56:523–528, 1963.
3. Agote, L. Nuevo procedimiento para la transfusión de sangre. *An. Inst. Modelo Clin. Méd.* (B. Aires) 1 (nos. 1 & 3), 1915.
4. Alexandre, G. P. J. In discussion: Organ Transplantation: The Practical Possibilities, by J. E. Murray. In Ciba Foundation Symposium, *Ethics in Medical Progress.* Boston: Little, Brown, 1966, pp. 68–71.
5. Arkansas, State of. Acts 1959, no. 482, 2, p. 1923.
6. Arkansas Statutes 1947 Annotated, 1960 Replacement. Vol. 7A, chap. 16, "Blood Transfusions."
7. Arnold, J. D., Martin, D. C., and Richart, R. H. A study of willingness to volunteer as human subjects in clinical research. Conference on *Ethical Aspects of Experimentation on Human Subjects,* American Academy of Arts and Sciences. Boston, Mass., Nov. 3–4, 1967.
8. Bailey, N. *An Universal Etymological English Dictionary.* London: Printed for E. Bell, J. Darby, A. Bettesworth, F. Favram, J. Pemberton, J. Hooke, C. Rivington, F. Clay, J. Batley, and E. Symon, 1724. (Anaesthesia: "A Defect of Sensation . . .")
9. Baldwin, A. L. The study of child behavior and development: Ethical problems of research. In P. H. Mussen (Ed.), *Handbook of*

Research Methods in Child Development. New York: Wiley, 1960, pp. 28–34.
10. Barcroft, J. Experiments on man. *Lancet* 1:1211–1216, 1934.
11. Bayley, N. Implicit and explicit values in science as related to human growth and development. *Merrill-Palmer Quart.,* pp. 121–126, 1956.
12. Beachboard, W. W. Federal and AMA policy on consents in the investigational use of drugs. Conference on *Ethical Aspects of Experimentation on Human Subjects,* American Academy of Arts and Sciences. Boston, Mass., Nov. 3–4, 1967.
13. Bean, W. B. A testament of duty. Some strictures on moral responsibilities in clinical research. *J. Lab. Clin. Med.* 39:3–9, 1952.
14. Bean, W. B. The ethics and morals of human experiments. University of London Lecture, St. Bartholomew's Hospital, London, July, 1967. Unpublished.
15. Beaumont, W. *Experiments and Observations on the Gastric Juice and the Physiology of Digestion.* Facsimile of the original edition of 1833 (Plattsburgh, printed by F. P. Allen), together with a biographical essay. Reprinted on the occasion of the XIIIth International Physiological Congress, Boston, 1929.
16. Beecher, H. K. Preparation of battle casualties for surgery. *Ann. Surg.* 121:769–792, 1945.
17. Beecher, H. K. Clinical impression and clinical investigation. *J.A.M.A.* 151:44–45, 1953.
18. Beecher, H. K. The powerful placebo. *J.A.M.A.* 159:1602–1606, 1955.
19. Beecher, H. K. Evidence for increased effectiveness of placebos with increased stress. *Amer. J. Physiol.* 187:163–169, 1956.
20. Beecher, H. K. The measurement of pain. Prototype for the quantitative study of subjective responses. *Pharmacol. Rev.* 9:59–209, 1957.
21. Beecher, H. K. *Experimentation in Man.* Springfield, Ill.: Thomas, 1959.
22. Beecher, H. K. *Measurement of Subjective Responses: Quantitative Effects of Drugs.* New York: Oxford, 1959.
23. Beecher, H. K. Research and common sense in a clinical specialty—anesthesia. *J.A.M.A.* 172:449–451, 1960.
24. Beecher, H. K. (Ed.) *Disease and the Advancement of Basic Science.* Cambridge: Harvard Univ. Press, 1960.
25. Beecher, H. K. Increased stress and effectiveness of placebos and "active" drugs. *Science* 132:91–92, 1960.
26. Beecher, H. K. Consent in clinical experimentation: myth and reality. *J.A.M.A.* 195:34–35, 1966.

27. Beecher, H. K. Some guiding principles for clinical investigation. *J.A.M.A.* 195:1135–1136, 1966.
28. Beecher, H. K. Ethics and clinical research. *New Eng. J. Med.* 274:1354–1360, 1966.
29. Beecher, H. K., McDonough, F. K., and Forbes, A. Effects of blood pressure changes on cortical potentials during anesthesia. *J. Neurophysiol.* 1:324–331, 1938.
29a. Beecher, H. K. Ethical problems created by the hopelessly unconscious patient. *New Eng. J. Med.* 278:1425–1430, 1968.
30. Beecher, H. K. (Chairman). A definition of irreversible coma. Report of the *ad hoc* committee of the Harvard Medical School to examine the definition of brain death. *J.A.M.A.* 205:337–340, 1968. (Other members of the *ad hoc* committee: R. D. Adams, M.D.; A. C. Barger, M.D.; W. J. Curran, LLM, SMHyg; D. Denny-Brown, M.D.; D. L. Farnsworth, M.D.; J. Folch-Pi, M.D.; E. I. Mendelsohn, Ph.D.; J. P. Merrill, M.D.; J. Murray, M.D.; R. Potter, Th.D.; R. Schwab, M.D.; and W. Sweet, M.D.)
31. Beecher, H. K. Scarce resources in the advancement of medicine: availability and allocation for experimentation. Conference on *Ethical Aspects of Experimentation on Human Subjects,* American Academy of Arts and Sciences. Boston, Mass., Sept. 26–28, 1968. *Daedalus* 98:275–313, 1969.
31a. Beecher, H. K. Protection for the investigator and his human subject. *Science,* in press.
31b. Beecher, H. K., and Curran, W. J. Ethical and legal problems arising in experimentation in children. *J.A.M.A.* In press.
32. Bell, J. *Proceedings of the National Medical Conventions* held in New York, May, 1846, and in Philadelphia, May, 1847.
33. Bennett, C. C. What price privacy? *Amer. Psychol.* 22:371–376, 1967.
34. Bentley, G. B. In discussion: Transplantation: The Clinical Problem, by M. F. A. Woodruff. In Ciba Foundation Symposium, *Ethics in Medical Progress.* Boston: Little, Brown, 1966, p. 19.
35. Bernard, C. *An Introduction to the Study of Experimental Medicine.* H. C. Greene (Transl.) New York: Macmillan, 1927, p. 191. Also, *Introduction à la Médecine Experimentale.* 2d ed. Paris: Velagrave, 1903.
36. Bernard, C. In C. J. Wiggers. Human experimentation: As exemplified by career of Dr. William Beaumont. *Alum. Bull., School of Med., West. Reserve Univ.,* 1950, pp. 60–65.
37. Blake, J. B. The development of American anatomy acts. *J. Med. Educ.* 30:431–439, 1955.
38. Blumgart, H. L. The ethical aspects of experimentation on hu-

man subjects. Conference on *Ethical Aspects of Experimentation on Human Subjects,* American Academy of Arts and Sciences. Boston, Mass., Nov. 3–4, 1967.
39. Blumgart, H. L. The medical framework for viewing the problem. Conference on *Ethical Aspects of Experimentation on Human Subjects,* American Academy of Arts and Sciences. Boston, Mass., Sept. 26–28, 1968. *Daedalus* 98:248–274, 1969.
40. Blundell, J. Cited by G. E. W. Wolstenholme in Ciba Foundation Symposium, *Ethics in Medical Progress.* Boston: Little, Brown, 1966, p. 27.
41. Board of Medical Registration and Examination *v.* Kaadt (1948). Sup. Ct. Ind., 1948, 76 N.E. 2d 669, 672. Cited in proceedings of conference of *Use of Human Subjects in Safety Evaluation of Food Chemicals.* Washington: National Academy of Sciences, National Research Council, 1967, pp. 113, 114, 161.
42. Bonhoeffer, D. Quoted by D. M. Jackson in I. Ladimer and R. W. Newman (Eds.), *Clinical Investigation in Medicine: Legal, Ethical and Moral Aspects.* Boston: Law-Medicine Research Inst., Boston University, 1963, p. 301.
43. Boylston, Z. *An Historical Account of the Small-Pox Inoculated in New England.* Boston: S. Gerish, 1730.
44. Brennan, W. *Life* 62:4, Apr. 21, 1967.
45. Bressler, B., Silverman, A. J., Cohen, S. I., and Shmavonian, B. Research in human subjects and the artificial traumatic neurosis: Where does our responsibility lie? *Amer. J. Psychiat.* 116:522–526, 1959.
46. Brieger, G. H. Some aspects of human experimentation in the history of nutrition. In proceedings of conference on *Use of Human Subjects in Safety Evaluation of Food Chemicals.* Washington: National Academy of Sciences, National Research Council, 1967, pp. 207–215.
47. Brinkley *v.* Hassig. 10th Cir. 1936, 83 F, 2d 351, 353. Cited in proceedings of conference on *Use of Human Subjects in Safety Evaluation of Food Chemicals.* Washington: National Academy of Sciences, National Research Council, 1967, pp. 113, 161.
48. British Medical Research Council. Memorandum, 1953.
49. British Medical Research Council. Memoranda, 1953, 1962, 1963.
50. Bronowski, J. *Science and Human Values.* New York: Harper & Row, 1965.
51. Brook Lodge Conference. Symposium for science writers sponsored by the Upjohn Co., Kalamazoo, Mich., March 22, 1965.

52. Brower, D. The role of incentive in psychological research. *J. Gen. Psychol.* 39:145–147, 1948.
53. Bukhartz, S. C. The Helsinki Declaration. *Hosp. Prac.* 2:24–25, 1967.
54. Bull. Quoted by D. M. Jackson in I. Ladimer and R. W. Newman (Eds.), *Clinical Investigation in Medicine: Legal, Ethical and Moral Aspects.* Boston: Law-Medicine Research Inst., Boston University, 1963, p. 298.
55. Cady, E. L., Jr. Medical malpractice: What about experimentation? *Ann. West. Med. Surg.* 6:164–170, 1952.
56. Cahn, E. Limits for experimentation. Excerpt from The lawyer as scientist and scoundrel: Reflections on Francis Bacon's quadricentennial. *N. Y. Univ. Law Rev.* 36:1–12, 1961.
57. Calabresi, G. Reflections on medical experimentation on humans. Conference on *Ethical Aspects of Experimentation on Human Subjects,* American Academy of Arts and Sciences. Boston, Mass., Nov. 3–4, 1967.
58. Calabresi, G. Reflections on medical experimentation in humans. Conference on *Ethical Aspects of Experimentation on Human Subjects,* American Academy of Arts and Sciences. Boston, Mass., Sept. 26–28, 1968. *Daedalus* 98:387–405, 1969.
59. Calne, R. Y. In Ciba Foundation Symposium, *Ethics in Medical Progress.* Boston: Little, Brown, 1966, pp. 16, 73.
60. Carpenter *v.* Blake (N. Y. 1871). 60 Barb. 488 rev'd other gnds. 50 N. Y. 696 (1872). Cited in proceedings of conference on *Use of Human Subjects in Safety Evaluation of Food Chemicals.* Washington: National Academy of Sciences, National Research Council, 1967, pp. 115, 161.
61. Cavers, D. F. Bonner *v.* Moran, 126 Fed. 2d 212 (D.C. Cir. 1941). In *Product and Environmental Hazards for 1965–1966.*
62. Cavers, D. F. Disclosure of the facts of consent in published reports of human experimentation. In conference on *Ethical Aspects of Experimentation on Human Subjects,* American Academy of Arts and Sciences. Boston, Mass., Nov. 3–4, 1967.
63. Cavers, D. F. Legal control of the clinical investigation of drugs: Some political, economic, and social questions. Conference on *Ethical Aspects of Experimentation on Human Subjects,* American Academy of Arts and Sciences. Boston, Mass., Sept. 26–28, 1968. *Daedalus* 98:427–448, 1969.
64. Cheever, D. W. The value and the fallacy of statistics in the observation of disease. *Boston Med. Surg. J.* 63:449–456, 1861.

65. Churchill, E. D. Wound shock and blood transfusion. Chap. IV in *Surgical Consultant, A.F.H.Q.* In preparation, 1969.
66. Clifford, W. K. In J. Bronowski, *Science and Human Values.* New York: Harper & Row, 1965, p. 65.
67. *Code,* American Hospital Association. *Statement of Principles Involved in the Use of Investigational Drugs in Hospitals.* Approved by Board of Trustees of the American Hospital Association, 1957. *Hospitals* 31:106–108, 1957.
68. *Codes,* American Medical Association. 1846, 1847, 1946, 1949, 1958, 1966, 1967.
69. *Code,* American Medical Association. *Transactions of the National Medical Conventions,* New York, May, 1846, and Philadelphia, May, 1847, pp. 84–106.
70. *Code,* American Medical Association. *Proceedings of the National Medical Conventions,* New York, May, 1846, and Philadelphia, May, 1847.
71. *Code,* American Medical Association. Principles of Medical Ethics. In F. J. L. Blasingame (Ed.), *1846–1958 Digest of Official Actions of the American Medical Association.* Chicago: American Medical Association, 1959, pp. 232–237.
72. *Code,* American Medical Association. Supplementary report of the judicial council. *J.A.M.A.* 132:1090, 1946. *Ibid.,* special edition, June 7, 1958, p. 11.
73. *Code,* American Medical Association. Resolutions on disapproval of participation in scientific experiments by inmates of penal institutions. Adopted by the House of Delegates, 1952.
74. *Code,* American Medical Association. Official opinions of the Judicial Council applicable in interpreting Section 2. *J.A.M.A.* 163:1158, 1957.
75. *Code,* American Medical Association. American Medical Association's patient consent guides added to Association's "Principles of Medical Ethics" support of 1964 World Medical Association Helsinki Declaration. Adopted by American Medical Association, June 1966.
76. *Code,* American Medical Association Guidelines (1967). *Blue sheet drug res. rep. 10* (no. 12).
77. *Code,* American Medical Association. *Ethical Guidelines for Organ Transplantation,* 1968.
78. *Code,* William Beaumont's, 1833. In C. J. Wiggers, Human experimentation. As exemplified by career of Dr. William Beaumont. *Alum. Bull. West. Reserve Univ.,* 1950, pp. 60–65.
79. *Code,* Beecher's, 1966. Some guiding principles for clinical investigation. *J.A.M.A.* 195:1135–1136, 1966.

80. *Code,* Claude Bernard's personal, 1856. In C. J. Wiggers, Human experimentation. As exemplified by career of Dr. William Beaumont. *Alum. Bull. West. Reserve Univ.,* 1950, p. 63.
81. *Code,* British Medical Association. Experimental research on human beings. Approved by the Representative Body of the British Medical Association, 1963.
82. *Code,* Catholic Hospitals Association. *Selections from Ethical and Religious Directives for Catholic Hospitals Related to Experimentation on Human Subjects.* 2d ed. St. Louis: Catholic Hospitals Assoc., 1955.
83. *Code,* Declaration of Geneva. Adopted at the Second General Assembly of the World Medical Association, Geneva, Switzerland, Sept., 1948. *World Med. Ass. Bull.* 1:35–38, 1949.
84. *Code,* Declaration of Helsinki, 1964. Recommendations guiding doctors in clinical research. Adopted by the World Medical Association in 1964.
85. *Code,* Food and Drug Administration Federal Regulation 11415, Aug. 30, 1966. Consent for use of investigational new drugs on humans: Statement of policy.
86. *Code,* Harvard University Health Services, 1963. Rules governing the participation of healthy human beings as subjects in research. Formulated by the University Health Services and adopted by the President and Fellows on April 1, 1963.
87. *Code,* Harvard Medical School, 1965. Rules governing the participation of medical students as experimental subjects. Office of the Dean, Harvard Medical School.
88. *Code,* A. Bradford Hill. Medical ethics and controlled trials. *Brit. Med. J.* 1:1043–1049, 1963.
89. *Code,* Hippocratic Oath. In A. Castiglioni, *A History of Medicine.* E. B. Krumbhaar (transl.) New York: Knopf, 1941, pp. 154–155.
90. *Code,* Medical Research Council, Great Britain, 1962–1963. *Responsibility in Investigations on Human Subjects.* (Cmnd. 2382), pp. 21–25.
91. *Code,* Medical Research Council, Great Britain, 1963. Responsibility in investigations on human subjects. *Brit. Med. J.* 2:178, 1964.
92. *Code,* National Academy of Sciences Board of Medicine, 1968. Cardiac transplantation in man.
93. *Code,* National Institutes of Health, July 1, 1966. Group consideration and informed consent in clinical research. Memo from J. A. Shannon, Dir.

94. *Code,* National Institutes of Health, 1968. A code for self-experimentation.
95. *Code,* Netherlands, 1955. Report on human experimentation. Adopted by the Public Health Council of the Netherlands. *World Med. J.* 4:299–300, 1957.
96. *Code,* Nuremberg. Nuremberg Military Tribunal: U.S. *v.* K. Brandt et al., 1946–1949.
97. *Code,* Percival's, 1803. *Medical Ethics.* London: S. Russell, 1803.
98. *Code,* Psychologists, ethical standards of. American Psychological Association, 1963. *Amer. Psychol.* 18:56–60, 1963.
99. *Code,* United Nations, Article Seven. Draft covenant on civil and political rights. Adopted by The Third Committee of the General Assembly of the United Nations, 1958. Reaffirmed by the General Assembly, 1966.
100. *Code,* United States Army. *Army regulation no. 70–25: Use of volunteers as subjects of research.* Washington: Department of the Army, 1962.
101. *Code,* United States Public Health Service. Requirement for review to insure the rights and welfare of individuals. U.S. Public Health Service Policy and Procedure Order No. 129, Revised July 1, 1966.
102. *Code,* United States Public Health Service. Requirements for review to insure the rights and welfare of individuals: Clarification. Washington: U.S. Public Health Service, Dec. 12, 1966.
103. *Code,* Wigger's, 1950. Human experimentation. As exemplified by career of Dr. William Beaumont. *Alum. Bull. Sch. of Med. West. Reserve Univ.,* 1950, pp. 60–65.
104. *Code,* Wolfensberger's, 1967. Ethical issues in research with human subjects. A rationale is formulated for a code of conduct in the recruitment of subjects for research. *Science* 155:47–51, 1967.
105. *Code,* World Medical Association. International code of medical ethics. Adopted at General Assembly of World Medical Association, London, England, 1949. *World Med. Ass. Bull.* 2:8–9, 1950.
106. *Code,* World Medical Association. Principles for those in research and experimentation. Adopted by the Eighth General Assembly of the World Medical Association, Rome, Italy, 1954. *World Med. J.* 2:14–15, 1955.
107. Conant, J. B. Scientific principles and moral conduct. *Amer. Sci.* 55:311–328, 1967.
108. Conference Report. The relation of the clinical investigator to the patient, pharmaceutical industry and Federal agencies. Fourth Bethesda conference of the American College of Cardiology, Aug. 27–28, 1966. *Amer. J. Cardiol.* 19:892–907.

109. Conrad, H. S. Clearance of questionnaires with respect to "invasion of privacy," public sensitivities, ethical standards, etc. *Amer. Psychol.* 22:356–359, 1967.
110. Consent. Group consideration and informed consent in clinical research at the National Institutes of Health, 1966.
111. Cooley, T. M. *A Treatise on the Law of Torts.* 2d ed. Chicago: Callaghan, 1888, p. 29.
112. Cortesini, R. In Ciba Foundation Symposium, *Ethics in Medical Progress.* Boston: Little, Brown, 1966, p. 16.
113. Cortesini, R. Outlines of a Legislation on Transplantation. In Ciba Foundation Symposium, *Ethics in Medical Progress.* Boston: Little, Brown, 1966, pp. 171–187.
114. Couch, N. P. Supply and demand in kidney and liver transplantation: A statistical survey. *Transplantation.* 4:587–595, 1966.
115. Coulston, F. Rationale and procedures in use of human subjects in safety evaluation. In proceedings of conference on *Use of Human Subjects in Safety Evaluation of Food Chemicals.* Washington: National Academy of Sciences, National Research Council, 1967, pp. 51–61.
116. Crime Commission, President's, 1967. *The Challenge of Crime in a Free Society. A Report by the President's Commission on Law Enforcement and Administration of Justice.* Washington: Govt. Printing Office, 1967.
117. Crime Commission, President's, 1967. *Wiretapping and Eavesdropping.* Washington: Govt. Printing Office, 1967, p. 201.
118. Crime Commission, President's, 1967. *People v. Berger.* Washington: Govt. Printing Office, 1967, p. 203.
119. Crime Commission, President's, 1967. *The Threat to Privacy.* Washington: Govt. Printing Office, 1967, p. 202.
120. Crime Commission, President's, 1967. *Present Law and Practice.* Washington: Govt. Printing Office, 1967, p. 202.
121. Crime Commission, President's, 1967. *Congressional Recommendations.* Washington: Govt. Printing Office, 1967, p. 203.
122. Curran, W. J. A problem of consent: Kidney transplantation in minors. *N. Y. Univ. Law Rev.* 34:891–898, 1959.
123. Curran, W. J. Legal codes in scientific research involving human subjects. Presented at the conference on *Law and Science,* International Academy of Law and Science, London, England, July 20, 1965.
124. Curran, W. J. The law and human experimentation. *New Eng. J. Med.* 275:323–325, 1966.
125. Curran, W. J. Legal principles concerning the use of human

subjects in clinical investigation. Conference on *Ethical Aspects of Experimentation on Human Subjects,* American Academy of Arts and Sciences. Boston, Mass., Nov. 3–4, 1967.

126. Curran, W. J. Current legal issues in clinical investigation with particular attention to the balance between the rights of the individual and the needs of society. Read at Sixth Annual Meeting, American College of Neuropsychopharmacology, San Juan, P. R., Dec. 12, 1967.
127. Curran, W. J. Governmental regulation of the use of human subjects in medical research: The approach of two Federal agencies. Conference on *Ethical Aspects of Experimentation on Human Subjects,* American Academy of Arts and Sciences, Boston, Mass., Sept. 26–28, 1968. *Daedalus* 98:542–594, 1969.
128. *Daedalus* and National Institutes of Health. Conference on *Ethical Aspects of Experimentation on Human Subjects,* American Academy of Arts and Sciences. Boston, Mass., Nov. 3–4, 1967.
129. *Daedalus* and National Institutes of Health. Conference on *Ethical Aspects of Experimentation on Human Subjects,* American Academy of Arts and Sciences, Boston, Mass., Sept. 26–28, 1968. *Daedalus* 98:i–xiv, 219–597, 1969.
130. Darwin, E. Quoted in Ciba Foundation Symposium, *Ethics in Medical Progress.* Boston: Little, Brown, 1966, p. 43.
131. Daube, D. Transplantation: Acceptability of Procedures and the Required Legal Sanctions. In Ciba Foundation Symposium, *Ethics in Medical Progress.* Boston: Little, Brown, 1966, pp. 188–201.
132. Davy, H. *Researches Chemical and Philosophical Chiefly Concerning Nitrous Oxide or Dephlogisticated Nitrous Air and Its Respiration.* Bristol: Biggs and Cottle, 1800.
133. De Bakey, M. E. Medical research and the golden rule. *J.A.M.A.* 203:132–134, 1968.
134. Denis, J. B. In Ciba Foundation Symposium, *Ethics in Medical Progress.* Boston: Little, Brown, 1966, pp. 26–27.
135. Denton, J. E., and Beecher, H. K. New analgesics: I. Methods in the clinical evaluation of new analgesics. *J.A.M.A.* 141:1051–1057, 1949.
136. De Senarclens, J. Human experimentation: A world problem from the standpoint of spiritual leaders. *World Med. J.* 7:80–81, 96, 1960.
137. de Wardener, H. E. Some Ethical and Economic Problems Associated with Intermittent Haemodialysis. In Ciba Foundation

Symposium, *Ethics in Medical Progress.* Boston: Little, Brown, 1966, pp. 104–125.

138. Dowling, H. F. Human dissection and experimentation with drugs. Some problems and parallels. *J.A.M.A.* 202:1132–1135, 1967.
139. *Duke Law Journal.* Editorial comment. 2:265–274, 1960.
140. Dyck, A. J., and Richardson, H. W. The moral justification for research using human subjects. Proceedings of conference on *Use of Human Subjects in Safety Evaluation of Food Chemicals.* Washington: National Academy of Sciences, National Research Council, 1967, pp. 229–247.
141. Dykstra, D. J. Invited discussion. Proceedings of conference on *Use of Human Subjects in Safety Evaluation of Food Chemicals.* Washington: National Academy of Sciences, National Research Council, 1967, pp. 183–184.
142. Editorial. Changing mores of biochemical research. A colloquium on ethical dilemmas from medical advances, held at the 48th annual session of American College of Physicians, San Francisco, April 12, 1967. *Ann. Int. Med.* 67 (suppl. 3): 1–83, 1967.
143. Editorial. What and when is death? *J.A.M.A.* 204:219–220, 1968.
144. E.D.R.S. and G.L.B.T. The moment of death: re Potter. *Medicoleg. J.* 31:195–196, 1963.
145. Edsall, G. A positive approach to the problem of human experimentation. Conference on *Ethical Aspects of Experimentation on Human Subjects,* American Academy of Arts and Sciences, Boston, Mass., Sept. 26–28, 1968. *Daedalus* 98:463–479, 1969.
146. Elkinton, J. R. Moral problems in the use of borrowed organs, artificial and transplanted. *Ann. Intern. Med.* 60:309–313, 1964.
147. Ernst, N. L., and Schwartz, A. U. *Privacy: The Right To Be Let Alone.* New York: Macmillan, 1962.
148. Esecover, H., Malitz, S., and Wilkens, B. Clinical profiles of paid normal subjects volunteering for hallucinogen drug studies. *Amer. J. Psychiat,* 117:910–915, 1961.
149. Ethics and the allocation of medical resources. Editorial by S. Gorovitz. *Med. Res. Engin.* 5:5–7, 1966.
150. Ethics in institutional setting. Editorial comment. *Med. Trib.* 8: No. 17, Feb. 15, 1967.
151. *Ethics in Medical Progress.* With special reference to transplantation. In G. E. W. Wolstenholme and M. O'Connor (Eds.), Ciba Foundation Symposium. Boston: Little, Brown, 1966.
152. Ethics, Medical. *Principles of Medical Ethics.* Chicago: American Medical Association, May 1955—present.

153. Fantus, B. Therapy of Cook County Hospital: blood preservation. *J.A.M.A.* 109:128–131, 1937.
154. Federal Food, Drug and Cosmetic Act. Secs. 505(1), 701(a); 52 Stat- 1053, as amended 1055; 21 U.S.C. 355(i) 371(a). 27 *Fed. Reg.* 7990, 1962.
155. Field, R. H. Personal communication, 1966.
156. Filatov, A. N. In Ciba Foundation Symposium, *Ethics in Medical Progress.* Boston: Little, Brown, 1966, p. 44.
157. Fink, B. R. Letter on patient consent. *Anesthesiology* 28:1109, 1967.
158. Finland, M. Ethics, consent and controlled clinical trial. *J.A.M.A.* 198:637–638, 1966.
159. Fiorentino *v.* Wenger (1966). Sup. Ct. App. Div. N.Y.. July 12, 1966 272 N.Y.S. 2d 557. Cited in proceedings of conference on *Use of Human Subjects in Safety Evaluation of Food Chemicals.* Washington: National Academy of Sciences, National Research Council, 1967, pp. 138, 172.
160. Fletcher, J. *Morals and Medicine.* Boston: Beacon Press, 1963.
161. Fletcher, J. *Situation Ethics.* Philadelphia: Westminster, 1966, p. 13.
161a. Fletcher, J. Human experimentation: Ethics in the consent situation. Medical Progress and the Law in Law and Contemporary Problems. Autumn, 1967. Duke Univ., Durham, N. C.
162. Fletcher, W. Rice and beri-beri. *Lancet* 1:1776–1779, 1907.
163. Food Protection: NAS/NRC Food Protection Committee on use of human subjects in evaluating safety of food chemicals, November, 1966, Conference. Washington.
164. Fortner *v.* Koch. Sup. Ct. Mich., 1935, 261 N.W. 762, 765. Cited in proceedings of conference on *Use of Human Subjects in Safety Evaluation of Food Chemicals.* Washington: National Academy of Sciences, National Research Council, 1967, pp. 113, 161.
165. Fox, R. C. Symposium on the study of drugs in man. IV. Some social and cultural factors in American society conducive to medical research on human subjects. *Clin. Pharmacol. Ther.* 1:423–443, 1960.
166. Fox, T. F. The ethics of clinical trials. *Medicoleg. J.* 28:132–141, 1960.
167. Frazer, A. C. Limitations in the value of studies in human subjects. In proceedings of conference on *Use of Human Subjects in Safety Evaluation of Food Chemicals.* Washington: National Academy of Sciences, National Research Council, 1967, pp. 63–69.

168. Freund, P. A. Ethical problems in human experimentation. *New End. J. Med.* 273:687–692, 1965.
169. Freund, P. A. Is the law ready for human experimentation? *Amer. Psychol.* 22:394–399, 1967.
170. Freund, P. A. Some reflections on consent. Conference on *Ethical Aspects of Experimentation on Human Subjects,* American Academy of Arts and Sciences, Boston, Mass., Nov. 3–4, 1967.
171. Freund, P. A. Legal frameworks for human experimentation. Conference on *Ethical Aspects of Experimentation on Human Subjects,* American Academy of Arts and Sciences, Boston, Mass., Sept. 26–28, 1968. *Daedalus* 98: 314–324, 1969.
172. Galdston, I. On the psychology of medical ethics. *New York J. Med.,* 4:19–21, 26, 1948.
173. Gale, J. The patients' association. *The Observer* (London), Feb. 3, 1963.
174. Garlick, Quoted by D. M. Jackson in I. Ladimer and R. W. Newman (Eds.), *Clinical Investigation in Medicine: Legal, Ethical and Moral Aspects.* Boston: Law-Medicine Research Inst., Boston University, 1963, pp. 300, 302.
175. Garrison, F. H. Footnote on Hippocratic Oath. In *History of Medicine.* Philadelphia: Saunders, 1914, p. 67.
176. Garrison, F. H. *An Introduction to the History of Medicine.* 4th ed. Philadelphia: Saunders, 1929.
177. Giertz, G. B. Ethical Problems in Medical Procedures in Sweden. In Ciba Foundation Symposium, *Ethics in Medical Progress.* Boston: Little, Brown, 1966, pp. 139–148.
178. Giuseppe, B. M. Human experimentation—A world problem from the standpoint of spiritual leaders. *World Med. J.* 7:80, 1960.
179. Glass, B. *Science and Ethical Values.* Chapel Hill: Univ. of North Carolina Press, 1965.
180. Goddard, J. L. Consent for use of investigational new drugs on humans: Proposed revision of statement of policy by the Food and Drug Administration. *Fed. Reg.* 32 (no. 118):8753–8754, (June 20) 1967.
181. Goddard, J. L. Regulation of human experimentation. Comments presented at the conference on *Ethical Aspects of Experimentation on Human Subjects,* American Academy of Arts and Sciences. Boston, Mass., Nov. 3–4, 1967.
182. Goldberger, J. Pellagra: Causation and a method of prevention. *J.A.M.A.* 66:471–476, 1916.
183. Goldberger, J., and Wheeler, G. A. Experimental pellagra in

the human subject brought about by a restricted diet. *Pub. Health Rep.* 30:3336–3339, 1915.

184. Goldberger, J., and Wheeler, G. A. Experimental pellagra in white male convicts. *Arch. Int. Med.* (Chicago). 25:451–471, 1920.
185. Goldman, S. *The Words of Justice Brandeis.* New York: Schuman, 1953, pp. 76–78.
186. Goodwin, W. E.: In Ciba Foundation Symposium, *Ethics in Medical Progress.* Boston: Little, Brown, 1966, p. 17.
187. Gorovitz, S. Ethics and the allocation of medical resources. *Med. Res. Engin.* 5:5–7, 1966.
188. *The Great Issues of Conscience in Modern Medicine.* The Dartmouth Convocation in Hanover, N.H. Sept., 8–10, 1960.
189. Green Committee Report. Ethics governing the service of prisoners as subjects in medical experiments. *J.A.M.A.* 136:457–458, 1948.
190. Green Committee Report. Resolutions on disapproval of participation in scientific experiments by inmates of penal institutions. Adopted by the House of Delegates of the American Medical Association, Dec. 1952:91–92, 109, 110. *Digest of Official Actions.* Chicago: American Medical Association, 1959, pp. 617–618.
191. Green, F. H. K. The clinical evaluation of remedies. *Lancet* II: 1085–1091, 1954.
192. Green, S. A. Centennial address delivered before Massachusetts Medical Society in Sanders Theatre, Cambridge, Mass., June 7, 1881.
193. Gregg, A. *The Furtherance of Medical Research.* New Haven: Yale Univ. Press, 1941.
194. Groen, J. J. Jewish view. *World Med. J.* 7:82–83, 96, 1960.
195. Grotius, H. De Jure Belli Au Pacis. Bk. 1, ch. 1, 10 (1). Publ. 1625.
196. Guttentag, O. E. The problem of experimentation on human beings. II. The physician's point of view. Symposium at the Medical Staff Conference, Division of Medicine, University of California School of Medicine, San Francisco, Oct. 10, 1951. *Science* 117: 207–210, 1953.
197. Guttentag, O. E. Introduction to *Physician · Patient · Pastor.* University of California Hospitals, San Francisco Medical Center, May, 1961.
198. Guttentag, O. E. Ethical Problems in Human Experimentation. In E. F. Torrey, *Ethical Issues in Medicine.* Boston: Little, Brown, 1968, pp. 195–226.
199. Guttentag, O. E. Organ transplantation from the deceased. *Linacre Quart.* 35:172–174, 1968.

200. Halley, M. M., and Harvey, W. F. Medical vs. legal definitions of death. *J.A.M.A.* 204:103–105, 1968.
201. Halpern, A. Discussion in proceedings of conference on *Use of Human Subjects in Safety Evaluation of Food Chemicals.* Washington: National Academy of Sciences, National Research Council, 1967, p. 72.
202. Hamburger, J. In Ciba Foundation Symposium, *Ethics in Medical Progress.* Boston: Little, Brown, 1966, pp. 14, 69, 134–138.
203. Hammond, J. The Willowbrook hepatitis project. *Med. Tribune* 8 (no. 19) 23, 1967.
204. Hatry, P. The physician's legal responsibility in clinical testing of new drugs. *Clin. Pharmacol. Therap.* 4:4–9, 1963.
205. Heller, C. G., and Clermont, Y. Kinetics of the germinal epithelium in man. *Recent Progr. Hormone Res.* 20:545–575, 1964.
206. Henderson, L. J. Physician and patient as a social system. *New Eng. J. Med.* 212:819–823, 1935.
206a. Henley, Lord. Vernon *v.* Bethell 28 Eng. Rep. 838, 839 (ch. 1762).
207. Hicks, J. B. Cases of transfusion, with some remarks on a new method of performing the operation. *Guy Hosp. Rep.,* Series 3, 14:1–14, 1869.
208. Hill, A. B. The clinical trial. *New Eng. J. Med.* 247:113–119, 1952.
209. Hill, A. B. Medical ethics and controlled trials. *Brit. Med. J.* 1:1043–1049, 1963.
210. Hill, A. B., Marshall, J., and Shaw, D. A. A controlled clinical trial of long-term anticoagulant therapy in cerebrovascular disease. *Quart. J. Med.* 29:597–609, 1960.
211. Hill, A. B., Marshall, J., and Shaw, D. A. Cerebrovascular disease: Trial of long-term anticoagulant therapy. *Brit. Med. J.* 2: 1003–1006, 1962.
212. Himsworth, Harold. In Ciba Foundation Symposium, *Ethics in Medical Progress.* Boston: Little, Brown, 1966, pp. 168–170.
213. Hippocrates "Aphorisms." In F. H. Garrison. *History of Medicine.* Philadelphia: Saunders, 1914, p. 67.
214. Hodges, R. E., and Bean, W. B. The use of prisoners for medical research. *J.A.M.A.* 202:513–515, 1967.
215. Hoff, H. E., and Guillemin, R. The tercentenary of transfusion in man. *Cardiov. Res. Cent. Bull.* 6:47–57, 1967.
216. Hogan, F. *Life,* Apr. 21, 1967. 62:4.
217. Hogben, L., and Sim, M. The self-controlled and self-recorded clinical trial for low-grade morbidity. *Brit. J. Prev. Soc. Med.* 7: 163–179, 1953.

218. Houde, R. W., and Wallenstein, S. L. A method for evaluating analgesics in patients with chronic pain. *Drug. Addic. Narc. Bull.,* App. F: 660–682, 1953.

219. Humphrey, H. H. *Life,* Apr. 21, 1967. 62:4.

220. Hustin, A. Principe d'une nouvelle méthode de transfusion muqueuse. *J. Med. Brux.* 12: 436, 1914.

221. Huxley, A. *Ends and Means.* New York: Harper, 1937.

222. Huxley, A. *Ape and Essence.* New York: Harper, 1948.

223. Hyman, W. A. In Human experimentation: Cancer studies at Sloan-Kettering stir public debate on medical ethics. *Science* 143: 551–553, 1964.

224. Hyman *v.* Jewish Hospital. *Science* 151:663–666, 1966. Also cited in proceedings of conference on *Use of Human Subjects in Safety Evaluation of Food Chemicals,* Washington: National Academy of Sciences, National Research Council, 1967, pp. 112, 160.

225. Minchew, B. H., and Gallogly, C. Informed consent, an American right. *FDA Papers* 1:8–11, Oct. 1967.

225a. Ingelfinger, F. J. *Yearbook of Medicine.* Chicago: Year Book Medical Publishers, 1967–1968, p. 430.

226. Ivy, A. C. The history and ethics of the use of human subjects in medical experiments. *Science* 108:1–5, 1948.

227. Jackson, D. M. *Moral Responsibility in Clinical Research.* London: Tyndale, 1958. Also *Lancet* 1:902–903, 1958.

228. Jaffe, L. L. Human experimentation. Conference on *Ethical Aspects of Experimentation on Human Subjects,* American Academy of Arts and Sciences. Boston, Mass., Nov. 3–4, 1967.

229. Jaffe, L. L. Law as a system of control. Conference on *Ethical Aspects of Experimentation on Human Subjects,* American Academy of Arts and Sciences. Boston, Mass., Sept. 26–28, 1968. *Daedalus* 98:406–426, 1969.

230. Jaffe, L. L. Personal communication, Nov. 5, 1968.

231. Jansky, J. *Shorn. Klin. Praha,* 8:95, 1907.

232. Jenkins, D. T. *The Doctor's Profession.* London: Student Christian Movement Press, 1949.

233. Johnson, W. H. The problem of experimentation on human beings. IV. Civil rights of military personnel regarding medical care and experimental procedures. *Science* 117:212–215, 1953.

234. Jonas, H. Philosophical reflections on experimenting with human subjects. Conference on *Ethical Aspects of Experimentation on Human Subjects,* American Academy of Arts and Sciences. Boston, Mass., Sept. 26–28, 1968. *Daedalus* 98:219–247, 1969.

235. Judicial Council, action of. Reported in *Opinions and Reports*

of the Judicial Council. Chicago: American Medical Association, 1960, p. 14. The action of the House of Delegates is reported in *Digest of Official Actions: 1846–1958.* Chicago: American Medical Association, 1959, p. 617.
236. Kalven, H., Jr., and Zeisel, H. *The American Jury.* Boston: Little, Brown, 1966.
237. Karsner, H. T. Clinical investigation in naval hospitals. *J.A.M.A.* 162:535–537, 1956.
238. Katz, J. The influence of human experimentation on the practice of medicine. Conference on *Ethical Aspects of Experimentation on Human Subjects,* American Academy of Arts and Sciences. Boston, Mass., Nov. 3–4, 1967.
239. Katz, J. The education of the physician-investigator. Conference on *Ethical Aspects of Experimentation on Human Subjects,* American Academy of Arts and Sciences. Boston, Mass., Sept. 26–28, 1968. *Daedalus* 98:480–501, 1969.
240. Katz, M. M. Ethical issues in the use of human subjects in psychopharmacologic research. *Amer. Psychol.* 22:360–363, 1967.
241. Keats, A. S., Beecher, H. K., and Mosteller, F. C. Measurement of pathological pain in distinction to experimental pain. *J. Appl. Physiol.* 3:35–44, 1950.
242. Kefauver-Harris Amendments to the Federal Food, Drug and Cosmetic Act, 1962. Proceedings *FDA Conference on the Kefauver-Harris Drug Amendments and Proposed Regulations,* Feb. 15, 1963. Washington: U.S. Department of Health, Education, and Welfare, Food and Drug Administration. 1963.
243. Kelsey, F. O. Patient consent provisions of the Federal Food, Drug, and Cosmetic Act. In I. Ladimer and R. W. Newman (Eds.), *Clinical Investigation in Medicine: Legal, Ethical and Moral Aspects.* Boston: Boston Univ. Law-Medicine Research Institute, 1963.
244. Kelsey, F. O. Statement in *Hearings Before the Subcommittee on Reorganization and International Organizations of the Committee on Government Operations, United States Senate, 88th Congress* [June 19, 1963, Part 5]. Washington: Govt. Printing Office, 1964, p. 2454.
245. Kennedy, D. A. Social issues in the conduct of clinical research. Conference on *Hazards to Children, Born and Unborn,* Training Center in Youth Development of Boston University Law-Medicine Institute, Nov. 13, 1964.
246. Kety, S. S. Personal communications, Nov. 6, 1957, Feb. 26, 1958.
247. Kevorkian, J. Capital punishment or capital gain. *J. Crim. Law Criminol. Police Sci.* 50:50–51, 1959.

248. Keynes, G. L. (Ed.) *Blood Transfusion.* Bristol: Wright, 1949.
249. Kidd, A. M. The problem of experimentation on human beings. III. Limits of the right of a person to consent to experimentation on himself. *Science* 117:211–212, 1953.
250. Kilbrandon, Lord. Chairman's opening remarks. In Ciba Foundation Symposium, *Ethics in Medical Progress.* Boston: Little, Brown, 1966, pp. 1–5.
251. Kinsey, A. Personal communication, 1955.
252. Krugman, S. The Willowbrook hepatitis project. *Med. Tribune 8* (no. 19) 23, 1967.
253. Krugman, S., Giles, J. P., and Hammond, J. Infectious hepatitis. *J.A.M.A.* 200:365–373, 1967.
253a. Krugman, S., Ward, R., Giles, J. P., Bodansky, O., and Jacobs, A. M. Infectious hepatitis: Detection of virus during the incubation period and in clinically inapparent infection. *New Eng. J. Med.* 261:729–734, 1959.
253b. Krugman, S., Ward, R., Giles, J. P., and Jacobs, A. M. Infectious hepatitis: Studies on the effect of gamma globulin and on the incidence of inapparent infection. *J.A.M.A.* 174:823–830, 1960.
254. Kvittingen, T. D., and Naess, A. Recovery from drowning in fresh water. *Brit. Med. J.* 1:1315–1317, 1963.
255. Ladimer, I. Ethical and legal aspects of medical research on human beings. *J. Publ. Law* 3:467–511, 1954.
256. Ladimer, I. Human experimentation: Medicolegal aspects. *New Eng. J. Med.* 257:18–24, 1957.
257. Ladimer, I. May physicians experiment? *Inter. Rec. Med.* 172: 586–598, 1959.
258. Ladimer, I. Survey of professional journals: Editorial responsibility in clinical research. Symposium under the direction of W. J. Curran, Boston University Law-Medicine Research Inst. Unpublished data, 1960.
259. Ladimer, I. Clinical research insurance. *J. Chronic Dis.* 16:1229–1235, 1963.
260. Ladimer, I. Report on the American Academy for the Advancement of Science symposium *Secrecy, Privacy, and Public Information,* Dec. 28–29, 1967.
261. Ladimer, I. Rights, responsibilities, and protection of patients in human studies. *J. Clin. Pharmacol.,* 7:125–130, 1967.
262. Ladimer, I. Human studies for safety evaluation: Medicolegal aspects. In proceedings of conference on *Use of Human Subjects in Safety Evaluation of Food Chemicals.* Washington: National

Academy of Sciences, National Research Council, 1967, pp. 97–104.

263. Ladimer, I., and Newman, R. W. (Eds.). *Clinical Investigation in Medicine: Legal, Ethical, and Moral Aspects.* Boston: Boston Univ. Law-Medicine Research Institute, 1963.

264. Langer, E. Human experimentation: Cancer studies at Sloan-Kettering stir public debate on medical ethics. *Science* 143:551–553, 1964.

265. Langer, E. Human experimentation: New York verdict affirms patient's rights. *Science* 151:663–666, 1966.

266. Larrick, G. P. Personal communication, Sept. 24, 1965.

267. Lasagna, L. *Life, Death, and the Doctor.* New York: Knopf, 1968, p. 255.

268. Lasagna, L. Special subjects in human experimentation. Conference on *Ethical Aspects of Experimentation on Human Subjects,* American Academy of Arts and Sciences. Boston, Mass., Sept. 26–28, 1968. *Daedalus* 98:449–462, 1969.

269. Lasagna, L., and Beecher, H. K. The optimal dose of morphine. *J.A.M.A.* 156:230–234, 1954.

270. Lasagna, L., and von Felsinger, J. M. The volunteer subject in research. *Science* 120:359–361, 1954.

271. Leach, G. A. Discussion in Ciba Foundation Symposium, *Ethics in Medical Progress.* Boston: Little, Brown, 1966, p. 35.

272. Lear, J. A realistic look at heart transplants. *Sat. Rev.* Feb. 3, 1968, pp. 53–60.

273. Legal implications of psychological research with human subjects. *Duke Law J.* 1960, pp. 265–274.

274. Leicester, R. *Decisions about Life and Death. A Problem in Modern Medicine.* Oxford: Church Army Press, 1965.

275. Leopold, N. F. *Life Plus 99 Years.* New York: Doubleday, 1958.

276. Lerner, D. In Ruebhausen and Brim, *Columbia Law Rev.* 65: 1185, 1965 (footnote 1).

277. Leviticus XVII:13, 14 and XVIII:5.

278. Lewisohn, R. New and greatly simplified method of blood transfusion: Preliminary report. *Med. Rec. N.Y.* 87:141–142, 1915.

279. Liberman, R. An experimental study of the placebo response under three different situations of pain. *J. Psychiat. Res.* 2:233–246, 1967.

280. Long, G., Dripps, R. D., and Price, H. L. Measurement of anti-arrhythmic potency of drugs in man: Effects of dehydrobenzperidol. *Anesthesiology* 28:318–323, 1967.

281. Lorenz, W. F. The treatment of pellagra. Clinical notes on pel-

lagrins receiving an excessive diet. *Pub. Health Rep.* 29:2357–2360, 1914.
282. Lorenz, W. F. The cerebrospinal fluid in pellagra. *Pub. Health Rep.* 29:2360–2363, 1914.
283. Louisell, D. W. Transplantation: Existing Legal Constraints. In Ciba Foundation Symposium, *Ethics in Medical Progress.* Boston: Little, Brown, 1966, pp. 78–103.
284. Lovell, V. R. The human use of personality tests: A dissenting view. *Amer. Psychol.* 22:383–393, 1967.
285. Lower, R. De corde. K. J. Franklin (Transl.). In R. W. T. Gunther, *Early Science in Oxford.* Vol. IX. London, Oxford Univ. Press, 1932, p. 172.
286. Lumbard, E. *Life* 62:4, Apr. 21, 1967.
287. Lynch, J. J. Human experimentation in medicine: Moral aspects. Part III, Symposium on the study of drugs in man. *Clin. Pharmacol. Ther.* 1:396–400, 1960.
288. MacKinney, A. C. Deceiving experimental subjects. *Amer. Psychol.* 10:133, 1955.
289. Mackintosh, J. M. Personal communication, Feb. 17, 1958.
290. Mainland, D. The clinical trial—some difficulties and suggestions. *J. Chronic Dis.* 11:484–496, 1960.
291. Maslow, A. H. Self-esteem (dominance-feeling) and sexuality in women. *J. Soc. Psychol.* 16:259–294, 1942.
292. Maslow, A. H., and Sakoda, J. M. Volunteer-error in the Kinsey study. *J. Abnorm. Soc. Psychol.* 47:259–262, 1952.
293. McCance, R. A. The practice of experimental medicine. *Proc. Roy. Soc. Med.* 44:189–194, 1951.
294. McDermott, W. Changing mores of biomedical research. Conference on *Ethical Aspects of Experimentation on Human Subjects,* American Academy of Arts and Sciences. Boston, Mass., Nov. 3–4, 1967.
295. McDonald, J. C. Why prisoners volunteer to be experimental subjects. *J.A.M.A.* 202:511–512, 1967.
296. Mead, M. The human study of human beings. *Science* 133:163, 1961.
297. Mead, M. Ethical aspects of experimentation on human subjects: From the standpoint of anthropology. Conference on *Ethical Aspects of Experimentation on Human Subjects,* American Academy of Arts and Sciences. Boston, Mass. Nov. 3–4, 1967.
298. Mead, M. Research with human beings: A model derived from anthropological field practice. Conference on *Ethical Aspects of Experimentation on Human Subjects,* American Academy of Arts

and Sciences. Boston, Mass., Sept. 26–28, 1968. *Daedalus* 98:361–386, 1969.

299. Medawar, P. B. *The Uniqueness of the Individual.* London: Methuen, 1957, p. 19.
300. Merrill, J. P. Clinical experience is tempered by genuine human concern. *J.A.M.A.* 189:626–627, 1964.
301. Miller, A. D. The Willowbrook hepatitis project. *Med. Tribune* 8(no. 17):24, 1967.
302. Miranda *v.* State of Arizona. 384 U.S. 436, 447 (1966).
303. Mitscherlich, A., and Mielke, F. *Doctors of Infamy.* H. Norden (Transl.) New York: Schuman, 1949.
304. Modell, W. Let each new patient be a complete experience. *J.A.M.A.* 174:1717–1719, 1960.
305. Modell, W. The primary ethical decision. *Med. Tribune* 1(22): 11, 1967.
306. Moore, F. D. Ethics in new medicine: Tissue transplants. *Nation,* April 5, 1965, pp. 358–362, and *Med. Coll. Va. Quart.* Fall, 1965, pp. 19–23.
307. Moore, F. D. Biologic and medical studies in human volunteer subjects: Ethics and safeguards. Part II, Symposium on the study of drugs in man. *Clin. Pharmacol. Ther.* 1:149–155, 1960.
308. Moore, F. D. Therapeutic innovation: ethical boundaries in the initial patient-trials of new drugs and surgical procedures. Conference on *Ethical Aspects of Experimentation on Human Subjects,* American Academy of Arts and Sciences. Boston, Mass., Sept. 26–28, 1968. *Daedalus* 98:502–522, 1969.
309. Moore, G. E. *Principia Ethica.* Quoted by J. Fletcher in *Situation Ethics.* Philadelphia: Westminster, 1966, p. 146.
310. Mores of biochemical research, changing. A colloquium on ethical dilemmas from medical advances, held at the 48th annual session of the American College of Physicians, San Francisco, April 12, 1967. *Ann. Intern. Med.* 67 (suppl. 3):1–83, 1967.
311. Morris, C. Human testing and the courtroom. In proceedings of conference on *Use of Human Subjects in Safety Evaluation of Food Chemicals.* Washington: National Academy of Sciences, National Research Council, 1967, pp. 105–174.
312. Morris, C. Personal communication, March 27, 1968.
313. Morton, W. J. *The X Ray.* New York: American Technical Book Co., 1896.
314. Mulvihill, J. J. The medical and moral difficulties of organ transplantation to humans. *Biol. J. Coll. of the Holy Cross* 8:7–17, 1965.

315. Murphy, G. What should be the relation of morals to law? V. The psychologist, the theologian. *J. Pub. Law,* 1:313–316, 1952.
316. Murray, J. E. Referred to by D. M. Jackson in I. Ladimer and R. W. Newman (Eds.), *Clinical Investigation in Medicine: Legal, Ethical and Moral Aspects.* Boston: Law-Medicine Research Inst., Boston Univ., 1963, p. 301.
317. Murray, J. E. Organ Transplantation: The Practical Possibilities. In Ciba Foundation Symposium, *Ethics in Medical Progress.* Boston: Little, Brown, 1966, pp. 54–77.
318. Nedey, R. Le coma dépassé (Stade IV). (Étude de quarante observations personelles). *Marseille Chir.* 18:137–146, 1966.
318a. National Research Council. *Manual on Shock.* Washington: National Academy of Sciences, 1943.
319. Newman, R. W. The participation of prisoners in clinical research. Address before the Wardens' Association of America, 92d American Correctional Congress, Philadelphia, Sept. 20, 1962, commenting on a paper presented by Joseph D. Boggs.
320. *New York Herald-Tribune.* Use of children in experimentation. Oct. 25, 1956.
321. New York (City) Department of Hospitals, General order no. 462 concerning research proposals. Oct. 27, 1949.
322. New York State Board of Regents. *Science* 151:664–665, 1966.
323. Niebuhr, H. R. *Radical Monotheism and Western Culture: with supplementary essays.* New York: Harper, 1960.
324. O'Donnell, T. J. Commentary according to the ethical insights of religion. In proceedings of conference on *Use of Human Subjects in Safety Evaluation of Food Chemicals.* Washington: National Academy of Sciences, National Research Council, 1967, pp. 253–254.
325. Ogilvie, H. See Pappworth, M. H., 1962.
326. Olmstead et al. *v.* United States (277 U.S. 438, 488. See Ruebhausen and Brim, 1965, p. 1188.
327. Osler, William. William Beaumont. A pioneer American physiologist. Address before the St. Louis Medical Society, Oct. 4, 1902. In *Beaumont's Experiments and Observations.* Cambridge: Harvard Univ. Press, 1902, pp. xii, xiii.
328. Page, I. H. Medical ethics. *Science* 153: p. 371, 1966.
329. Pappworth, M. H. Human guinea pigs. A warning. *20th. Cent.* 171:66–75 (Autumn) 1962.
330. Pappworth, M. H. Personal communication, Jan., 1965.
331. Parsons, T. Some sociological considerations bearing upon research with human subjects. Conference on *Ethical Aspects of Experimentation on Human Subjects,* American Academy of Arts

and Sciences. Boston, Mass., Sept. 26–28, 1968. *Daedalus* 98:325–360, 1969.

332. Pellier de Quengsy (1784). Cited by P. V. Rycroft in Ciba Foundation Symposium, *Ethics in Medical Progress*. Boston: Little, Brown, 1966, p. 49.
333. Pendras, J. P. Experience with patient selection. Unpublished data, 1967.
334. Pendras, J. P., and Erickson, R. V. Hemodialysis: A successful therapy for chronic uremia. *Ann. Intern. Med.* 64:293–311, 1966.
335. Pepys, S. *Diary:* Nov. 14, 1666, Nov. 21, 1667.
336. Percival, T. *Medical Ethics*. London: Russell, 1803.
337. Perlin, S., Pollin, W., and Butler, R. N. The experimental subject: The psychiatric evaluation and selection of a volunteer population. *Arch. Neurol. Psychiat.* 80:65–70, 1958.
338. Pfeiffer, C. C. Request for formulation of experimental procedures for human experimentation. Letter to R. Stormont, Secretary of the Council on Pharmacy and Chemistry, Committee on Research, American Medical Association, Sept. 18, 1951.
339. Pfeiffer, C. C. Personal communication, Feb. 24, 1958.
340. Pickering, George W. Concepts of medical education abroad as they relate to cardiovascular teaching. *Fifth Conference of Cardiovascular Training Grants Program Directors,* Williamsburg, Va., June 7–8. Washington: U.S. Public Health Service, 1958.
341. Pickering, G. W. Quoted in Ciba Foundation Symposium, *Ethics in Medical Progress*. Boston: Little, Brown, 1966, pp. 100–101.
342. Pickering, G. W. Personal communication, Nov. 16, 1967.
343. Pius XII. The moral limits of medical research and treatment. Address to the First International Congress on the Histopathology of the Nervous System, Sept. 14, 1952. Translated from the original French by the N.C.W.C. News Service and distributed as "Editorial Information" on Sept. 26, 1952; published in *Acta Apostolicae Sedis,* 44:779, 1952.
344. Pius XII. The Pope Speaks—The Prolongation of Life. An address to an International Congress of Anesthesiologists on Nov. 24, 1957. *Osservatore Romano,* 4:393–398, 1958.
345. Platt, R. *Doctor and Patient. Ethics, Morale, Government*. London: Nuffield Provincial Hospitals Trust, 1963, pp. 62–63.
346. Platt, R. Ethical Problems in Medical Procedures. In Ciba Foundation Symposium, *Ethics in Medical Progress*. Boston: Little, Brown, 1966, pp. 149–170.
347. Platt, R. The ethical basis of medical science. *Sci. Basis Med. Ann. Rev.,* 1966.
348. Pollock, T. M., and Reid, D. Assessment of British gamma globu-

lin in preventing infectious hepatitis. *Brit. Med. J.* 3:451–454, 1968.

349. Privacy and behavioral research. Preliminary summary of the report of the panel on privacy and behavioral research under chairmanship of Kenneth E. Clark, Dean, College of Arts and Sciences, Univ. of Rochester, Rochester, N.Y. *Science* 155:535–538, 1967. Also: Washington: Government Printing Office, 1967. Also: *Amer. Psychol.* 22:345–349, 1967.
350. Rabbi and the physician and the whole man. Report of Committee on Judaism and Medicine of the Central Conference of American Rabbis, 1965. Unpublished.
351. Rabbis, Report of Central Conference of American. Committee on Judaism and Medicine. *Yearbook* 63:153, 1953.
352. Rabbis, Report of Central Conference of American. Committee on Judaism and Medicine. *Yearbook* 66:106, 1956.
353. Ramsey, P. Freedom and responsibility in medical and sex ethics. A Protestant view. *N. Y. Univ. Law Rev.* 31:1189–1204, 1956.
354. Ramsey, P. The sanctity of life. In the first of it. *Dublin Rev.* Spring, 1967, p. 121.
355. Reemtsma, K. In Ciba Foundation Symposium, *Ethics in Medical Progress.* Boston: Little, Brown, 1966, pp. 158, 163–167, 206.
356. Reisinger. Referred to by P. V. Rycroft in Ciba Foundation Symposium, *Ethics in Medical Progress.* Boston: Little, Brown, 1966, pp. 43, 44.
357. Reports and opinions of the Judicial Council which are applicable in interpreting Section 2. *J.A.M.A.* 167: 1958.
358. Reston, J. Washington: The capital and the Easter story. *New York Times,* April 18, 1965.
359. Revillard, J. P. In Ciba Foundation Symposium, *Ethics in Medical Progress.* Boston: Little, Brown, 1966, pp. 70–71.
360. Richmond, J. B. Patient reaction to the teaching and research situation. *J. Med. Educ.* 36:347–352, 1961.
361. Ritts, R. E., Jr. Consent and participation by minors and incompetents: A suggestion. Conference on *Ethical Aspects of Experimentation on Human Subjects, American Academy of Arts and Sciences.* Boston, Mass.: Nov. 3–4, 1967.
362. Robertson, O. H. Transfusion with preserved red blood cells. *Brit. Med. J.* 1:691–695, 1918.
363. Robin, E. D. Rapid scientific advances bring new ethical questions. *J.A.M.A.* 189:624–625, 1964.
364. Robinson, K. House of Commons Written Answers, nos. 820, 821, 823, 1964/65. Cited in Ciba Foundation Symposium, *Ethics in Medical Progress.* Boston: Little, Brown, 1966, p. 125.

365. Rosoff, S. D., and Schwab, R. S. The EEG in establishing brain death. A 10-year report, with criteria and legal safeguards in the 50 states. Presented at the American Electroencephalographic Society, Atlantic City, N.J., June 8, 1967.
366. Rubin, G. Placental blood for transfusion. *N. Y. Med. J.* 100:421, 1914.
367. Ruebhausen, O. M.: Comment made at the American Association for the Advancement of Science symposium *Secrecy, Privacy, and Public Information,* Dec. 28–29, 1967.
368. Ruebhausen, O. M., and Brim, O. G., Jr. Privacy and behavioral research. *Columbia Law Rev.* 65:1184–1211, 1965.
369. Ruff, G. E. In *Duke Law Journal* 2:265–274, 1960.
370. Rusk, H. A. Aid to kidney patients. *New York Times,* June 2, 1968, p. 90.
371. Russell, Lord. Quoted by D. M. Jackson in I. Ladimer and R. W. Newman (Eds.), *Clinical Investigation in Medicine: Legal, Ethical and Moral Aspects.* Boston: Boston University Law-Medicine Research Institute, 1963, p. 303.
372. Rycroft, P. V. A Recently Established Procedure: Corneal Transplantation. In Ciba Foundation Symposium, *Ethics in Medical Progress,* Boston: Little, Brown, 1966, pp. 43–53.
372a. Sadler, A. M., Sadler, B. L., and Stason, E. B. The Uniform Anatomical Gift Act. *J.A.M.A.:* 206, 2501–2506, 1968.
373. Sanhedrin 74a.
374. Saron, Admr. *v.* State of New York. Sup. Ct. App. Div. 1965, 263 N.Y.S. 2nd 591. Cited in proceedings of conference on *Use of Human Subjects in Safety Evaluation of Food Chemicals.* Washington: National Academy of Sciences, National Research Council, 1967, pp. 113, 161.
375. Schreiner, G. E. In Ciba Foundation Symposium, *Ethics in Medical Progress.* Boston: Little, Brown, 1966, pp. 100, 118.
376. Schrödinger, E. The Mystery of the Sensual Qualities in *Mind and Matter.* Cambridge: Cambridge Univ. Press, 1958, pp. 88–104.
377. Schwitzgebel, R. K. Law-Medicine Notes: Positive concepts of privacy in research. *New Eng. J. Med.* 276:282–283, 1967.
378. *Science,* 3:512, 1896. Comment.
379. Sessoms, S. M. Guiding principles in medical research involving humans. *Hospitals* 32:44, 58–64, 1958.
380. Shaldon, S. Referred to by H. E. de Wardener in Ciba Foundation Symposium, *Ethics in Medical Progress.* Boston: Little, Brown, 1966, pp. 115–116.
381. Sharpe, D. J. Responsibilities in medical experimentation on hu-

man beings. Presented at the National Lawyers' Club, Washington, May 8, 1967.

382. Shils, E. A. Social inquiry and the autonomy of the individual. In D. Lerner (Ed.), *The Human Meaning of the Social Sciences.* New York: Meridian, 1959, pp. 114–157.

383. Shimkin, M. B. The problem of experimentation on human beings: I. The research worker's point of view. *Science* 117:205–207, 1953.

384. Shimkin, M. B. Scientific investigations on man: A medical research worker's viewpoint. Proceedings of a conference on *Use of Human Subjects in Safety Evaluation of Food Chemicals.* Washington: National Academy of Sciences, National Research Council, 1967, pp. 217–227.

385. Shuster, A. Why human 'guinea pigs' volunteer. *N.Y. Times Magazine,* April 13, 1958, pp. 62, 65, 67.

386. Shusterman, A. Commentary according to the ethical insights of religion. In proceedings of conference on *Use of Human Subjects in Safety Evaluation of Food Chemicals.* Washington: National Academy of Sciences, National Research Council, 1967, pp. 249–251.

387. Simmel, G. *The Sociology of Georg Simmel.* K. H. Wolff (Ed. and Transl.). Glencoe, Ill.: Free Press, 1950, pp. 307–344.

388. Slater *v.* Baker. 2 Wils. K.B. 359 95 Eng. Rep. 860, 1767. Cited in proceedings of conference on *Use of Human Subjects in Safety Evaluation of Food Chemicals.* Washington: National Academy of Sciences, National Research Council, 1967, pp. 115–116.

389. Sloane, H. An account of inoculation by Sir Hans Sloane, Bart., given to Mr. Ranby, to be published, Anno 1736. Communicated by Thomas Birch, D.D. Sec. *Roy. Soc. Phil. Trans.* 49:516–520, 1756.

390. Smith, E. E. Obtaining subjects for research. *Amer. Psychol.* 17:577–578, 1962.

391. Smith, G. M., Egbert, L. D., Markowitz, R. A., Mosteller, F., and Beecher, H. K. An experimental pain method sensitive to morphine in man: The submaximum effort tourniquet technique. *J. Pharmacol. Exp. Ther.* 154:324–332, 1966.

392. Smith, J. Science and ethics. In *Ethical Problems for the Sixties.* New Britain, Conn.: Central Connecticut State College, 1962, pp. 43–52.

393. Smith, M. B. Conflicting values affecting behavioral research with children. *Amer. Psychol.* 22:377–382, 1967.

394. Starzl, T. E. In Ciba Foundation Symposium, *Ethics in Medical Progress*. Boston: Little, Brown, 1966, p. 98.
395. Stason, E. B. The role of law in medical progress. *Med. Prog. Law* 32:563–596, 1967.
396. Stevenson, L. G. Science down the drain. *Bull. Hist. Med.* 29:1–26, 1955.
397. Stewart, W. H. An invitation to open dialogue. *Sat. Review*, July 22, 1966, pp. 43–44.
398. Strong, R. P., and Crowell, B. C. The etiology of beriberi. *Philipp. J. Sci.* 7:271–411, 1912.
399. Studies with children based on medical, ethical grounds. *Med. Tribune* 8: Feb. 20, 1967.
400. Stumpf, S. E. Some moral dimensions of medicine. *Ann. Intern. Med.* 64:460–470, 1966.
401. Stumpf, S. E. A critique and summary. Proceedings of a conference on *Use of Human Subjects in Safety Evaluation of Food Chemicals*. Washington: National Academy of Sciences, National Research Council, 1967, pp. 255–264.
402. Sugar, O., and Gerard, R. W. Anoxia and brain potentials. *J. Neurophysiol.* 1:558–572, 1938.
403. Supreme Court of Massachusetts. Masden *v.* Harrison, No. 68651 Eq., Mass. Sup. Jud. Ct., June 12, 1957. Cited by W. J. Curran in I. Ladimer and R. W. Newman (Eds.), *Clinical Investigation in Medicine: Legal, Ethical and Moral Aspects*. Boston: Law-Medicine Research Institute, Boston University, 1966, pp. 239–240.
404. Swetlow, G. I., and Florman, M. G. Your liability in experimental treatment. *Med. Econ.* 27:54–56, 1949.
405. Taft, E. Report on the American Academy for the Advancement of Science symposium *Secrecy, Privacy, and Public Information*, Dec. 28–29, 1967.
406. Temple, W. *Mens Creatrix*, p. 206. Quoted by J. Fletcher, in *Situation Ethics*. Philadelphia: Westminster, 1966, foreword.
407. Thomson, W. A. R. Editorial responsibility in relation to human experimentation. *World Med. J.* 2:153–154, 1955.
408. Thulborne, T., and Young, M. H. Prophylactic penicillin and postoperative chest infections. *Lancet* 2:907–909, 1962.
409. Thymus experimentation. Letter from B. H. Waksman. *New Eng. J. Med.* 270:1018, 1964. Editorial concerning letter, p. 1014.
410. Tommasi, M. Documents anatomiques concernant les comas "prolongés" et "dépassés." *Marseille Chir.* 18:147–149, 1966.
411. United States Supreme Court. Mapp decision. Mapp *v.* Ohio, 1967.

412. United States Supreme Court. People *v.* Berger. 388 U.S. 41, 1967.
412a. *Use of Human Subjects in Safety Evaluation of Food Chemicals,* proceedings of conference on. Washington: National Academy of Sciences, National Research Council, 1967, 273 pp.
413. Van Rood, J. J. In Ciba Foundation Symposium, *Ethics in Medical Progress.* Boston: Little, Brown, 1966, p. 120.
414. Vedder, E. B. In proceedings of a conference on *Use of Human Subjects in Safety Evaluation of Food Chemicals.* Washington: National Academy of Sciences, National Research Council, 1967, p. 211.
415. von Weizsaecker, V. "Euthanasie" und Menschenversuche. *Psyche* 1:68–102, 1947–1948.
416. Waksman, B. H. Thymus experimentation. *New Eng. J. Med.* 270:1018, 1964.
417. Warren, S. D., and Brandeis, L. D. The right to privacy. *Harv. Law Rev.* 4:193–220, 1890.
418. Wasmuth, C. E. Law for the physician: Legal aspects of organ transplantation. *Anesth. Analg.* 46:25–27, 1967.
419. Wasmuth, C. E., and Stewart, B. H. Medical and legal aspects of human organ transplantation. *Cleveland-Marshall Law Rev.* 14: 442–471, 1965.
420. Waterhouse, B. *A Prospect of Exterminating the Small-Pox.* Printed for the author at the Cambridge Press by William Hilliard, 1800.
421. Ways to control snooping. Editorial. *Life,* 62:4, Apr. 21, 1967.
422. Weaver, W. Comment on the problem of statistical morality. The Dartmouth Convocation of Great Issues of Conscience in Modern Medicine, Sept. 8, 9, 10, 1960. *Dartmouth Alumni Mag.* (Suppl.), Nov. 1960, p. 4.
423. Welt, L. G. Reflections on the problems of human experimentation. *Conn. Med.* 25:75–78, 1961.
424. Westin, A. *Life,* Apr. 21, 1967, p. 4.
424a. Whitehead, A. N. Modes of thought. Quoted by J. Fletcher, *Situation Ethics.* Philadelphia: Westminster, 1966, foreword.
425. Wiggers, C. J. Human experimentation. As exemplified by career of Dr. William Beaumont. *Alum. Bull. Sch. of Med. West. Reserve Univ.* pp. 60–65, 1950.
426. Wiretapping legal with warrant. *Boston Herald-Traveler,* Dec. 19, 1967.
427. Wilkins, E. W. Personal communication, 1967.
428. Wolfensberger, W. Ethical issues in research with human sub-

jects. A rationale is formulated for a code of conduct in the recruitment of subjects for research. *Science* 155:47–51, 1967.

429. Wolfle, D. Research with human subjects. *Science* 132:989, 1960.
430. Wolstenholme, G. E. W. An old-established procedure: The development of blood transfusion. In Ciba Foundation Symposium, *Ethics in Medical Progress.* Boston: Little, Brown, 1966, pp. 24–42.
431. Woodruff, M. F. A. Transplanation: The clinical problem. In Ciba Foundation Symposium, *Ethics in Medical Progress.* Boston: Little, Brown, 1966, pp. 6–23. Also in discussion of Organ Transplantation: The Practical Possibilities, by J. E. Murray. *Ibid.* pp. 71–72.
432. Zirm. Cited by P. V. Rycroft in Ciba Foundation Symposium, *Ethics in Medical Progress.* Boston: Little, Brown, 1966, p. 44.
433. Zolich, J. Laudatory invasion of privacy. *Cleveland-Marshall Law Rev.,* 16:532–540, 1967.

Index